Acute Pain Management: Scientific Evidence

Australian and New Zealand College of Anaesthetists and Faculty of Pain Medicine

Endorsed by:

Australasian Faculty of Rehabilitation Medicine

Royal Australasian College of Physicians

Royal Australasian College of Surgeons

Royal Australian and New Zealand College of Psychiatrists

Australian Pain Society

International Association for the Study of Pain

Royal College of Anaesthetists (UK)

Approved by the NHMRC on 9 June 2005

Australian Government
National Health and Medical Research Council

ISBN Print: 0-9585208-6-0 Online: 0-9585208-7-9

Acknowledgements

The production of a document such as this requires a considerable amount of time over a long period. Although institutional support in terms of time and resources came from a number of centres, in particular the working party would like to thank the Department of Anaesthesia, Hyperbaric Medicine and Pain Medicine at the Royal Adelaide Hospital for its assistance as well as acknowledge the support of the Department of Anaesthesia and Pain Medicine at the Royal Perth Hospital, the Department of Anaesthesia, St Vincent's Hospital, Melbourne, The Portex Department of Anaesthesia, Great Ormond Street Hospital, London and the Department of Anaesthesia, Critical Care and Pain Medicine, Royal Infirmary, Edinburgh.

Printing of this document was supported by unconditional education grants from Pfizer Inc, Mundipharma Pty Limited, Bristol-Myers Squibb Australia, CSL Pharmaceuticals and Grünenthal GmbH.

NHMRC approval

These guidelines were approved by the National Health and Medical Research Council at its 157th Session on 9 June 2005, under section 14A of the National Health and Medical Research Council Act 1992. Approval for the guidelines by NHMRC is granted for a period not exceeding five years, at which date the approval expires. The NHMRC expects that all guidelines will be reviewed no less than once every five years. Readers should check with the Australian and New Zealand College of Anaesthetists for any reviews or updates of these guidelines.

Disclaimer

This document is a general guide to appropriate practice, to be followed subject to the clinician's judgement and the patient's preference in each individual case.

The guidelines are designed to provide information to assist decision-making and are based on the best evidence available at the time of publication.

These guidelines can be downloaded from the National Health and Medical Research Council website: www.nhmrc.gov.au/publications. Copies of the document can be ordered through the Australian and New Zealand College of Anaesthetists on +61 3 9150 6299.

FOREWORD

In 1994 I was invited by the National Health and Medical Research Council (NHMRC) of Australia to chair a Working Party whose brief would be to develop an evidence-based-medicine (EBM) clinical practice guideline on all aspects of the broad field of acute pain management. Previously a guideline had been published in the United States but this was limited to postoperative and trauma acute pain management. The task proved to be even more challenging than I had estimated, not the least because of the very diverse range of health professionals who made contributions, and the sometimes very divergent views and data that were presented to the Working Party.

Although there was strong evidence available for some aspects of acute pain management, in other areas it was necessary to utilise 'best available evidence' and to rely on a consensus of the experts; after sometimes robust discussions, in all cases it was possible to reach consensus and the document was warmly received. Indeed it is my understanding that this document has been the subject of more requests in Australia and overseas than any other NHMRC report.

The first edition of *Acute Pain Management: Scientific Evidence* occupied a substantial amount of my time, and that of the Working Party, over more than four years. During the last two years of this time, I was a Councillor on the NHMRC Council and became aware that the NHMRC was unlikely to be able to provide the resources that would be needed to update this document in a more timely period than the original four years. Thus in my capacity as a Councillor of the Australian & New Zealand College of Anaesthetists (ANZCA) and Founding Dean of ANZCA's Faculty of Pain Medicine, I began to encourage ANZCA to provide resources and to set up a working party capable of meeting the NHMRC's standards for an NHMRC-endorsed revised document. I am very proud that ANZCA has taken up this challenge. This document represents ANZCA's first major EBM document; there will be more to follow.

It has been my privilege to provide reviewer input to the Chair, Dr Pam Macintyre. Without doubt this document builds in a major way on the prior document and this is largely due to the enormous dedication, knowledge and sheer hard work of Dr Macintyre, ably assisted by many high calibre individuals in the Working Party. This document will be of great assistance to a very broad range of health professionals and patients. In an era where pain management is beginning to have the priority that it clearly deserves, acute pain management must surely be **the top priority.**

At the time of the publication of the prior document I called for **acute pain management to be a basic human right**. Encouragingly, very recently the International Association for the Study of Pain and the World Health Organization have co-sponsored a 'Global Day Against Pain' with the main theme being 'Pain relief: a basic human right'. ANZCA and its two Faculties (Pain Medicine and Intensive Care Medicine) have recently promulgated a professional document entitled *Patients' Rights to Pain Management*. Thus the scene is set for the current document to provide the up-to-date evidence for health professionals to deliver effective and safe acute pain management.

Michael J Cousins AM
President, Australian and New Zealand College Anaesthetists

INTRODUCTION

This is the second edition of the report *Acute Pain Management: Scientific Evidence*. The first edition was written by a multidisciplinary committee headed by Professor Michael Cousins and published by the National Health and Medical Research Council (NHMRC) in 1999. In accord with the NHMRC requirement that guidelines should be revised as further evidence accumulates, and with the move towards development of guidelines by external bodies, the Australian and New Zealand College of Anaesthetists (ANZCA) took responsibility for revising and updating the first edition.

Since the first edition there has been an enormous increase in the quantity of information available about acute pain management. However, there have also been recent publications showing that the management of acute pain is still sometimes less than optimal (Dolin et al 2002; Apfelbaum et al 2003; Dix et al 2004).

In addition, as outlined in the Foreword, there has been increasing international acknowledgement, including by the International Association for the Study of Pain and the World Health Organization, that pain relief should be a 'basic human right'. In 2001 The Australian and New Zealand College of Anaesthetists also published its *Statement on Patients' Rights to Pain Management* (ANZCA 2001) which included: the rights of a patient to be believed; to be properly assessed; to access appropriate effective pain management strategies; to have education about effective pain management options; and to be cared for by health professionals with training and experience in the management of pain.

It was therefore seen as timely to reassess the evidence available for the management of acute pain.

A working party was convened to coordinate and oversee the development process. A large panel of contributors was appointed to draft sections of the document and a multidisciplinary consultative committee was chosen to review the early drafts of the document and contribute more broadly as required. To ensure general applicability and inclusiveness, there was a very wide range of experts on the contributor and multidisciplinary committee, including medical, nursing, allied health and complementary medicine clinicians and consumers.

The working party also included a representative from the Royal College of Anaesthetists in the United Kingdom. Rather than developing a similar document itself, the College will be promulgating this document, which will be used throughout the UK. Other professional bodies have also endorsed the document (see title page).

A list of members of the working party is attached at Appendix A, together with a list of contributing authors and working party members. Through the NHMRC Guidelines Assessment Register (GAR), the working party was provided with expert advice on the use of evidence-based findings and the application of NHMRC criteria by Professor Karen Grimmer from the University of South Australia.

Acute Pain Management: Scientific Evidence covers a wide range of clinical topics. The aim of the report is, as with the first edition, to combine the best available evidence for acute pain management with current clinical and expert practice. Accordingly, the report aims to summarise the substantial amount of evidence currently available for the management of acute pain in a concise and easily readable form to assist the practising clinician. The development process is summarised in Appendix B.

Excellent and recent evidence-based guidelines exist in the areas of acute musculoskeletal pain and of cancer pain and recommendations relevant to the management of acute pain in these areas have been drawn directly from these.

Key messages for each topic are given with the highest level of evidence available to support them, or with a symbol indicating that they are based on clinical experience or expert opinion. In the key messages, Level I evidence from the Cochrane Database is identified.

Levels of evidence are documented according to the NHMRC designation (1999).

Levels of evidence

I	Evidence obtained from a systematic review of all relevant randomised controlled trials.
II	Evidence obtained from at least one properly designed randomised controlled trial
III-1	Evidence obtained from well-designed pseudo-randomised controlled trials (alternate allocation or some other method)
III-2	Evidence obtained from comparative studies with concurrent controls and allocation not randomised (cohort studies), case-controlled studies or interrupted time series with a control group
III-3	Evidence obtained from comparative studies with historical control, 2 or more single-arm studies, or interrupted time series without a parallel control group
IV	Evidence obtained from case series, either post-test or pre-test and post-test

Clinical practice points

☑ Recommended best practice based on clinical experience and expert opinion

This document is not intended to be a textbook but rather a compilation of the highest levels of evidence available relevant to acute pain management in a large number of areas. In making this information available to clinicians in a short and succinct form, the working party hopes that *Acute Pain Management: Scientific Evidence* will be a useful resource for all involved in the management of acute pain. Feedback on any aspect of this document will be welcomed.

The field of acute pain medicine is a rapidly changing one. New information arising in areas considered to be of importance will be posted periodically on the website of the Australian and New Zealand College of Anaesthetists (www.anzca.edu.au). A link to this site will be provided in the preamble to the document from the NHMRC website. This information will not yet have been approved by the NHMRC but will be included, as appropriate, in future editions of this document.

Dr Pam Macintyre
on behalf of the Working Party

INTRODUCTION

References

ANZCA (2001) *Patients' Rights to Pain Management.* ANZCA professional document PS45. Australian and New Zealand College of Anaesthetists and Faculty of Pain Medicine. (www.anzca.edu.au/publications/profdocs/profstandards/ps45_2001.htm)

Apfelbaum JL, Chen C, Mehta SS et al (2003) Postoperative pain experience: results from a national survey suggest postoperative pain continues to be under managed. *Anesth Analg* 97: 534–40.

Dix P, Sandhar B, Murdoch J et al (2004) Pain on medical wards in a district general hospital. *Br J Anaesth* 92: 235–37.

Dolin SJ, Cashman JN, Bland JM (2002) Effectiveness of acute postoperative pain management: I. Evidence from published data. *Br J Anaesth* 89: 409–23.

NHMRC (1999) *A Guide to the Development, Implementation and Evaluation of Clinical Practice Guidelines.* National Health and Medical Research Council, Canberra.

CONTENTS

Contents

List of tables and figures

Tables

Figures

SUMMARY OF KEY MESSAGES

A description of the levels of evidence and associated symbols can be found in the introduction (see page vi).

1. Physiology and psychology of acute pain

Psychological aspects of acute pain

1. Preoperative anxiety, catastrophising, neuroticism and depression are associated with higher postoperative pain intensity (**Level IV**).
2. Preoperative anxiety and depression are associated with an increased number of patient-controlled analgesia (PCA) demands and dissatisfaction with PCA (**Level IV**).

☑ Pain is an individual, multifactorial experience influenced by culture, previous pain events, beliefs, mood and ability to cope.

Progression of acute to chronic pain

1. Some specific early analgesic interventions reduce the incidence of chronic pain after surgery (**Level II**).
2. Chronic postsurgical pain is common and may lead to significant disability (**Level IV**).
3. Risk factors that predispose to the development of chronic postsurgical pain include the severity of pre and postoperative pain, intraoperative nerve injury and psychological vulnerability (**Level IV**).
4. Many patients suffering chronic pain relate the onset to an acute incident (**Level IV**).

Pre-emptive and preventive analgesia

1. The timing of a single analgesic intervention (preincisional versus postincisional), defined as pre-emptive analgesia, does not have a clinically significant effect on postoperative pain relief (**Level I**).
2. There is evidence that some analgesic interventions have an effect on postoperative pain and/or analgesic consumption that exceeds the expected duration of action of the drug, defined as preventive analgesia (**Level I**).
3. NMDA (n-methyl-D-aspartate) receptor antagonist drugs in particular may show preventive analgesic effects (**Level I**).

2. Assessment and measurement of acute pain and its treatment

Measurement

1. Regular assessment of pain leads to improved acute pain management (**Level III-3**).
2. There is good correlation between the visual analogue and numerical rating scales (**Level IV**).

☑ Self-reporting of pain should be used whenever appropriate as pain is by definition a subjective experience.

☑ The pain measurement tool chosen should be appropriate to the individual patient; developmental, cognitive, emotional and cultural factors should be considered.

☑ Scoring should incorporate different components of pain. In the postoperative patient this should include static (rest) and dynamic (eg pain on sitting, coughing) pain.

☑ Uncontrolled or unexpected pain requires a reassessment of the diagnosis and consideration of alternative causes for the pain (eg new surgical/ medical diagnosis, neuropathic pain).

SUMMARY

Outcome measures in acute pain management

☑ Multiple outcome measures are required to adequately capture the complexity of the pain experience and how it may be modified by pain management interventions.

3. Provision of safe and effective acute pain management

1. Preoperative education improves patient or carer knowledge of pain and encourages a more positive attitude towards pain relief (**Level II**).
2. Implementation of an acute pain service may improve pain relief and reduce the incidence of side effects (**Level III-3**).
3. Staff education and the use of guidelines improve pain assessment, pain relief and prescribing practices (**Level III-3**).
4. Even 'simple' techniques of pain relief can be more effective if attention is given to education, documentation, patient assessment and provision of appropriate guidelines and policies (**Level III-3**).

☑ Successful management of acute pain requires close liaison with all personnel involved in the care of the patient.

☑ More effective acute pain management will result from appropriate education and organisational structures for the delivery of pain relief rather than the analgesic techniques themselves.

4. Systemically administered analgesic drugs

Opioids

1. Dextropropoxyphene has low analgesic efficacy (**Level I** [Cochrane Review]).
2. Tramadol is an effective treatment in neuropathic pain (**Level I** [Cochrane Review]).
3 Droperidol, dexamethasone and ondansetron are equally effective in prophylaxis of postoperative nausea and vomiting (**Level I**).
4. Naloxone, naltrexone, nalbuphine and droperidol are effective treatments for opioid-induced pruritus (**Level I**).
5. In the management of acute pain, one opioid is not superior over others but some opioids are better in some patients (**Level II**).
6. The incidence of clinically meaningful adverse effects of opioids is dose-related (**Level II**).
7. Tramadol has a lower risk of respiratory depression and impairs gastrointestinal motor function less than other opioids at equianalgesic doses (**Level II**).

8. Pethidine is not superior to morphine in treatment of pain of renal or biliary colic (**Level II**).

9. Supplemental oxygen in the postoperative period improves oxygen saturation and reduces tachycardia and myocardial ischaemia (**Level II**).

10. In adults, patient age rather than weight is a better predictor of opioid requirements, although there is a large interpatient variation (**Level IV**).

11. Impaired renal function and the oral route of administration result in higher levels of the morphine metabolites M3G and M6G (**Level IV**).

☑ Assessment of sedation level is a more reliable way of detecting early opioid-induced respiratory depression than a decreased respiratory rate.

☑ The use of pethidine should be discouraged in favour of other opioids.

Paracetamol, non-steroidal anti-inflammatory drugs and COX-2 selective inhibitors

1. Paracetamol is an effective analgesic for acute pain (**Level I** [Cochrane Review]).

2. NSAIDs and COX-2 inhibitors are effective analgesics of similar efficacy for acute pain (**Level I** [Cochrane Review]).

3. NSAIDs given in addition to paracetamol improve analgesia (**Level I**).

4. With careful patient selection and monitoring, the incidence of NSAID-induced perioperative renal impairment is low (**Level I** [Cochrane Review]).

5. Aspirin and some NSAIDs increase the risk of perioperative bleeding after tonsillectomy (**Level I**).

6. COX-2 inhibitors and NSAIDs have similar adverse effects on renal function (**Level I**).

7. COX-2 selective inhibitors do not appear to produce bronchospasm in individuals known to have aspirin-exacerbated respiratory disease (**Level I**).

8. Paracetamol, NSAIDs and COX-2 inhibitors are valuable components of multimodal analgesia (**Level II**).

9. COX-2 inhibitors do not impair platelet function (**Level II**).

10. Short-term use of COX-2 inhibitors results in gastric ulceration rates similar to placebo (**Level II**).

11. Use of parecoxib followed by valdecoxib after coronary artery bypass surgery increases the incidence of cardiovascular events (**Level II**).

☑ Adverse effects of NSAIDs are significant and may limit their use.

☑ The risk of adverse renal effects of NSAIDs and COX-2 inhibitors is increased in the presence of factors such as pre-existing renal impairment, hypovolaemia, hypotension, use of other nephrotoxic agents and ACE inhibitors.

☑ Serious cardiovascular complications have been reported with the use of COX-2 inhibitors in some settings and the use of these agents is currently being assessed; no recommendation about their use can be made until further evidence is available.

SUMMARY

Adjuvant drugs

Nitrous oxide

1. Nitrous oxide is an effective analgesic during labour (**Level I**).
2. Nitrous oxide is an effective analgesic agent in a variety of other acute pain situations (**Level II**).

☑ Neuropathy and bone marrow suppression are rare but potentially serious complications of nitrous oxide use, particularly in at-risk patients.

☑ The information about the complications of nitrous oxide comes from case reports only. There are no controlled studies that evaluate the safety of repeated intermittent exposure to nitrous oxide in humans and no data to guide the appropriate maximum duration or number of times a patient can safely be exposed to nitrous oxide. The suggestions for use of nitrous oxide are extrapolations only from the information above. Consideration should be given to duration of exposure and supplementation with vitamin B_{12}, methionine, and folic or folinic acid.

☑ If nitrous oxide is used with other sedative or analgesic agents, appropriate clinical monitoring should be used.

N-methyl-D-aspartate receptor (NMDA) antagonists

1. Ketamine has an opioid-sparing effect in postoperative pain although there is no concurrent reduction in opioid-related side effects (**Level I**).
2. NMDA receptor antagonist drugs may show preventive analgesic effects (**Level I**).
3. Ketamine improves analgesia in patients with severe pain that is poorly responsive to opioids (**Level II**).
4. Ketamine may reduce opioid requirements in opioid-tolerant patients (**Level IV**).

☑ Ketamine may be a useful adjunct in conditions of allodynia, hyperalgesia and opioid tolerance.

Antidepressant drugs

1. Tricyclic antidepressants are effective in the treatment of chronic neuropathic pain states, chronic headaches and chronic back pain (**Level I**).
2. In neuropathic pain, tricyclic antidepressants are more effective than selective serotonergic re-uptake inhibitors (**Level I**).
3. Antidepressants reduce the incidence of chronic neuropathic pain after acute zoster and breast surgery (**Level II**).

☑ Based on the experience in chronic neuropathic pain states, it would seem reasonable to use tricyclic antidepressants in the management of acute neuropathic pain.

☑ To minimise adverse effects, particularly in elderly people, it is advisable to initiate treatment with low doses.

Anticonvulsant drugs

1. Anticonvulsants are effective in the treatment of chronic neuropathic pain states (**Level I**).
2. Perioperative gabapentin reduces postoperative pain and opioid requirements (**Level I**).

☑ Based on the experience in chronic neuropathic pain states, it would seem reasonable to use anticonvulsants in the management of acute neuropathic pain.

Membrane stabilisers

1. Membrane stabilisers are effective in the treatment of chronic neuropathic pain states, particularly after peripheral nerve trauma (**Level I**).
2. Perioperative intravenous lignocaine (lidocaine) reduces pain on movement and morphine requirements following major abdominal surgery (**Level II**).

☑ Based on the experience in chronic neuropathic pain states, it would seem reasonable to use membrane stabilisers in the management of acute neuropathic pain.

☑ Lignocaine (lidocaine) (intravenous or subcutaneous) may be a useful agent to treat acute neuropathic pain.

Alpha-2 agonists

1. The use of systemic alpha-2-agonists consistently improves perioperative opioid analgesia, but frequency and severity of side effects may limit their clinical usefulness (**Level II**).

Calcitonin

1. Calcitonin is effective in the treatment of acute pain after osteoporosis-related vertebral fractures (**Level I**).

Cannabinoids

1. Current evidence does not support the use of cannabinoids in acute pain management (**Level I**).

5. Regionally and locally administered analgesic drugs

Local anaesthetics

1. Continuous perineural infusions of lignocaine (lidocaine) result in less effective analgesia and more motor block than long-acting local anaesthetic agents (**Level II**).
2. There are no consistent differences between ropivacaine, levobupivacaine and bupivacaine when given in low doses for regional analgesia in terms of quality of analgesia or motor blockade (**Level II**).
3. Cardiovascular and central nervous system effects of the stereospecific isomers ropivacaine and levobupivacaine are less severe than those resulting from racemic bupivacaine (**Level II**).

☑ Case reports following accidental overdose with ropivacaine and bupivacaine suggest that resuscitation is likely to be more successful with ropivacaine.

SUMMARY

Opioids

1. Intrathecal morphine produces better postoperative analgesia than intrathecal fentanyl after caesarean section (**Level I**).
2. The combination of an opioid with an epidural local anaesthetic improves analgesic efficacy and reduces the dose requirements of both drugs (**Level I**).
3. Morphine injected as a single dose into the intra-articular space produces analgesia that lasts up to 24 hours (**Level I**).
4. Evidence for a clinically relevant peripheral opioid effect at non-articular sites, including perineural, is inconclusive (**Level I**).
5. Epidural pethidine produces better pain relief and less sedation than IV pethidine after caesarean section (**Level II**).

☑ No neurotoxicity has been shown at normal clinical intrathecal doses of morphine, fentanyl and sufentanil.

☑ Neuraxial administration of bolus doses of hydrophilic opioids carries an increased risk of delayed sedation and respiratory depression compared with lipophilic opioids.

Adjuvant drugs

1. Evidence that the addition of clonidine to an epidural or intrathecal opioid is more effective than clonidine or the opioid alone is weak and inconsistent (**Level I**).
2. Epidural ketamine (without preservative) added to opioid-based epidural analgesia regimens improves pain relief without reducing side effects (**Level I**).
3. Epidural neostigmine combined with an opioid reduces the dose of epidural opioid that is required for analgesia (**Level I**).
4. Intrathecal neostigmine prolongs the analgesic effect of intrathecal morphine and bupivacaine but increases the incidence of nausea and vomiting unless given in low doses (**Level I**).
5. Epidural and intrathecal clonidine prolong the effects of local anaesthetics (**Level II**).
6. Epidural adrenaline (epinephrine) in combination with a local anaesthetic improves the quality of postoperative thoracic epidural analgesia (**Level II**).

☑ There is conflicting evidence of analgesic efficacy for the addition of clonidine to brachial plexus blocks.

6. Routes used for systemic drug administration in management of acute pain

1. NSAIDs (including COX-2 selective inhibitors) given parenterally or rectally are not more effective and do not result in fewer side effects than the same drug given orally (**Level I** [Cochrane Review]).
2. Intermittent subcutaneous morphine injections are as effective as intramuscular injections and have better patient acceptance (**Level II**).
3. Continuous intravenous infusion of opioids in the general ward setting are associated with an increased risk of respiratory depression compared with other methods of parenteral opioid administration (**Level IV**).
4. Transdermal fentanyl should not be used in the management of acute pain because of safety concerns and difficulties in short-term dose adjustments needed for titration (**Level IV**).

☑ Other than in the treatment of severe acute pain, and providing there are no contraindications to its use, the oral route is the route of choice for the administration of most analgesic drugs.

☑ Titration of opioids for severe acute pain is best achieved using intermittent intravenous bolus doses as it allows more rapid titration of effect and avoids the uncertainty of drug absorption by other routes.

☑ Controlled-release opioid preparations should only be given at set time intervals.

☑ Immediate-release opioids should be used for breakthrough pain and for titration of controlled-release opioids.

☑ The use of controlled-release opioid preparations as the sole agents for the early management of acute pain is discouraged because of difficulties in short-term dose adjustments needed for titration.

☑ Rectal administration of analgesic drugs may be useful when other routes are unavailable but bioavailability is unpredictable and consent should be obtained.

7. Techniques used for drug administration in the management of acute pain

Patient-controlled analgesia (PCA)

1. Intravenous opioid PCA provides better analgesia than conventional parenteral opioid regimens (**Level I**).
2. Patient preference for intravenous PCA is higher when compared with conventional regimens (**Level I**).
3. Opioid administration by IV PCA does not lead to lower opioid consumption, reduced hospital stay or a lower incidence of opioid-related adverse effects compared with traditional methods of intermittent parenteral opioid administration (**Level I**).
4. The addition of ketamine to PCA morphine does not improve analgesia or reduce the incidence of opioid-related side effects (**Level I**).

5. Patient-controlled epidural analgesia for pain in labour results in the use of lower doses of local anaesthetic, less motor block and fewer anaesthetic interventions compared with continuous epidural infusions (**Level I**).
6. There is little evidence that one opioid via PCA is superior to another with regards to analgesic or adverse effects in general; on an individual patient basis one opioid may be better tolerated than another (**Level II**).
7. There is no analgesic benefit in adding naloxone to the PCA morphine solution, however the incidence of nausea and pruritus may be decreased (**Level II**).
8. The addition of a background infusion to intravenous PCA does not improve pain relief or sleep, or reduce the number of PCA demands (**Level II**).
9. Subcutaneous PCA opioids can be as effective as intravenous PCA (**Level II**).
10. Intranasal PCA opioids can be as effective as intravenous PCA (**Level II**).
11. Patient-controlled epidural analgesia results in lower cumulative doses of the drugs compared with continuous epidural infusions without any differences in pain relief or side effects (**Level II**).
12. The risk of respiratory depression is increased when a background infusion is used (**Level IV**).

☑ Adequate analgesia needs to be obtained prior to commencement of PCA. Initial orders for bolus doses should take into account individual patient factors such as a history of prior opioid use and patient age. Individual PCA prescriptions may need to be adjusted.

☑ The routine addition of anti-emetics to PCA opioids is not encouraged, as it is of no benefit compared with selective administration.

☑ PCA infusion systems must incorporate antisyphon valves and in non-dedicated lines, antireflux valves.

☑ Drug concentrations should be standardised within institutions to reduce the chance of programming errors.

Epidural analgesia

1. All techniques of epidural analgesia for all types of surgery provide better postoperative pain relief compared with parenteral opioid administration (**Level I** [Cochrane Review]).
2. Epidural local anaesthetics improve oxygenation and reduce pulmonary infections and other pulmonary complications compared with parenteral opioids (**Level I**).
3. Thoracic epidural analgesia utilising local anaesthetics improves bowel recovery after abdominal surgery (**Level I**).
4. Thoracic epidural analgesia extended for more than 24 hours reduces the incidence of postoperative myocardial infarction (**Level I**).
5. Epidural analgesia is not associated with increased risk of anastomotic leakage after bowel surgery (**Level I**).
6. Thoracic epidural analgesia reduces incidence of pneumonia and need for ventilation in patients with multiple rib fractures (**Level II**).

7. The combination of thoracic epidural analgesia with local anaesthetics and nutritional support leads to preservation of total body protein after upper abdominal surgery (**Level II**).
8. Lumbar epidural analgesia reduces graft occlusion rates after peripheral vascular surgery (**Level II**).
9. Combinations of low concentrations of local anaesthetics and opioids provide better analgesia than either component alone (**Level II**).
10. The risk of permanent neurologic damage in association with epidural analgesia is very low; the incidence is higher where there have been delays in diagnosing an epidural haematoma or abscess (**Level IV**).
11. Immediate decompression (within 8 hours of the onset of neurological signs) increases the likelihood of partial or good neurological recovery (**Level IV**).

☑ The provision of epidural analgesia by continuous infusion or patient-controlled administration of local anaesthetic-opioid mixtures is safe on general hospital wards, as long as supervised by an anaesthesia-based pain service with 24-hour medical staff cover. and monitored by well-trained nursing staff.

SUMMARY

Intrathecal analgesia

1. Combination of spinal opioids with local anaesthetics reduces dose requirements for either drug alone (**Level I**).
2. Intrathecal morphine at doses of 100–200 microgram offers effective analgesia with a low risk of adverse effects (**Level II**).

☑ Clinical experience with morphine, fentanyl and sufentanil has shown no neurotoxicity or behavioural changes at normal clinical intrathecal doses.

Regional analgesia and concurrent anticoagulant medications

1. Anticoagulation is the most important risk factor for the development of epidural haematoma after neuraxial blockade (**Level IV**).

☑ Consensus statements of experts guide the timing and choice of regional anaesthesia and analgesia in the context of anticoagulation, but do not represent a standard of care and will not substitute the risk/benefit assessment of the individual patient by the individual anaesthetist.

Other regional and local analgesic techniques

1. Intra-articular local anaesthetics reduce postoperative pain only minimally (**Level I**).
2. Intra-articular opioids following knee arthroscopy provide analgesia for up to 24 hours (**Level I**).
3. Wound infiltration with long-acting local anaesthetics provides effective analgesia following inguinal hernia repair but not open cholecystectomy or hysterectomy (**Level I**).
4. Topical EMLA® cream (eutectic mixture of lignocaine [lidocaine] and prilocaine) is effective in reducing the pain associated with venous ulcer debridement (**Level I** [Cochrane Review]).

5. Continuous interscalene analgesia provides better analgesia, reduced opioid-related side effects and improved patient satisfaction compared with IV PCA after open shoulder surgery (**Level II**).
6. Continuous femoral nerve blockade provides postoperative analgesia and functional recovery superior to IV morphine, with fewer side effects, and comparable to epidural analgesia following total knee joint replacement surgery (**Level II**).
7. Continuous posterior lumbar plexus analgesia is as effective as continuous femoral analgesia following total knee joint replacement surgery (**Level II**).
8. Wound infiltration with continuous infusions of local anaesthetics improves analgesia and reduces opioid requirements following a range of non-abdominal surgical procedures (**Level II**).

SUMMARY

8. Non-pharmacological techniques

Psychological interventions

1. Combined sensory-procedural information is effective in reducing pain and distress (**Level I**).
2. Training in coping methods or behavioural instruction prior to surgery reduces pain, negative affect and analgesic use (**Level I**).
3. Hypnosis and attentional techniques reduce procedure-related pain (**Level II**).

Transcutaneous electrical nerve stimulation (TENS)

1. Certain stimulation patterns of TENS may be effective in some acute pain settings (**Level I**).

Acupuncture

1. Acupuncture may be effective in some acute pain settings (**Level I**).

Physical therapies

A summary of findings relating to manual and massage therapies can be found in *Evidence-based Management of Acute Musculoskeletal Pain*, published by the Australian Acute Musculoskeletal Pain Guidelines Group (2003) and endorsed by the National Health and Medical Research Council.

9. The management of acute pain in specific clinical situations

Postoperative pain

Risks of neuropathic pain

1. Acute neuropathic pain occurs after trauma and surgery (**Level IV**).

☑ Diagnosis and subsequent appropriate treatment of acute neuropathic pain might prevent development of chronic pain.

Acute postamputation pain syndromes

1. There is little evidence from randomised controlled trials to guide specific treatment of postamputation pain syndromes (**Level I**)
2. Continuous regional blockade via nerve sheath catheters provides effective postoperative analgesia after amputation, but has no preventive effect on phantom limb pain (**Level II**).
3. Calcitonin, morphine, ketamine, gabapentin and sensory discrimination training reduce phantom limb pain (**Level II**).
4. Ketamine and lignocaine (lidocaine) reduce stump pain (**Level II**).
5. Perioperative epidural analgesia reduces the incidence of severe phantom limb pain (**Level III-2**).

☑ Perioperative ketamine may prevent severe phantom limb pain.

Day surgery

1. The use of NSAIDs or clonidine as adjuncts to local anaesthetic agents in intravenous regional anaesthesia improves postoperative analgesia (**Level I**).
2. Infiltration of the wound with local anaesthetic agents provides good and long-lasting analgesia after ambulatory surgery (**Level II**).
3. Peripheral nerve blocks with long-acting local anaesthetic agents provide long-lasting postoperative analgesia after ambulatory surgery (**Level II**).
4. Continuous peripheral nerve blocks provide extended analgesia after ambulatory surgery and have been shown to be safe if adequate resources and patient education are provided (**Level II**).
5. Optimal analgesia is essential for the success of ambulatory surgery (**Level IV**).

Acute spinal cord injury

1. Intravenous opioids, ketamine and lignocaine (lidocaine) decrease acute spinal cord injury pain (**Level II**).
2. Gabapentin is effective in the treatment of acute spinal cord injury pain (**Level II**).

☑ Treatment of acute spinal cord pain is largely based on evidence from studies of other neuropathic and nociceptive pain syndromes.

Acute burns injury pain

1. Opioids, particularly via patient-controlled analgesia, are effective in burns pain, including procedural pain (**Level IV**).

☑ Acute pain following burns injury can be nociceptive and/or neuropathic in nature and may be constant (background pain), intermittent or procedure-related.

☑ Acute pain following burns injury requires aggressive multimodal and multidisciplinary treatment.

SUMMARY

Acute back pain

A summary of findings relating to acute back pain can be found in *Evidence-based Management of Acute Musculoskeletal Pain*, published by the Australian Acute Musculoskeletal Pain Guidelines Group (2003) and endorsed by the National Health and Medical Research Council. The following are selected key messages from these guidelines.

1. Acute low back pain is non-specific in about 95% of cases and serious causes are rare; common examination and investigation findings also occur in asymptomatic controls and may not be the cause of pain (**Level I**).
2. Advice to stay active, heat wrap therapy, 'activity-focused' printed and verbal information and behavioural therapy interventions are beneficial in acute low back pain (**Level I**).
3. Advice to stay active, exercises, multimodal therapy and pulsed electromagnetic therapy are effective in acute neck pain (**Level I**).
4. Soft collars are not effective for acute neck pain (**Level I**).
5. Appropriate investigations are indicated in cases of acute low back pain when alerting features ('red flags') of serious conditions are present (**Level III-2**).
6. Psychosocial and occupational factors ('yellow flags') appear to be associated with progression from acute to chronic back pain; such factors should be assessed early to facilitate intervention (**Level III-2**).

Acute musculoskeletal pain

A summary of findings relating to acute musculoskeletal pain can be found in *Evidence-based Management of Acute Musculoskeletal Pain*, published by the Australian Acute Musculoskeletal Pain Guidelines Group (2003) and endorsed by the National Health and Medical Research Council. The following are selected key messages from these guidelines.

1. Topical and oral NSAIDs improve acute shoulder pain (**Level I**).
2. Subacromial corticosteroid injection relieves acute shoulder pain in the early stages (**Level I**).
3. Exercises improve acute shoulder pain in patients with rotator cuff disease (**Level I**).
4. Therapeutic ultrasound may improve acute shoulder pain in calcific tendonitis (**Level I**).
5. Advice to stay active, exercises, injection therapy and foot orthoses are effective in acute patellofemoral pain (**Level I**).
6. Low-level laser therapy is ineffective in the management of patellofemoral pain (**Level I**).

☑ A management plan for acute musculoskeletal pain should comprise the elements of assessment (history and physical examination, but ancillary investigations are not generally indicated), management (information, assurance, advice to resume normal activity, pain management) and review to reassess pain and revise management plan.

☑ Information should be provided to patients in correct but neutral terms with the avoidance of alarming diagnostic labels to overcome inappropriate expectations, fears or mistaken beliefs.

☑ Regular paracetamol, then if ineffective, NSAIDs, may be used for acute musculoskeletal pain.

☑ Oral opioids, preferably short-acting agents at regular intervals, may be necessary to relieve severe acute musculoskeletal pain; ongoing need for such treatment requires reassessment.

☑ Adjuvant agents such as anticonvulsants, antidepressants and muscle relaxants are not recommended for the routine treatment of acute musculoskeletal pain.

Acute medical pain

Abdominal pain

1. Provision of analgesia does not interfere with the diagnostic process in acute abdominal pain (**Level I**).
2. NSAIDs are superior to parenteral opioids in the treatment of renal colic (**Level I** [Cochrane Review]).
3. The onset of analgesia is faster when NSAIDs are given IV for the treatment of renal colic (**Level I**).
4. Antispasmodics and peppermint oil are effective in the treatment of acute pain in irritable bowel syndrome (**Level I**).
5. NSAIDS and vitamin B_1 are effective in the treatment of primary dysmenorrhoea (**Level I** [Cochrane Review]).
6. There is no difference between pethidine and morphine in the treatment of renal colic (**Level II**).
7. Parenteral NSAIDs are as effective as parenteral opioids in the treatment of biliary colic (**Level II**).

Acute herpes zoster infection

1. Antiviral agents started within 72 hours of onset of rash accelerate acute pain resolution and may reduce severity and duration of postherpetic neuralgia (**Level I**).
2. Amitriptyline use in low doses from onset of rash for 90 days reduces incidence of postherpetic neuralgia (**Level II**).
3. Topical aspirin is an effective analgesic in acute zoster (**Level II**).

☑ Provision of early and appropriate analgesia is an important component of the management of acute zoster and may have benefits in reducing postherpetic neuralgia.

Cardiac pain

1. Morphine is an effective and appropriate analgesic for acute cardiac pain (**Level II**).
2. Nitroglycerine is an effective and appropriate agent in the treatment of acute ischaemic chest pain (**Level IV**).

☑ The mainstay of analgesia in acute coronary syndrome is the restoration of adequate myocardial oxygenation, including the use of supplemental oxygen, nitroglycerine, beta blockers and strategies to improve coronary vascular perfusion.

Acute pain in haematological disorders

1. Hydroxyurea is effective in decreasing the frequency of acute crises, life-threatening complications and transfusion requirements in sickle cell disease (**Level I**).
2. Intravenous opioid loading optimises analgesia in the early stages of an acute sickle cell crisis. Effective analgesia may be continued with intravenous (including PCA) opioids such as morphine, however pethidine should be avoided (**Level II**).
3. Methylprednisolone decreases acute pain in sickle cell crises (**Level II**).
4. Oxygen supplementation during a sickle cell crisis does not decrease pain (**Level II**).

Acute headache

1. Triptans are effective in the treatment of severe migraine (**Level I**).
2. Aspirin-metoclopramide is effective in the treatment of migraine with mild symptoms (**Level I**).
3. Parenteral metoclopramide is effective in the treatment of acute migraine (**Level I**).
4. Parenteral prochlorperazine, chlorpromazine and droperidol are effective in the treatment of acute migraine (**Level II**).
5. Addition of caffeine to aspirin or paracetamol improves analgesia in acute tension type headaches (TTH) (**Level I**).
6. The incidence of post dural puncture headache (PDPH) may be reduced by using small gauge needles with a non-cutting edge (**Level I**).
7. There is no evidence that bed rest is beneficial in the prevention of PDPH (**Level I**).
8. Ibuprofen and paracetamol are effective in the treatment of mild to moderate migraine (**Level II**).
9. A 'stratified care strategy' is effective in treating migraine (**Level II**).
10. Simple analgesics such as aspirin, paracetamol, NSAIDs, either alone or in combination, are effective in the treatment of episodic tension-type headache (**Level II**).
11. Sumatriptan is effective in the treatment of cluster headache (**Level II**).
12. Oxygen is effective in the treatment of cluster headache (**Level II**).
13. Epidural blood patch administration may be effective in the treatment of PDPH (**Level IV**).

☑ Opioids should be used with extreme caution in the treatment of headaches, pethidine should be avoided.

☑ Frequent use of analgesics, triptans and ergot derivatives in the treatment of recurrent acute headache may lead to medication overuse headache.

Neurological disorders

☑ Treatment of acute pain associated with neurological disorders is largely based on evidence from trials for the treatment of a variety of chronic neuropathic pain states.

Orofacial pain

1. NSAIDs, COX-2 selective inhibitors, paracetamol, opioids and tramadol provide effective analgesia after dental extraction (**Level I**).
2. NSAIDS and COX-2 selective inhibitors provide better analgesia with less adverse effects than paracetamol, paracetamol/opioid, paracetamol/tramadol, tramadol or weaker opioids after dental extraction (**Level I**).
3. Perioperative local anaesthetic infiltration does not improve analgesia after tonsillectomy (**Level I** [Cochrane Review]).
4. Aspirin and NSAIDs increase reoperation rates for post-tonsillectomy bleeding (**Level I**).
5. PCA and continuous opioid infusions are equally effective in the treatment of pain in mucositis, but opioid consumption is less with PCA (**Level I** [Cochrane Review]).
6. Perioperative dexamethasone administration reduces acute pain, nausea and swelling after third molar extraction (**Level II**).
7. Topical treatments may provide analgesia in acute oral ulceration (**Level II**).

☑ Recurrent or persistent orofacial pain requires biopsychosocial assessment and appropriate multidisciplinary approaches. Neuropathic orofacial pain (atypical odontalgia, phantom pain) may be exacerbated by repeated dental procedures, incorrect drug therapy or psychological factors.

Acute pain in patients with HIV infection

☑ Neuropathic pain is common in patients with HIV/AIDS.

☑ In the absence of specific evidence, the treatment of pain in patients with HIV/AIDS should be based on similar principles to those for the management of cancer and chronic pain.

☑ Interaction between anti-retroviral and antibiotic medications and opioids should be considered in this population.

Acute cancer pain

1. Oral transmucosal fentanyl is effective in treating acute breakthrough pain in cancer patients (**Level II**).
2. Analgesic medications prescribed for cancer pain should be adjusted to alterations of pain intensity (**Level III**).
3. Opioid doses for individual patients with cancer pain should be titrated to achieve maximum analgesic benefit with minimal adverse effects (**Level III**).

☑ Acute pain in patients with cancer often signals disease progression; sudden severe pain in patients with cancer should be recognised as a medical emergency and immediately assessed and treated.

☑ Cancer patients receiving controlled-release opioids need access to immediate-release opioids for breakthrough pain; if the response is insufficient after 30–60 minutes, administration should be repeated.

☑ Breakthrough analgesia should be one-sixth of the total regular daily opioid dose in patients with cancer pain (except when methadone is used, because of its long and variable half life).

☑ If nausea and vomiting accompany acute cancer pain, parenteral opioids are needed.

Acute pain management in intensive care

1. Daily interruptions of sedative infusions reduce duration of ventilation and ICU stay without causing adverse psychological outcomes (**Level II**).
2. Gabapentin and carbamazepine are effective in reducing the pain associated with Guillain-Barre syndrome (**Level II**).
3. Patients should be provided with appropriate sedation and analgesia during potentially painful procedures (**Level III**).

☑ Observation of behavioural and physiological responses permits assessment of pain in unconscious patients.

Acute pain management in emergency departments

1. Provision of analgesia does not interfere with the diagnostic process in acute abdominal pain (**Level I**).
2. In patients with renal colic, NSAIDs provide better pain relief with fewer adverse effects compared with opioids (**Level I** [Cochrane Review]).
3. Pethidine does not provide better pain relief than morphine in the treatment of renal colic (**Level II**).
4. Parenteral NSAIDs provide pain relief in biliary colic that is comparable to opioids and superior to hyoscine-N-butylbromide (**Level II**).
5. Triptan and phenothiazines (prochlorperazine, chlorpromazine) are effective in at least 75% of patients presenting to the emergency department with migraine (**Level II**).
6. Femoral nerve blocks in combination with IV opioids are superior to IV opioids alone in the treatment of pain from a fractured neck of femur (**Level II**).

☑ To ensure optimal management of acute pain, emergency departments should adopt systems to ensure adequate assessment of pain, provision of timely and appropriate analgesia, frequent monitoring and reassessment of pain.

10. The management of acute pain in specific patient groups

The paediatric patient

Characteristics of pain in children

☑ Even the most premature neonate responds to nociceptive stimuli.

☑ In early development more generalised reflex nociceptive responses occur in response to lower intensity stimuli.

☑ Due to the increased plasticity of the developing nervous system, pain and injury in early life may have adverse long-term consequences.

Paediatric pain assessment

☑ Pain assessment and measurement are important components of paediatric pain management.

☑ Pain measurement tools are available for children of all ages.

☑ Pain measurement tools must be matched to the age and development of the child, be appropriate for the clinical context and be explained and used consistently.

Managing procedural pain in children

1. Sucrose reduces the behavioural response to heel stick in neonates (**Level I** [Cochrane Review]).
2. Topical local anaesthetic application, inhalation of nitrous oxide (50%) or the combination of both provides effective and safe analgesia for minor procedures (**Level I**).
3. Psychological interventions (cognitive-behavioural techniques, hypnosis) reduce procedure-related distress (**Level II**).
4. A combination of pharmacological and psychological interventions reduces pain and distress (**Level II**).
5. Combinations of hypnotic and analgesic agents are effective for procedures of moderate and major severity (**Level II**).

☑ Inadequate monitoring of the child, lack of adequate resuscitation skills and equipment, and the use of multiple drug combinations (particularly three or more) have been associated with major adverse outcomes.

Analgesic agents for use in children

1. Aspirin and NSAIDs increase the risk of reoperation for post-tonsillectomy bleeding (**Level I**).
2. Paracetamol and NSAIDs are effective for moderately severe pain and decrease opioid requirements after major surgery (**Level II**).
3. The efficacy of oral codeine in children is variable, particularly in individuals with a reduced ability to generate active metabolites (**Level II**).
4. Safe dosing of paracetamol requires consideration of the age and body weight of the child, and the duration of therapy.

5. Aspirin should be avoided in children, but serious adverse events after NSAIDs are rare in children over 6 months of age. Evidence for safety of NSAIDs following tonsillectomy is inconclusive.

Opioid infusions and patient-controlled analgesia in children

1. Effective PCA prescription in children incorporates a bolus that is adequate for control of movement-related pain, and may include a low dose background infusion to improve efficacy and sleep (**Level II**).
2. Intermittent intramuscular injections are distressing for children and are less effective for pain control than intravenous infusions (**Level III-1**).

☑ Intravenous opioids can be used safely and effectively in children of all ages.

☑ Initial doses of opioid should be based on the age and weight of the child and then titrated against the individual's response.

Regional analgesia in children

1. Topical local anaesthetic does not adequately control pain associated with circumcision in awake neonates (**Level I** [Cochrane Review]).
2. Perioperative local anaesthetic infiltration does not improve analgesia after tonsillectomy (**Level I** [Cochrane Review]).
3. Clonidine prolongs analgesia when added to caudal local anaesthetic blocks (**Level I**)
4. Clonidine improves analgesia when added to epidural local anaesthetic infusions (**Level II**).
5. Wound infiltration, peripheral nerve blocks, and caudal local anaesthetic provide effective analgesia after day case surgery (**Level II**).
6. Caudal local anaesthetic and dorsal penile nerve block provide perioperative analgesia for circumcision (**Level II**).
7. Epidural infusions of local anaesthetic provide similar levels of analgesia as systemic opioids (**Level II**).
8. Epidural opioids alone are less effective than local anaesthetic or combinations of local anaesthetic and opioid (**Level II**).

☑ Caudal local anaesthetic blocks provide effective analgesia for lower abdominal, perineal and lower limb surgery and have a low incidence of serious complications.

☑ Continuous epidural infusions provide effective postoperative analgesia in children of all ages and are safe if appropriate doses and equipment are used by experienced practitioners, with adequate monitoring and management of complications.

Managing acute pain in children with cancer

1. PCA and continuous opioid infusions are equally effective in the treatment of pain in mucositis, but opioid consumption is less with PCA (**Level I** [Cochrane Review]).
2. PCA morphine and hydromorphone are equally effective for the control of pain associated with oral mucositis (**Level II**).

☑ Procedure and treatment related pain are significant problems for children with cancer.

The pregnant patient

Managing acute pain during pregnancy

1. Use of non-steroidal anti-inflammatory drugs during pregnancy is associated with increased risk of miscarriage (**Level III-2**).
2. Use of opioids in pregnancy does not cause fetal malformations, but may result in neonatal abstinence syndrome (**Level III-2**).

☑ For pain management in pregnancy non-pharmacological treatment options should be considered where possible before analgesic medications are used.

☑ Use of medications for pain in pregnancy should be guided by published recommendations; ongoing analgesic use requires close liaison between the obstetrician and the medical practitioner managing the pain.

☑ NSAIDs should be used with caution in the last trimester of pregnancy and should be avoided after the 32nd week.

Pain management during delivery

1. Continuous or one-to-one support by a midwife or trained layperson during labour reduces analgesic use, operative delivery and dissatisfaction (**Level I**).
2. Epidural and combined spinal-epidural analgesia provide superior pain relief for labour and delivery compared with systemic analgesics (**Level I**).
3. Combined spinal-epidural in comparison with epidural analgesia reduces time to effective analgesia and improves maternal satisfaction but increases the incidence of pruritus (**Level I** [Cochrane Review]).
4. Epidural analgesia does not increase the incidence of caesarean section and long-term backache (**Level I**).
5. Epidural analgesia is associated with increased duration of labour and may increase rate of instrumental vaginal delivery (**Level I**).
6. There is no significant difference in any outcome between use of bupivacaine and ropivacaine for epidural labour analgesia (**Level I**).
7. Patient-controlled epidural analgesia without background infusion reduces local anaesthetic use and motor block compared with continuous epidural infusion (**Level I**).
8. Single-injection intrathecal opioids provide comparable early labour analgesia to epidural local anaesthetics with increased pruritus (**Level I**).
9. Systemic opioids in labour increase the need for neonatal resuscitation and worsen acid-base status compared with regional analgesia (**Level I**).
10. Nitrous oxide has some analgesic efficacy and is safe during labour (**Level I**).
11. Acupuncture reduces analgesic requirements in labour (**Level I** [Cochrane Review]**)**.
12. Hypnosis used in labour reduces analgesic requirements and use of labour augmentation and increases the incidence of spontaneous vaginal delivery (**Level I**).
13. TENS does not reduce labour pain (**Level I**).
14. Systemic opioids are less effective than regional analgesia for pain in labour (**Level II**).

SUMMARY

15. Paracervical block is more effective than intramuscular opioid analgesia but there is insufficient evidence to support its safety (**Level II**).

16. Lumbosacral intradermal injection of sterile water is painful, but reduces labour pain (**Level II**).

Pain management during lactation

☑ Prescribing medications during lactation requires consideration of possible transfer into breast milk, uptake by the baby and potential adverse effects for the baby; it should follow available prescribing guidelines.

☑ Local anaesthetics, paracetamol and several NSAIDs, in particular ibuprofen, are considered to be safe in the lactating patient.

☑ Morphine, fentanyl and oxycodone are also considered safe in the lactating patient and should be preferred over pethidine.

SUMMARY

Pain in the puerperium

1. Routine episiotomy does not reduce perineal pain (**Level I**).
2. Paracetamol and NSAIDs are effective in treating perineal pain after childbirth (**Level I**).
3. The use of codeine for perineal pain after childbirth leads to more side effects than the use of NSAIDs (**Level II**).
4. Paracetamol and NSAIDs are equally, but only modestly effective in treating uterine pain (**Level II**).
5. The application of cooling, in particular with cooling gel pads, and the use of warm baths is effective in treatment of perineal pain after childbirth (**Level II**).
6. Bromocriptine should be avoided for the treatment of breast pain in puerperium because of the potential for serious adverse effects (**Level II**).

☑ Pain after childbirth requires appropriate treatment as it coincides with new emotional, physical and learning demands and may trigger postnatal depression.

☑ Management of breast and nipple pain should target the cause.

The elderly patient

1. Experimental pain thresholds to a variety of noxious stimuli are increased in elderly people but there is also a reduction in tolerance to pain (**Level I**).
2. PCA and epidural analgesia are more effective in elderly people than conventional opioid regimens (**Level II**).
3. Reported frequency and intensity of acute pain in clinical situations may be reduced in the elderly person (**Level III-2**).
4. Common unidimensional self-report measures of pain can be used in the elderly patient in the acute pain setting; in the clinical setting, the verbal descriptor scale may be more reliable than others (**Level III-2**).
5. There is an age-related decrease in opioid requirements; significant interpatient variability persists (**Level IV**).

6. The use of NSAIDs and COX-2 inhibitors in elderly people requires extreme caution; paracetamol is the preferred non-opioid analgesic (**Level IV**).

☑ The assessment of pain and evaluation of pain relief therapies in the elderly patient may present problems arising from differences in reporting, cognitive impairment and difficulties in measurement.

☑ Measures of present pain may be more reliable than past pain, especially in patients with some cognitive impairment.

☑ The physiological changes associated with ageing are progressive. While the rate of change can vary markedly between individuals, these changes may decrease the dose (maintenance and/or bolus) of drug required for pain relief and may lead to increased accumulation of active metabolites.

SUMMARY

Aboriginal and Torres Strait Islander peoples

1. The verbal descriptor scale may be a better choice of pain measurement tool than verbal numerical rating scales (**Level III-3**).
2. Medical comorbidities such as renal impairment are more common in Aboriginal and Torres Strait Islander peoples and New Zealand Maoris, and may influence the choice of analgesic agent (**Level IV**).
3. Clinicians should be aware that pain may be under-reported by this group of patients (**Level IV**).

☑ Communication may be hindered by social, language and cultural factors.

Other ethnic groups and non-English speaking patients

1. Multilingual printed information and pain measurement scales are useful in managing patients from different cultural or ethnic backgrounds (**Level IV**).
2. With appropriate instruction, PCA may help overcome some of the barriers to postoperative analgesia provision in a multicultural environment (**Level IV**).

☑ Ethnic and cultural background can significantly affect the ability to assess and treat acute pain.

The patient with obstructive sleep apnoea (OSA)

1. Patients with OSA may be at higher risk of complications after surgery and from opioid analgesia (**Level III-3**).
2. Continuous positive airway pressure (CPAP) does not increase the risk of anastomotic leak after upper gastrointestinal surgery (**Level III-2**).

☑ Management strategies that may increase the efficacy and safety of pain relief in patients with OSA include the provision of appropriate multimodal opioid-sparing analgesia, CPAP, monitoring and supervision (in a high-dependency area if necessary) and supplemental oxygen.

SUMMARY

The patient with concurrent hepatic or renal disease

☑ Consideration should be given to choice and dose regimen of analgesic agents in patients with hepatic and particularly renal impairment.

The opioid-tolerant patient

1. Opioid-tolerant patients report higher pain scores and have a lower incidence of opioid-induced nausea and vomiting (**Level III-2**).
2. Ketamine may reduce opioid requirements in opioid-tolerant patients **(Level IV)**.

☑ Usual preadmission opioid regimens should be maintained where possible or appropriate substitutions made.

☑ Opioid-tolerant patients are at risk of opioid withdrawal if non-opioid analgesic regimens or tramadol alone are used.

☑ PCA settings may need to include a background infusion to replace the usual opioid dose and a higher bolus dose.

☑ Neuraxial opioids can be used effectively in opioid-tolerant patients although higher doses may be required and these doses may be inadequate to prevent withdrawal.

☑ Liaison with all clinicians involved in the treatment of the opioid-tolerant patient is important.

Patients with a substance abuse disorder

☑ Naltrexone should be stopped at least 24 hours prior to elective surgery.

☑ Patients who have completed naltrexone therapy should be regarded as opioid naïve; in the immediate post-treatment phase they may be opioid-sensitive.

☑ Maintenance methadone regimens should be continued where possible.

☑ Buprenorphine maintenance may be continued; if buprenorphine is ceased prior to surgery conversion to an alternative opioid is required.

☑ There is no cross-tolerance between CNS stimulants and opioids.

I. PHYSIOLOGY AND PSYCHOLOGY OF ACUTE PAIN

1.1 APPLIED PHYSIOLOGY OF PAIN

1.1.1 Definition of acute pain

Pain is defined by the International Association for the Study of Pain (IASP) as 'an unpleasant sensory and emotional experience associated with actual or potential tissue damage, or described in terms of such damage' (Merskey 1979). In addition, it is noted that the inability to communicate verbally does not negate the possibility that an individual is experiencing pain and is in need of suitable pain-relieving treatment. This emphasises the need for appropriate assessment and management of pain when caring for unconscious patients, preverbal or developmentally delayed children, and individuals with impaired communication skills due to disease or language barriers.

Acute pain is defined as 'pain of recent onset and probable limited duration. It usually has an identifiable temporal and causal relationship to injury or disease' (Ready & Edwards 1992). Chronic pain 'commonly persists beyond the time of healing of an injury and frequently there may not be any clearly identifiable cause' (Ready & Edwards 1992).

It is increasingly recognised that acute and chronic pain may represent a continuum rather than distinct entities and that features of inflammatory, visceral, neuropathic or cancer pain may be components of pain of varying duration. Increased understanding of the mechanisms of acute pain has led to improvements in clinical management and in the future it may be possible to more directly target the pathophysiological processes associated with specific pain syndromes.

For detailed descriptions of the pathophysiology of acute pain arising from specific structures (eg viscera, muscle, bone) or related to specific conditions (eg orofacial pain, back pain, cancer pain, Complex Regional Pain Syndrome), see the appropriate specialised texts.

1.1.2 Pain perception and pain pathways

The ability of the somatosensory system to detect noxious and potentially tissue-damaging stimuli (ie nociception) is an important protective mechanism that involves multiple interacting peripheral and central mechanisms. In addition to these sensory effects, the perception and experience of pain is multifactorial and will be influenced by psychological and environmental factors in every individual.

Peripheral nociceptors

The detection of noxious stimuli requires activation of peripheral sensory organs (nociceptors) and transduction of the energy into electrical signals for conduction to the central nervous system. Nociceptive afferents are widely distributed throughout the body (skin, muscle, joints, viscera, meninges) and comprise both medium-diameter lightly myelinated A-delta fibres and small-diameter, slow conducting unmyelinated

CHAPTER 1

C-fibres. The most numerous subclass of nociceptor is the C-fibre polymodal nociceptor, which responds to a broad range of physical (heat, cold, pressure) and chemical stimuli. Tissue damage, such as that associated with infection, inflammation or ischaemia, produces an array of chemical mediators that act either directly via ligand-gated ion channels or via metabotropic receptors linked to second messenger systems to activate and/or sensitise nociceptors (see Table 1.1). Non-steroidal anti-inflammatory drugs (NSAIDs) modulate peripheral pain by reducing prostaglandin production and opioids can also have a peripheral effect following transport of opioid receptors to the periphery during inflammation. Neuropeptides (substance P and calcitonin gene-related peptide) released from the peripheral terminals also contribute to the recruitment of serum factors and inflammatory cells at the site of injury (neurogenic oedema). In the presence of ongoing stimuli, the excitability of nociceptors is increased (ie the threshold for activation is reduced and the response to suprathreshold stimuli is enhanced). This increase in sensitivity within the area of injury due to peripheral mechanisms is termed peripheral sensitisation or primary hyperalgesia (Snider & McMahon 1998).

Table 1.1 Examples of primary afferent and dorsal horn receptors and ligands

Ionotropic receptor	Subtype	Ligand
TRP channels	TRPV1	heat (>42C), capsaicin, H^+
	TRPV2	heat (>53C)
	TRPA	noxious cold (<17C)
acid sensing	DRASIC, ASIC	protons
purine	P2X3	ATP
serotonin	5HT3	5HT
NMDA	NR1	glutamate
AMPA	iGluR1	glutamate
kainate	iGluR5	glutamate
Metabotropic receptor	**Subtype**	**Ligand**
metabotropic glutamate	$mGluR_{1,2/3,5}$	glutamate
prostanoids	EP1-4	PGE2
	IP	PGI2
histamine	H1	HA
serotonin	5HT1A, 5HT4, 5HT2A	5HT
bradykinin	Bl, B2	BK
cannabinoid	CB1-2	anandamide
tachykinin	neurokinin-1 (NK1)	substance P, neurokinin A
opioid	mu, delta, kappa	enkephalin, dynorphin, beta-endorphin

Notes: 5HT: serotonin; ASIC: acid sensing ion channel; ATP: adenosine triphosphate; BK: bradykinin; DRASIC: subtype of acid sensing ion channel; iGluR: ionotropic glutamate receptor; P2X3: purinergic receptor subtype; PGE2: prostaglandin E2; PGI2: prostacyclin; TRP: transient receptor potential; NK1: neurokinin-1 Others (eg H1; EP1-4, TRPV2) are designated subtypes of receptors rather than abbreviations.

Once transduced into electrical stimuli, conduction of neuronal action potentials is dependent on voltage-gated sodium channels. A rapidly inactivating fast sodium current which is blocked by tetrodotoxin is present in all sensory neurons. This is the principal site of action for local anaesthetics, but as the channel is present in all nerve fibres, conduction in sympathetic and motor neurons may also be blocked. Subtypes of slowly activating and inactivating tetrodotoxin-resistant sodium currents are selectively present on nociceptive fibres. Following injury, changes in sodium channel kinetics contribute to hyperexcitability, and specific alterations in the expression of sodium channels (upregulation or downregulation) occur in different pain states (Lai et al 2003). Agents specific for different subtypes of sodium channel are not yet available for clinical use.

The cell bodies of nociceptive afferents that innervate the trunk, limbs and viscera are found in the dorsal root ganglia, while those innervating the head, oral cavity and neck are in the trigeminal ganglia and project to the brain stem trigeminal nucleus. The central terminals of C- and A-delta fibres convey information to nociceptive-specific areas within lamina I and II of the superficial dorsal horn and also to wide dynamic range neurons in lamina V, which encode both innocuous and noxious information. By contrast, large myelinated A-beta fibres transmit light touch or innocuous mechanical stimuli to deep laminae III and IV.

Pain transmission in the spinal cord

Primary afferent terminals contain both excitatory amino acid (eg glutamate) and peptide (eg substance P) neurotransmitters. Depolarisation of the primary afferent terminal results in glutamate release, which activates postsynaptic ionotropic AMPA receptors and rapidly signals information relating to the location and intensity of noxious stimuli. In this 'normal mode' a high intensity stimulus elicits brief localised pain, and the stimulus-response relationship between afferent input and dorsal horn neuron output is predictable and reproducible (Woolf & Salter 2000).

Summation of repeated C-fibre inputs results in a progressively more depolarised postsynaptic membrane and removal of the magnesium block from the N-methyl-D-aspartate (NMDA) receptor. This is mediated by glutamate acting on ionotropic NMDA receptors and metabotropic glutamate receptors (mGluR), and by substance P acting on neurokinin-1 (NK1) receptors. A progressive increase in action potential output from the dorsal horn cell is seen with each stimulus, and this rapid increase in responsiveness during the course of a train of inputs has been termed 'wind-up'. A behavioural correlate of this electrophysiological phenomenon is seen in human volunteers, as repeated stimuli of the same intensity elicit progressive increases in reported pain. Blockade of this excitatory mechanism offers potential benefits for the management of pain.

Intense and ongoing stimuli further increase the excitability of dorsal horn neurons, leading to central sensitisation. Increases in intracellular calcium due to influx through the NMDA receptor and release from intracellular stores activate a number of intracellular kinase cascades. Subsequent alterations in ion channel and/or receptor activity and trafficking of additional receptors to the membrane increase the efficacy of synaptic transmission. As a result of the increased excitability of central nociceptive neurons, the threshold for activation is reduced, pain can occur in response to low intensity previously non-painful stimuli (ie allodynia), and sensitivity spreads beyond the area of tissue injury (ie secondary hyperalgesia) (Ji et al 2003).

The intracellular changes associated with sensitisation may also activate a number of transcription factors both in dorsal root ganglion (DRG) and dorsal horn neurons, with resultant changes in gene and protein expression. Unique patterns of either upregulation or downregulation of neuropeptides, G-protein coupled receptors, growth factors and their receptors, and many other messenger molecules occur in the spinal cord and DRG in inflammatory, neuropathic and cancer pain (Ji & Woolf 2001). Further elucidation of changes specific to different pain states may allow more accurate targeting of therapy in the future.

In addition to the excitatory processes outlined above, inhibitory modulation also occurs within the dorsal horn and can be mediated by: non-nociceptive peripheral inputs; local inhibitory GABAergic and glycinergic interneurones; descending bulbospinal projections; and higher order brain function (eg distraction, cognitive input). These inhibitory mechanisms are activated endogenously to reduce the excitatory responses to persistent C-fibre activity and are also targets for many exogenous analgesic agents. Thus, analgesia may be achieved by either enhancing inhibition (eg clonidine acting at alpha-2 adrenergic receptors, opioids) or by reducing excitatory transmission (eg local anaesthetics, ketamine). Drugs may be administered epidurally or intrathecally to enhance access to spinal sites of action and are often given in combination with the aim of improving analgesia or reducing side effects (Walker et al 2002, **Level I**).

Central projections of pain pathways

Different qualities of the overall pain experience are subserved by projections of multiple parallel ascending pathways from the spinal cord to the midbrain, forebrain and cortex. The spinothalamic pathway ascends from primary afferent terminals in lamina I and II, via connections in lamina V of the dorsal horn, to the thalamus and then to the somatosensory cortex. This pathway provides information on the sensory-discriminative aspects of pain (ie the site and type of painful stimulus). The spinoparabrachial pathway projects to central areas mediating the emotional or affective component of pain. This pathway originates from superficial dorsal horn lamina I neurons that express the NK1 receptor and projects to the ventromedial hypothalamus (which coordinates autonomic and sensory information) and central nucleus of the amygdala. Multiple further connections include those with: cortical areas involved in the affective and motivational components of pain (eg cingulate cortex, insula and prefrontal cortex); projections back to the periaqueductal grey (PAG) region of the midbrain and rostroventromedial medulla (RVM) which are crucial for fight or flight responses and stress induced analgesia; and projections to the reticular formation which are important for the regulation of descending pathways to the spinal cord (Hunt & Mantyh 2001) (see Figure 1.1).

Figure 1.1 The main ascending and descending spinal pain pathways

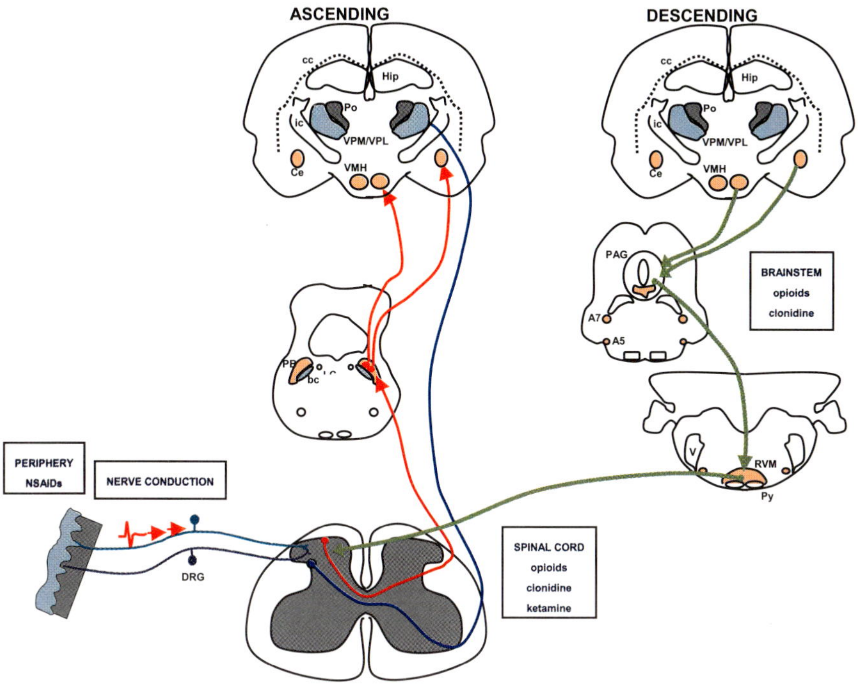

Notes: (a) There are 2 primary ascending nociceptive pathways. The spinoparabrachial pathway (red) originates from the superficial dorsal horn and feeds areas of the brain concerned with affect. The spinothalamic pathway (blue) originates from deeper dorsal horn (lamina V) after receiving input from the superficial dorsal horn and predominantly distributes nociceptive information to areas of the cortex concerned with discrimination.

(b) The descending pathway highlighted originates from the amygdala and hypothalamus and terminates in the periaqueductal grey (PAG). Neurons project from here to the lower brainstem and control many of the antinociceptive and autonomic responses that follow noxious stimulation.

Other less prominent pathways are not illustrated.

The site of action of some commonly utilised analgesics are included.

Legend A: adrenergic nucleus; bc: brachium conjunctivum; cc: corpus collosum; Ce: central nucleus of the amygdala; DRG: dorsal root ganglion; Hip: hippocampus; ic: internal capsule; LC: locus coeruleus; PAG: periaqueductal grey; PB: parabrachial area; Po: posterior group of thalamic nuclei; Py: pyramidal tract; RVM: rostroventrmedial medulla; V: ventricle; VMH: ventral medial nucleus of the hypothalamus; VPL: ventral posterolateral nucleus of the thalamus; VPM: ventral posteromedial nucleus of the thalamus

Source: Modified from Hunt & Mantyh (2001).

Descending modulatory pain pathways

Descending pathways contribute to the modulation of pain transmission in the spinal cord via presynaptic actions on primary afferent fibres, postsynaptic actions on projection neurons, or via effects on intrinsic interneurones within the dorsal horn. Sources include: direct corticofugal and indirect (via modulatory structures such as the PAG) pathways from the cortex; the hypothalamus, which is important for coordinating autonomic and sensory information; and brainstem regions such as the parabrachial nucleus, nucleus tractus solitarius, RVM and PAG. This complex system of multiple pathways, transmitters and receptor subtypes can lead to either excitatory (descending facilitation) or inhibitory (descending inhibition) effects on pain transmission. The relative balance of effect can vary with time and the type of painful stimulus.

Acutely, facilitation further enhances excitatory responses to provide warning of tissue injury and encourage protective behaviours; whereas inhibition may provide analgesia at times of danger so that pain does not compromise performance. With persistent pain, progressive reinforcement of descending inhibition may dampen excessive sensitivity and return the system to a 'normal' state. Alterations in descending modulation contribute to chronic pathological pain states, as descending inhibitory mechanisms may have limited efficacy or be subject to progressive exhaustion, or descending facilitation may be persistently activated. Descending inhibitory controls are an important therapeutic target for analgesic agents such as opioids, clonidine and tricyclic antidepressants, and the analgesia produced by nitrous oxide is at least in part due to effects on descending inhibition. As yet it is unclear if altering descending facilitation will produce analgesia or be clinically feasible (Millan 2002; Table 1.2).

1.1.3 Neuropathic pain

Neuropathic pain has been defined by the IASP as 'pain initiated or caused by a primary lesion or dysfunction in the nervous system' (Merskey 1994). Although commonly a cause of chronic symptoms, neuropathic pain can also be a component of acute pain (eg following surgery or trauma). In addition, Complex Regional Pain Syndrome (CRPS) may be the consequence of acute, often minor trauma (CRPS Type I) or nerve injury (CRPS Type II); it can be associated with sympathetically maintained pain (SMP), but can also manifest as sympathetically independent pain (Birklein et al 2001).

The mechanisms of neuropathic pain and its treatment differ significantly from nociceptive pain (Dworkin et al 2003). In the periphery, the threshold for activation of injured primary afferents is lowered and ectopic discharges may arise from the injury site or the DRG due to changes in sodium channel expression. Within the spinal cord, the increased peripheral input induces central sensitisation. Loss of inhibitory mechanisms, reparatory processes in damaged nerves and reactive changes in adjacent tissues (particularly glial and immune cells) may further increase central excitability. Functional (altered neurotransmitter expression) and anatomical (sprouting into superficial laminae in the dorsal horn) changes in A-beta fibres contribute to the tactile allodynia (ie pain induced by light touch) that is a frequent feature of neuropathic pain.

Table 1.2 Transmitters involved in descending pain pathways

1. **Transmitters predominantly contained in descending pathways**
   a. monoamines
      ii. noradrenaline
      ii. serotonin
      iii. dopamine
   b. histamine
   c. vasopressin and oxytocin
2. **Transmitters in descending pathways and predominantly in intrinsic dorsal horn neurons**
   a. acetylcholine
   b. GABA and glycine
   c. opioid peptides
   d. others: neuropeptide FF; cholecystokinin (CCK), neurotensin, galanin
3. **Transmitters in descending pathways and predominantly in primary afferent fibres**
   a. substance P
   b. glutamate
4. **Modulators not generated in specific classes of neuronal pathways**
   a. cannabinoids
   b. adenosine

Source: Adapted from Millan (2002).

1.2 PSYCHOLOGICAL ASPECTS OF ACUTE PAIN

Pain is an individual, multifactorial experience influenced by culture, previous pain events, beliefs, mood and ability to cope. It may be an indicator of tissue damage but may also be present in the absence of an identifiable cause. The degree of disability in relation to the experience of pain varies; similarly there is individual variation in response to methods of pain relief (Eccleston 2001). Knowledge of nociception and somatic contributors is important in understanding pain. However, it is often not enough to adequately explain the pain experience and an appreciation of psychosocial contributors is also required.

Pain is not a directly observable or measurable phenomenon, but rather a subjective experience with sensory and affective elements (Merskey & Bogduk 1994) which has a variable relationship with tissue damage. In this sense, pain is a psychological phenomenon. The task of researchers and clinicians is to identify the factors that contribute to pain as an experience. These may include somatic (physical) and psychological processes, as well as contextual factors, such as situational and cultural considerations.

From the perspective of Engel's (1977) biopsychosocial model of illness, pain experience may be seen as the result of a dynamic interaction between psychological, social and pathophysiological variables. This model of pain, elaborated by Turk (1995) and others, proposes that biological factors can influence physiological changes and that psychological variables are reflected in the appraisal and perception of internal physiological phenomena. These appraisals and behavioural responses are, in turn, influenced by social or environmental factors. At the same time, psychological and social factors can influence biological variables, such as hormone production, activity in the autonomic nervous system and physical deconditioning. Flor et al (2004) reviewed experimental evidence in support of these propositions.

Particular psychological contributors to the experience of pain include the process of attention, other cognitive processes (eg memory/learning, thought processing, beliefs, mood), behavioural responses, and interactions with the person's environment.

1.2.1 Attention

Attention is an active process and the primary mechanism by which nociception accesses awareness and disrupts current activity. The degree to which pain interrupts attention depends on factors such as: the intensity, novelty, unpredictability and emotional significance of the pain stimulus; the degree of awareness of bodily information; catastrophic thinking; and environmental demands (Eccleston & Crombez 1999).

1.2.2 Learning/memory

The role of learning or memory mechanisms has been studied primarily with experimentally-induced pain. Pain severity ratings can be operantly conditioned by their consequences (ie positive or negative reinforcement can influence pain behaviours). This effect can also be reflected in changes in skin conductance, facial activity and cortical responses (Flor et al 2002; Jolliffe & Nicholas 2004). Taken together, these studies support the hypothesis that the experience of pain is not solely due to noxious input, but that environmental factors may also contribute.

1.2.3 Beliefs and thought processes

Fear and anxiety influence the experience of pain (Vlaeyen & Linton 2000). Fear of pain may contribute to the development of avoidance behaviours that ultimately lead to disability in many people with persisting pain (Vlaeyen & Linton 2000). Negative appraisals of internal and external stimuli, high negative affectivity (hypervigilance for threats) and the personality characteristic of 'anxiety sensitivity' contribute to the development of pain-related fear. This in turn can lead to escape and avoidance behaviours which may be appropriate in the short term, but in the long term contribute to physical disuse. Increases in muscular reactivity due to fear can increase levels of pain (Vlaeyen & Linton 2000).

Evidence from experimental work with healthy human subjects receiving either noxious or innocuous stimulation has indicated that anticipation of pain appears to influence cortical nociceptive systems. This suggests that the activity of cortical nociceptive networks may be directly influenced by cognitive factors. The possible clinical relevance of these findings is that if there is a widespread 'priming' effect of nociceptive circuits during anticipation, it would provide support for an appropriate psychological approach to predictable or potentially noxious events (Porro et al 2002).

1.2.4 Acute pain settings

The contribution of psychosocial factors to the pain experience is important in acute and chronic pain settings as well as in the transition from acute to chronic pain (Linton 2000, **Level IV**; Pincus et al 2002, **Level IV**).

Preoperative anxiety has been shown to be associated with higher pain intensities in the first hour after a variety of different operations (Kalkman et al 2003, **Level IV**), the first day after abdominal (Caumo et al 2002, **Level IV**) and coronary artery bypass surgery (Nelson et al 1998, **Level IV**) and 1 year after total knee replacement (Brander et al 2003, **Level IV**).

In patients who underwent repair of their anterior cruciate ligament, those with high Pain Catastrophizing Scale scores (assessed prior to surgery) reported more pain immediately after surgery and when walking at 24 hours compared with those with low scores, but there was no difference in analgesic consumption (Pavlin et al 2005, **Level IV**). After breast surgery, catastrophising was associated with increased pain intensity and analgesic use (Jacobsen & Butler 1996, **Level IV**).

Similarly, preoperative depression (Kudoh et al 2001, **Level III-2**; Caumo et al 2002, **Level IV**) and neuroticism (Bisgaard et al 2001, **Level IV**) were predictors of postoperative pain early after surgery; preoperative depression is also associated with pain 1 year after total knee replacement (Brander et al 2003, **Level IV**). Strong information-seeking behaviour was associated with a reduction in the incidence of severe pain (Kalkman et al 2003, **Level IV**).

Preoperative anxiety and moderate to severe postoperative pain are, in turn, predictors of postoperative anxiety (Caumo et al 2001, **Level IV**).

Patient-controlled analgesia

A number of studies have looked specifically at the relationship between pain relief and psychological factors in patients using patient-controlled analgesia (PCA) in the postoperative period.

In general, anxiety seems to be the most important psychological variable that affects PCA use. Preoperative anxiety correlates with increased postoperative pain intensity, the number of PCA demands made by the patient (often 'unsuccessful', that is, during the lockout interval), degree of dissatisfaction with PCA and lower self-reports of quality of analgesia (Jamieson et al 1993, **Level IV**; Perry et al 1994, **Level IV**; Thomas et al 1995, **Level III-1**; Brandner et al 2002, **Level IV**; Ozalp et al 2003, **Level IV**). Evidence regarding PCA opioid consumption is contradictory; both no change (Gil et al 1990, **Level IV**; Gil et al 1992, **Level IV**; Jamieson et al 1993, **Level IV**) and an increase (Ozalp et al 2003, **Level IV**) have been reported. There appears to be no relationship between locus of control and postoperative pain intensity, satisfaction with PCA or PCA dose-demand ratio (Brandner et al 2002, **Level IV**).

Preoperative depression is associated with increased pain intensity, morphine requirements, PCA demands and degree of dissatisfaction (Ozalp et al 2003, **Level IV**).

Key messages

1. Preoperative anxiety, catastrophising, neuroticism and depression are associated with higher postoperative pain intensity (Level IV).
2. Preoperative anxiety and depression are associated with an increased number of PCA demands and dissatisfaction with PCA (Level IV).

The following tick box ☑ represents conclusions based on clinical experience and expert opinion.

☑ Pain is an individual, multifactorial experience influenced by culture, previous pain events, beliefs, mood and ability to cope.

1.3 Progression of acute to chronic pain

The importance of addressing the link between acute and chronic pain has been emphasised by recent studies. To highlight this link, chronic pain is increasingly referred to as persistent pain. A survey of the incidence of chronic pain-related disability in the community concluded that patients often relate the onset of their pain to an acute injury, drawing attention to the need to prevent the progression from acute to chronic pain (Blyth et al 2003, **Level IV**).

The association between acute and chronic pain is well-defined, but few randomised controlled studies have addressed the aetiology, time course, prevention or therapy of the transition between the two pain states.

Acute pain states that may progress to chronic pain include postoperative and post-traumatic pain, acute back pain (see Section 9.4) (Carey et al 2000, **Level IV**) and acute zoster (see Section 9.6.2).

Chronic pain is common after surgery (see Table 1.3) (Perkins & Kehlet 2000, **Level IV**; Macrae 2001) and represents a significant source of ongoing disability, often with considerable economic consequences. Such pain frequently has a neuropathic element and may appear early in the postoperative period (see Section 9.1.1).

There is some evidence that specific early analgesic interventions may reduce the incidence of chronic pain after surgery. Epidural analgesia initiated prior to thoracotomy and continued into the postoperative period resulted in significantly fewer patients reporting pain 6 months later compared with patients who had received IV PCA opioids for postoperative analgesia (45% vs 78% respectively) (Senturk et al 2002, **Level II**)). Evidence of any benefit for epidural analgesia established before surgery compared with at the end of the operation is mixed; it may (Obata et al 1999, **Level II**) or may not (Ochroch et al 2002 **Level II**; Senturk et al 2002, **Level II**) lead to a lower incidence of pain 6 months after thoracotomy.

Morphine injected into the site of iliac bone harvest resulted in a lower incidence of pain at 1 year compared with the same dose of IM morphine (Reuben et al 2001, **Level II**). Infusion of ropivacaine into the site of iliac crest bone graft harvest resulted in significantly less pain in the iliac crest during movement at 3 months (Blumenthal et al 2005, **Level II**).

See Section 9.1.2 for comments on prevention of phantom pain after limb amputation.

Table 1.3 Incidence of chronic pain after surgery

Type of operation	Incidence of chronic pain (%)
Amputation	30–85
Thoracotomy	5–67
Mastectomy	11–57
Cholecystectomy	3–56
Inguinal hernia	0–63
Vasectomy	0–37
Dental surgery	5–13

Sources: Adapted from Perkins & Kehlet (2000) and Macrae (2001).

1.3.1 Predictive factors for chronic postsurgical pain

A number of risk factors for the development of chronic postsurgical pain have been identified (Perkins & Kehlet 2000, **Level IV**).

Table 1.4 Risk factors for chronic postsurgical pain

Preoperative factors	Pain, moderate to severe, lasting more than 1 month
	Repeat surgery
	Psychologic vulnerability
	Workers' compensation
Intraoperative factors	Surgical approach with risk of nerve damage
Postoperative factors	Pain (acute, moderate to severe)
	Radiation therapy to area
	Neurotoxic chemotherapy
	Depression
	Psychologic vulnerability
	Neuroticism
	Anxiety

Source: Perkins & Kehlet (2000).

1.3.2 Mechanisms of the progression from acute to chronic pain

The pathophysiological processes that occur after tissue or nerve injury mean that acute pain may become persistent (Cousins et al 2000). Such processes include inflammation at the site of tissue damage with a barrage of afferent nociceptor activity that produces changes in the peripheral nerves, spinal cord, higher central pain pathways and the sympathetic nervous system (see Section 1.1).

After limb amputation, reorganisation or remapping of the somatosensory cortex and other cortical structures may be a contributory mechanism in the development of phantom-limb pain (Flor et al 1995; Grusser et al 2004). There is preclinical and clinical evidence of a genetic predisposition for chronic pain (Mogil 1999), although one study found that an inherited component did not feature in the development of phantom pain in members of the same family who all had a limb amputation (Schott 1986).

Key messages

1. Some specific early analgesic interventions reduce the incidence of chronic pain after surgery (**Level II**).
2. Chronic postsurgical pain is common and may lead to significant disability (**Level IV**).
3. Risk factors that predispose to the development of chronic postsurgical pain include the severity of pre and postoperative pain, intraoperative nerve injury and psychological vulnerability (**Level IV**).
4. Many patients suffering chronic pain relate the onset to an acute incident (**Level IV**).

CHAPTER 1

1.4 PRE-EMPTIVE AND PREVENTIVE ANALGESIA

In laboratory studies, administration of an analgesic prior to an acute pain stimulus more effectively minimises dorsal horn changes associated with central sensitisation than the same analgesic given after the pain state is established (see Section 1.1) (Woolf 1983). This led to the hypothesis that pain relief prior to surgery may enhance postoperative pain management (ie 'pre-emptive preoperative analgesia') (Wall 1988). However, clinical studies have failed to confirm a significant effect of timing of analgesia when comparing preincisional (ie 'pre-emptive') and postincisional interventions (Møiniche et al 2002, **Level I**). This in part relates to variability in definitions, deficiencies in clinical trial design and differences in the outcomes available to laboratory and clinical investigators (Kissin 1994; Katz & McCartney 2002).

As the process of central sensitisation relates not only to skin incision but also to the extent of intraoperative tissue injury and postoperative inflammation, the focus has shifted from the timing of a single intervention to the concept of 'preventive' analgesia (Kissin 1994) (See Table 1.5).

Table 1.5 Definitions of pre-emptive and preventive analgesia

Pre-emptive analgesia	Preoperative treatment is more effective than the identical treatment administered after incision or surgery. The only difference is the timing of administration.
Preventive analgesia	Postoperative pain and/or analgesic consumption is reduced relative to another treatment, a placebo treatment, or no treatment as long as the effect is observed at a point in time that exceeds the expected duration of action of the target agent. The intervention may or may not be initiated before surgery.

Sources: Møiniche et al (2002) and Katz (2002).

A systematic review (Katz 2002, **Level I**) reported benefit with preventive analgesia but equivocal or no benefit from pre-emptive treatment (Table 1.6).

Table 1.6 Summary of studies according to target agent administered

Agent(s)	No. of studies	Pre-emptive studies Positive	Pre-emptive studies Negative	Preventive effects Positive	Preventive effects Negative	Opposite effects	Total no. effects
Local anaesthetics[a]	59	7 (10.1)	16 (23.2)	26 (37.7)	14 (20.3)	6 (8.7)	69 (100)
Opioids	21	4 (16.7)	5 (20.8)	9 (37.5)	3 (12.5)	3 (12.5)	24 (100)
NSAIDs	20	1 (4.2)	10 (41.7)	3 (12.5)	8 (33.3)	2 (8.3)	24 (100)
NMDA antagonists	24	4 (12.9)	6 (19.4)	15 (48.4)	5 (16.1)	1 (3.2)	31 (100)
LAs and opioids	19	3 (14.3)	4 (19.0)	7 (33.3)	6 (28.6)	1 (4.8)	21 (100)
Multimodal	5	1 (14.3)	0 (0)	2 (28.6)	3 (42.9)	1 (14.3)	7 (100)
Total [b]	**148**	**20 (11.4)**	**41 (23.3)**	**62 (35.2)**	**39 (22.2)**	**14 (7.9)**	**176 (100)**

Notes: Table shows the total number of studies and number (%) with positive and negative pre-emptive and preventive effects. Also shown is the number (%) of studies reporting effects opposite to those predicted and the total number of effects (positive, negative and opposite). The total number of effects exceeds the number of studies because some studies were designed to evaluate both pre-emptive and preventive effects. See text for definition of pre-emptive and preventive effects.

a. P = 0.01 for the number of positive preventive effects by Fisher's exact test.

b. = P = 0.0001 for the number of positive preventive effects by chi-squared test

Source: Reproduced from Katz J (2003); Reprinted by permission of Hodder Arnold.

As activation of the NMDA receptor plays an important role in central sensitisation, many studies have focussed on the ability of NMDA receptor antagonists to produce pre-emptive or preventive analgesic effects.

In another review, 14 of 24 ketamine studies and 8 of 12 dextromethorphan studies reported a preventive analgesic effect, although no clear dose response could be identified; no positive effect was seen in four studies using magnesium (McCartney et al 2004, **Level I**).

Key messages

1. The timing of a single analgesic intervention (preincisional versus postincisional), defined as pre-emptive analgesia, does not have a clinically significant effect on postoperative pain relief (**Level I**).
2. There is evidence that some analgesic interventions have an effect on postoperative pain and/or analgesic consumption that exceeds the expected duration of action of the drug, defined as preventive analgesia (**Level I**).
3. NMDA receptor antagonist drugs in particular show preventive analgesic effects (**Level I**).

1.5 Adverse physiological and psychological effects of pain

Acute pain is a symptom that signals real or imminent tissue damage (Ready & Edwards 1992). Effective management of acute pain is required not only for ethical reasons (Cousins 2000; Cousins et al 2004) but to modify the response to injury. The magnitude of the injury response, while influenced by a variety of factors (Figure 1.2), is proportional to the degree of tissue damage (Chernow 1987; Cousins 1989). This response leads in turn to a number of physiological changes that promote catabolism, increased sympathetic activity, immunosuppression and other adverse effects.

The psychological effects of acute pain are just as harmful although they may be less obvious. They interact with the physical changes and often form part of a vicious cycle (Dianrello 1984; Cousins & Phillips 1986).

Figure 1.2 The injury response

		Injury response
Postoperative pain	Acute phase 'cytokines' (eg Interleukin 1,6)	Inflammation
Surgical trauma	Neural	Hyperalgesia
Psychological, environmental factors	Humoral	Catabolism
Other factors (eg drugs)	Metabolic	Other systemic adaptations
	Immune	Physical, mental deactivation

Note: Pain is only one of the factors, including psychological and environmental factors, that trigger complex intermediates (neural, humoral etc) leading to the 'injury response'. Thus acute pain and the injury response are inevitably inter-related. The end result is physical and mental deactivation.

Source: *Acute Pain Management: the Scientific Evidence* (NHMRC 1999); © Commonwealth of Australia, reproduced with permission.

1.5.1 Physiological changes

The physiological changes that result from pain and injury are a result of activation of both the peripheral and central nervous systems (Woolf 1989; Kehlet 1997). The 'stress response' evoked by injury includes a systemic metabolic response due to the release of neuroendocrine hormones and the local release of cytokines (eg interleukins, tumour necrosis factor) at the site of injury, leading to physiological alterations in all major organ systems (see Table 1.7).

Table 1.7 Metabolic and endocrine responses to surgery

Endocrine	↑ Catabolic hormones	↑ ACTH, cortisol, ADH, growth hormone, catecholamines, angiotensin II, aldosterone, glucagons, IL-1, TNF, IL-6
	↓ Anabolic hormones	↓ Insulin, testosterone
Metabolic		
carbohydrate	Hyperglycaemia, glucose intolerance, insulin resistance	↑ Glycogenolysis, gluconeogenesis (cortisol, glucagon, growth hormone, adrenaline, free fatty acids) ↓ Insulin secretion/activation
protein	Muscle protein catabolism, ↑ synthesis of acute phase proteins	↑Cortisol, adrenaline, glucagons, IL-1, IL-6, TNF
lipid	↑ Lipolysis and oxidation	↑ Catecholamines, cortisol, glucagon, growth hormone
Water and electrolyte flux	Retention of water and sodium, ↑ excretion of potassium and ↓ functional ECF with shifts to ICF	↑ Catecholamine, aldosterone, ADH, cortisol, angiotensin II, prostaglandins and other factors

Note: ACTH = adrenocorticotrophic hormone, ADH = antidiuretic hormone, IL = interleukin, TNF = tumour necrosis factor, ECF = extracellular fluid, ICF = intracellular fluid

Source: *Acute Pain Management: the Scientific Evidence* (NHMRC 1999); copyright Commonwealth of Australia, reproduced with permission.

Pain from surgical stimuli can activate sympathetic efferent nerves and increase heart rate, inotropy, and blood pressure. As sympathetic activation increases myocardial oxygen demand and reduces myocardial oxygen supply, the risk of cardiac ischaemia, particularly in patients with pre-existing cardiac disease, is increased. Increased sympathetic activity can also reduce gastrointestinal motility and contribute to ileus. Severe pain after upper abdominal and thoracic surgery contributes to an inability to cough and a reduction in functional residual capacity, resulting in atelectasis and ventilation-perfusion abnormalities, hypoxaemia and an increased incidence of pulmonary complications. The stress response also contributes to a suppression of cellular and humoral immune function and a hypercoagulable state following surgery, both of which can contribute to postoperative complications (Liu et al 1995). Patients at greatest risk of adverse outcomes from acute unrelieved pain include the very young or elderly patient, those with concurrent medical illnesses and those undergoing major surgery.

Effective analgesia is capable of modifying many of the pathophysiological responses to injury, thereby assisting recovery (Kehlet 1999; Kehlet & Dahl 2003). Current studies comparing analgesic techniques have shown a reduction in respiratory complications and improved pain relief with epidural analgesia, but an association between modifying the stress response and improved outcome or reduction in mortality is difficult to confirm (Ballantyne et al 1998, **Level I**; Liu et al 2004, **Level I**) (see Section 7.2).

CHAPTER 1

1.5.2 Psychological changes

Psychological changes associated with acute pain have received less attention than those associated with chronic pain, however they are no less important. Persistent nociceptive input, as occurs after surgery, trauma or burns can have a major influence on psychological function, which may in turn alter pain perception. Failure to relieve acute pain may result in increasing anxiety, inability to sleep, demoralisation, a feeling of helplessness, loss of control, inability to think and interact with others — in the most extreme situations, where patients can no longer communicate, effectively they have lost their autonomy (Cousins et al 2004). In some forms of acute pain (eg low back pain), psychological and environmental responses in the acute phase may be major determinants of progression to a persistent phase. An animal model of nerve injury produces consistent sensory disturbances in the affected limb, but only a subpopulation (about 30%) have persistent disturbance of sleep and social interactions, such as those observed in patients with chronic pain (Monassi 2003). It is not yet known if such disturbances indicate different behavioural responses per se, or a genetically determined difference in severity of pain due to the nerve injury.

References

Ballantyne JC, Carr DB, deFerranti S et al (1998) The comparative effects of postoperative analgesic therapies on pulmonary outcome: cumulative meta-analyses of randomized, controlled trials. *Anesth Analg* 86: 598–612.

Birklein F, Kunzel W, Sieweke N (2001) Despite clinical similarities there are significant differences between acute limb trauma and complex regional pain syndrome I (CRPS I). *Pain* 93: 165–71.

Bisgaard T, Klarskov B, Rosendberg J et al (2001) Characteristics and prediction of early pain after laparoscopic cholecystectomy. *Pain* 90: 261–69.

Blumenthal S, Dullenkopf A, Rentsch K et al (2005). Continuous infusion of ropivacaine for pain relief after iliac crest bone grafting for shoulder surgery. *Anesthesiology* 102: 392–97.

Blyth F M, March L M, Cousins M J (2003) Chronic pain-related disability and use of analgesia and health services in a Sydney community. *Med J Aust* 179: 84–87.

Brander VA, Stulberg SD, Adams AD et al (2003) Predicting total knee replacement pain: a prospective, observational study. *Clin Orthop* 416: 27–36.

Brandner B, Bromley L, Blagrove M (2002) Influence of psychological factors in the use of patient controlled analgesia. *Acute Pain* 4: 53–56.

Carey TS, Garrett JM, Jackman AM (2000) Beyond the good prognosis. Examination of an inception cohort of patients with chronic low back pain. *Spine* 25: 115–20.

Caumo W, Schmidt AP, Schneider CN et al (2001) Risk factors for postoperative anxiety in adults. *Anaesthesia* 56: 720–28.

Caumo W, Schmidt AP, Schneider CN et al (2002) Preoperative predictors of moderate to intense acute postoperative pain in patients undergoing abdominal surgery. *Acta Anaesthesiol Scand* 46: 1265–71.

Chernow B (1987) Hormonal responses to a graded surgical stress. *Arch Int Med* 147: 1273–78.

Cousins MJ & Phillips GD (1986) *Acute Pain Management. Clinics in Critical Care Medicine.* New York: Churchill Livingstone, p8.

Cousins MJ (1989) J.J.Bonica Lecture. Acute pain and the injury response: immediate and prolonged effects. *Reg Anesth Pain Med* 14: 162–78.

Cousins MJ (2000) Relief of acute pain: a basic human right? *Med J Aust* 172: 3–4.

Cousins MJ, Power I, Smith G (2000) 1996 Labat lecture: pain — a persistent problem. *Reg Anesth Pain Med* 25: 6–21.

Cousins MJ, Brennan F, Carr DB (2004) Editorial. Pain relief: a universal human right. *Pain* 112: 1–4.

Dinarello C (1984) Interleukin-I. *Rev Infect Dis* 6: 51–95.

Dworkin RH, Backonja M, Rowbotham MC et al (2003). Advances in neuropathic pain: diagnosis, mechanisms, and treatment recommendations. *Arch Neurol* 60:1524–34.

Eccleston C & Crombez G (1999) Pain demands attention: a cognitive-affective model of the interruptive function of pain. *Psych Bull* 125: 356–66.

Eccleston C (2001) Role of psychology in pain management. *Br J Anaesth* 87: 144–52.

Engel CL (1997) The need for a new medical model: a challenge for biomedical science. *Science* 196: 129–36.

Flor H, Elbert T, Knecht S et al (1995) Phantom-limb pain as a perceptual correlate of cortical reorganization following arm amputation. *Nature* 375: 482–84.

Flor H, Knost B, Birbaumer N (2002) The role of operant conditioning in chronic pain: an experimental investigation. *Pain* 95: 111–18.

Flor H & Hermann C (2004).Biopsychosocial models of pain In: Dworkin RH & Breitbart WS (Eds) *Psychosocial Aspects of Pain: a Handbook for Health Care Providers. Progress in Pain Research and Management.* Vol 27 Seattle: IASP Press.

Gil KM, Ginsberg B, Muir M et al (1990) Patient-controlled analgesia in postoperative pain: the relation of psychological factors to pain and analgesic use. *Clin J Pain* 6: 137–42.

Gil KM, Ginsberg B, Muir M et al (1992) Patient-controlled analgesia: the relation of psychological factors to pain and analgesic use in adolescents with postoperative pain. *Clin J Pain* 6: 215–21.

Grusser S M, Muhlnickel W, Schaefer M et al (2004) Remote activation of referred phantom sensation and cortical reorganization in human upper extremity amputees. *Exp Brain Res* 154: 97–102.

Hunt SP & Mantyh PW (2001). The molecular dynamics of pain control. *Nat Rev Neurosci* 2: 83–91.

Jacobsen PB & Butler RW (1996) Relation of cognitive coping and catastrophizing to acute pain and analgesic use following breast surgery. *J Behav Med* 19: 17–29.

Jamieson RN, Taft K, O'Hara JP et al (1993) Psychosocial and pharmacological predictors of satisfaction with intravenous patient-controlled analgesia. *Anesth Analg* 77: 121–25.

Ji RR & Woolf CJ (2001). Neuronal plasticity and signal transduction in nociceptive neurons: implications for the initiation and maintenance of pathological pain. *Neurobiol Dis* 8:1–10.

Ji RR, Kohno T, Moore KA et al (2003). Central sensitization and LTP: do pain and memory share similar mechanisms? *Trends Neurosci* 26: 696–705.

Jolliffe CD & Nicholas MK (2004) Verbally reinforcing pain reports: an experimental test of the operant model of chronic pain. *Pain* 107: 167–75.

Kalkman CJ, Visser K, Moen J et al (2003) Preoperative prediction of severe postoperative pain. *Pain* 105: 415–23.

Katz J & McCartney CJ (2002) Current status of pre-emptive analgesia. *Curr Opin Anaesthesiol* 15: 435–41.

Katz J (2003) Timing of treatment and preemptive analgesia. In: Rowbotham DJ & Macintyre PE (Eds) *Clinical Pain Management: Acute Pain*. London: Arnold.

Kehlet H (1997) Multimodal approach to control postoperative pathophysiology and rehabilitation. *Br J Anaesth* 78: 606–17.

Kehlet H (1999) Acute pain control and accelerated postoperative surgical recovery. *Surg Clin North Am* 79: 431–43.

Kehlet H & Dahl JB (2003) Anaesthesia, surgery and challenges in postoperative recovery. *Lancet* 362: 1921–28.

Kissin I (1994) Preemptive analgesia: terminology and clinical relevance. *Anesth Analg* 79: 809–10.

Kudoh A, Katagai H, Takazawa T (2001) Increased postoperative pain scores in chronic depression patients who take antidepressants. *J Clin Anesth* 14: 421–25.

Lai J, Hunter JC, Porreca F (2003). The role of voltage-gated sodium channels in neuropathic pain. *Curr Opin Neurobiol* 13: 291–97.

Linton SJ (2000) A Review of psychological risk factors in back and neck pain. *Spine* 25: 1148–56.

Liu S, Carpenter RL, Neal JM (1995) Epidural anesthesia and analgesia: their role in postoperative outcome. *Anesthesiology* 82: 1474–506.

Liu SS, Block BM, Wu CL (2004) Effects of perioperative central neuraxial analgesia on outcome after coronary artery bypass surgery: a meta-analysis. *Anesthesiology* 101: 153–56.

Macrae WA (2001) Chronic pain after surgery. *Br J Anaesth* 87: 88–98.

McCartney CJ, Sinha A, Katz J (2004) A qualitative systematic review of the role of N-methyl-D-aspartate receptor antagonists in preventive analgesia. *Anesth Analg* 98: 1385–400.

Merskey H (1979) Pain terms: a list with definitions and notes on usage. Recommended by the Subcommittee on Taxonomy. *Pain* 6: 249–52

Merskey H (1994) Logic, truth and language in concepts of pain. *Qual Life Res* 3 (Suppl 1): S69–76.

Merskey H & Bogduk N (Eds) (1994) *Classification of Chronic Pain. Descriptions of Chronic Pain Syndromes and Definitions of Pain Terms*. 2nd edn. Seattle: IASP Press.

Millan MJ (2002) Descending control of pain. *Prog Neurobiol* 66: 355–474.

Mogil JS (1999) The genetic mediation of individual differences in sensitivity to pain and its inhibition. *Proc Natl Acad Sci* 96: 7744–51.

Møiniche S, Kehlet H, Dahl JB (2002) A qualitative and quantitative systematic review of preemptive analgesia for postoperative pain relief: the role of timing of analgesia. *Anesthesiology* 96: 725–41.

Nelson FV, Zimmerman L, Barnason S et al (1998) The relationship and influence of anxiety on post-operative pain in the coronary artery bypass patients. *J Pain Sympt Manage* 15: 102–09.

Obata H, Saito S, Fujita N et al (1999) Epidural block with mepivacaine before surgery reduces long-term post-thoracotomy pain. *Can J Anaesth* 46: 1127–32.

Ochroch EA, Gottschalk A, Augistides J et al (2002) Long-term pain and activity during recovery from major thoracotomy using thoracic epidural analgesia. *Anesthesiology* 97: 1234–44.

Ozalp G, Sarioglu R, Tuncel G et al (2003) Preoperative emotional states in patients with breast cancer and postoperative pain. *Acta Anaesthesiol Scand* 47: 26–29.

Pavlin JD, Sullivan MJL, Freund PR et al (2005) Catastrophizing: a risk factor for postsurgical pain. *Clin J Pain* 21: 83–90.

Perkins FM & Kehlet H (2000) Chronic pain as an outcome of surgery — A review of predictive factors. *Anesthesiology* 93: 1123–33.

Perry F, Parker RK, White PF et al (1994) Role of psychological factors in postoperative pain control and recovery with patient-controlled analgesia. *Clin J Pain* 10: 57–63.

Pincus T, Vlaeyen JW, Kendall NA et al (2002)Cognitive-behavioral therapy and psychosocial factors in low back pain: directions for the future. *Spine* 27: E133–38.

Porro CA, Baraldi P, Pagnoni G et al (2002) Does anticipation of pain affect cortical nociceptive systems? *J Neurosci* 22: 3206–14.

Ready LB & Edwards WT (1992) *Management of Acute Pain: A Practical Guide*. Taskforce on Acute Pain. Seattle: IASP Publications.

Reuben SS, Vieriap P, Faruqi S et al (2001) Local administration of morphine for analgesia after iliac bone graft harvest. *Anesthesiology* 95: 390–94.

Schott GD (1986) Pain and its absence in an unfortunate family of amputees. *Pain* 25: 229–31.

Senturk M, Ozcan PE, Talu GK et al (2002) The effects of three different analgesia techniques on long-term postthoracotomy pain. *Anesth Analg* 94: 11–15.

Snider WD & McMahon SB (1998) Tackling pain at the source: new ideas about nociceptors. *Neuron* 20: 629–32.

Thomas V, Heath M, Rose D et al (1995) Psychological characteristics and the effectiveness of patient-controlled analgesia. *Br J Anaesth* 74: 271–76.

Turk DC (1995) Biopsychosocial perspective on chronic pain. In: Gatchel RJ & Turk DC (Eds) *Psychological Approaches to Pain Management.* New York: Guilford Press.

Vlaeyen JWS & Linton SJ (2000) Fear-avoidance and its consequences in chronic musculoskeletal pain: a state of the art. *Pain* 85: 317–32.

Walker SM, Goudas LC, Cousins MJ et al (2002) Combination spinal analgesic chemotherapy: a systematic review. *Anesth Analg* 95: 674–715.

Wall PD (1988) The prevention of post-operative pain. *Pain* 33: 289–90.

Woolf CJ (1983) Evidence for a central component of post-injury pain hypersensitivity. *Nature* 306: 686–88.

Woolf CJ (1989) Recent advances in the pathophysiology of acute pain. *Br J Anaesth* 63: 139–46.

Woolf CJ & Salter MW (2000) Neuronal plasticity: increasing the gain in pain. *Science* 288: 1765–69.

2. ASSESSMENT AND MEASUREMENT OF ACUTE PAIN AND ITS TREATMENT

2.1 Assessment

The assessment and measurement of pain are fundamental to the process of assisting in the diagnosis of the cause of a patient's pain, selecting an appropriate analgesic therapy and evaluating then modifying that therapy according to the patient's response. Pain should be assessed within a biopsychosocial model which recognises that physiological, psychological and environmental factors influence the overall pain experience.

The assessment of acute pain should include a thorough general medical history and physical examination, a specific 'pain history' (see Table 2.1) and an evaluation of associated disability (see Section 2.3). A complete pain history provides important diagnostic information that may help distinguish different underlying pain states such as nociceptive (somatic and visceral) or neuropathic pain (Hobbs & Hodgkinson 2003).

Somatic pain may be described as sharp, hot or stinging, is generally well localised and is associated with local and surrounding tenderness. By contrast, visceral pain may be described as dull, cramping, or colicky, is often poorly localised and may be associated with tenderness locally or in the area of referred pain, or with symptoms such as nausea, sweating and cardiovascular changes (Hobbs & Hodgkinson 2003).

While nociceptive pain is more common in the acute pain setting, neuropathic pain may also be present (see Section 1.3). Features in the pain history that may suggest a diagnosis of neuropathic pain include (Hobbs & Hodgkinson 2003):

- pain descriptors such as burning, shooting and stabbing;
- the paroxysmal or spontaneous nature of the pain which may have no clear precipitating factors;
- the presence of dysaesthesias (spontaneous or evoked unpleasant abnormal sensations), hyperalgesia (increased response to a normally painful stimulus), allodynia (pain due to a stimulus that does not normally evoke pain such as light touch) or areas of hypoaesthesia; and
- regional autonomic features (changes in colour, temperature and sweating) and phantom phenomena.

Table 2.1 Fundamentals of a pain history

1 **Site of pain**
   a primary location : description ± body map diagram
   b radiation
2 **Circumstances associated with pain onset**
3 **Character of pain**
   a sensory descriptors eg sharp, throbbing, aching
   b McGill Pain Questionnaire: includes sensory and affective descriptors (Melzack 1987)
4 **Intensity of pain**
   a at rest
   b on movement
   c temporal factors
      i duration
      ii current pain; during last week; highest level
      iii continuous or intermittent
   d aggravating or relieving factors
5 **Associated symptoms (eg nausea)**
6 **Effect of pain on activities and sleep**
7 **Treatment**
   a current and previous medications – dose, frequency of use, efficacy, side effects
   b other treatment eg transcutaneous electrical nerve stimulation
   c health professionals consulted
8 **Relevant medical history**
   a prior or coexisting pain conditions and treatment outcomes
   b prior or coexisting medical conditions
9 **Factors influencing the patient's symptomatic treatment**
   a belief concerning the causes of pain
   b knowledge, expectations and preferences for pain management
   c expectations of outcome of pain treatment
   d reduction in pain required for patient satisfaction or to resume 'reasonable activities'
   e typical coping response for stress or pain, including presence of anxiety or psychiatric disorders (eg depression or psychosis)
   f family expectations and beliefs about pain, stress and postoperative course

It is useful to draw the distinction between the different types of pain because the likely duration of the pain and the response to analgesic strategies may vary. The concept of 'mechanism-based pain diagnosis' has been promoted (Woolf & Max 2001) but currently the correlation between symptoms, mechanisms and response to therapy is not fully defined.

2.2 Measurement

The definition of pain underlies the complexity of its measurement. Pain is an individual and subjective experience modulated by physiological, psychological and environmental factors such as previous events, culture, prognosis, coping strategies, fear and anxiety. Therefore, most measures of pain are based on self-report. These measures lead to sensitive and consistent results if done properly (Moore et al 2003). Self-report measures may be influenced by mood, sleep disturbance and medications (Hobbs & Hodgkinson 2003).

In some instances it may not be possible to obtain reliable self-reports of pain (eg patients with impaired consciousness or cognitive impairment, young children, or where there are failures of communication due to language difficulties, inability to understand the measures, unwillingness to cooperate or severe anxiety). In these circumstances other methods of pain assessment will be needed.

There are no objective measures of 'pain' but associated factors such as hyperalgesia (eg mechanical withdrawal threshold), the stress response (eg plasma cortisol), behavioural responses (eg facial expression), functional impairment (eg coughing, ambulation) or physiological responses (eg changes in heart rate) may provide additional information (Hobbs & Hodgkinson 2003). Analgesic requirements (eg patient-controlled opioid doses delivered) are commonly used as *post hoc* measures of pain experienced (Moore et al 2003).

Recording pain intensity as 'the fifth vital sign' aims to increase awareness and utilisation of pain assessment (JCAHO 2001) and may lead to improved acute pain management (Gould et al 1992, **Level III-3**). Regular and repeated measurements of pain should be made to assess ongoing adequacy of analgesic therapy. An appropriate frequency of reassessment will be determined by the duration and severity of the pain, patient needs and response, and the type of drug or intervention (JCAHO 2001). Such measurements should incorporate different components of pain. For example, in the postoperative patient this should include assessments of static (rest) and dynamic (on sitting, coughing or moving the affected part) pain. Whereas static measures may relate to the patient's ability to sleep, dynamic measures can provide a simple test for mechanical hyperalgesia (Katz 2003) and determine whether analgesia is adequate for recovery of function (Hobbs & Hodgkinson 2003).

Uncontrolled pain should always trigger a reassessment of the diagnosis and consideration of alternatives such as developing surgical or other complications, or the presence of neuropathic pain. Review by an acute pain service or other specialist group should be considered.

2.2.1 Unidimensional measures of pain

A number of scales are available that measure either pain intensity, or the degree of pain relief following an intervention. Pain relief scales have some advantage when comparing the response to different treatments as all patients start with the same baseline relief score (zero), whereas they may have differing levels of baseline pain intensity (Hobbs & Hodgkinson 2003; Moore et al 2003).

Categorical scales

Categorical scales use words to describe the magnitude of pain or the degree of pain relief (Moore et al 2003). The verbal descriptor scale (VDS) is the most common example (eg using terms such as none, mild, moderate and severe). Pain relief may also be graded using a VDS — none, mild, moderate and complete.

There is a good correlation between descriptive verbal categories and visual analogue scales (Banos et al 1989, **Level III-2**), but the VDS is a less sensitive measure of pain treatment outcome than the visual analogue scale (VAS) (Jensen et al 2002, **Level IV**).

Categorical scales have the advantage of being quick and simple and may be useful in the elderly or visually impaired patient and in some children. However, the limited number of choices in categorical compared with numerical scales may make it more difficult to detect differences between treatments (Breivik et al 2000, **Level II**).

Numerical rating scales

Numerical rating scales have both written and verbal forms. Patients rate their pain intensity on the scale of 0 to 10 where 0 represents 'no pain' and 10 represents 'worst pain imaginable', or their degree of pain relief from 0 representing 'no relief' to 10 representing 'complete relief'.

Visual analogue scales consist of a 100 mm horizontal line with verbal anchors at both ends. The patient is asked to mark the line and the 'score' is the distance in millimetres from the left side of the scale to the mark. VAS are the most commonly used scales for rating pain intensity, with the words 'no pain' at the left end and 'worst pain possible' at the right, while VAS used to rate pain relief have the verbal anchors 'no pain relief' and 'complete pain relief'. VAS can also be used to measure other aspects of the pain experience (eg affective components, patient satisfaction, side effects).

VAS ratings of greater than 70 mm are indicative of 'severe pain' (Aubrun et al 2003, **Level IV**; Jensen et al 2003, **Level IV**) and 0-5 mm 'no pain', 5–44 mm 'mild pain' and 45–74 'moderate pain' (Aubrun et al 2003, **Level IV**).

These scales have the advantage of being simple and quick to use, allow for a wide choice of ratings and avoid imprecise descriptive terms (Hobbs & Hodgkinson 2003). However, the scales require more concentration and coordination, are unsuitable for children under 5 years and may also be unsuitable in up to 26% of adult patients (Cook et al 1999).

The VAS has been shown to be a linear scale for patients with acute postoperative pain of mild-moderate intensity (Myles et al 1999, **Level IV**). Therefore, results are equally distributed across the scale, such that the difference in pain between each successive increment is equal.

Verbal numerical rating scales (VNRS) where patients are asked to imagine that 0 represents 'no pain' and 10 represents 'worst pain imaginable' are simple to administer, give consistent results and correlate well with the VAS (Murphy et al 1988, **Level IV**; DeLoach et al 1998, **Level IV**; Breivik et al 2000, **Level IV**).

2.2.2 Multidimensional measures of pain

Rather than assessing only pain intensity, multidimensional tools provide further information about the characteristics of the pain and its impact on the individual. Examples include the Brief Pain Inventory which assesses pain intensity and associated disability (Daut et al 1983) and the McGill Pain Questionnaire which assesses the sensory, affective and evaluative dimensions of pain (Melzack 1987).

Unidimensional tools such as the VAS are inadequate when it comes to quantifying neuropathic pain. Specific scales have been developed that identify (and/or quantify) descriptive factors specific for neuropathic pain (Galer & Jensen 1997, **Level IV**; Bennett 2001, **Level IV**; Bouhassira et al 2004, **Level IV**) and which may also include bedside sensory examination (Bennett 2001) and allow evaluation of response to treatment (Bouhassira et al 2004).

Global scales are designed to measure the effectiveness of overall treatment (see Section 2.3.1). They are more suited to outcome evaluation at the end of treatment than to modifying treatment in the acute stage (Moore et al 2003). Questions such as 'How effective do you think the treatment was?' recognise that unimodal measures of pain intensity cannot adequately represent all aspects of pain perception.

2.2.3 Patients with special needs

Validated tools are available for measuring pain in neonates, infants and children, but must be both age and developmentally appropriate (see Section 10.1). Patients who have difficulty communicating their pain (eg cognitively impaired patients) require special attention as do patients whose language or cultural background differs significantly from that of their health care team. In such patients, pain measurement scales must be modified to suit individual patient needs (see Sections 10.3 to 10.5).

Key messages

1. Regular assessment of pain leads to improved acute pain management (**Level III-3**).
2. There is good correlation between the visual analogue and numerical rating scales (**Level III-2**).

The following tick boxes ☑ represent conclusions based on clinical experience and expert opinion.

☑ Self-reporting of pain should be used whenever appropriate as pain is by definition a subjective experience.

☑ The pain measurement tool chosen should be appropriate to the individual patient; developmental, cognitive, emotional, language and cultural factors should be considered.

☑ Scoring should incorporate different components of pain. In the postoperative patient this should include static (rest) and dynamic (eg pain on sitting, coughing) pain.

☑ Uncontrolled or unexpected pain requires a reassessment of the diagnosis and consideration of alternative causes for the pain (eg new surgical/ medical diagnosis, neuropathic pain).

2.3 Outcome measures in acute pain management

The aims of this section are to define outcome measures and related terms and describe their use in acute pain management.

Table 2.2 Definitions of outcome measures

Outcome	A result or evident effect of an action, event or process. One action may have several outcomes. Outcomes may be valued as desired or adverse.
Clinical outcome	A clinically meaningful endpoint that reflects directly how a patient ultimately feels, functions or survives as the result of a medical intervention in a specific disease process (examples: resolution of postoperative pain and suffering, return to usual vocation after an episode of acute back pain, the rate of serious irreversible adverse events following epidural analgesia, all-cause mortality resulting from use of COX-2 inhibitors). It may be difficult to measure clinical outcomes and to show changes or differences over a relatively short study period.
Intermediate outcome	A clinical outcome but one that is not the ultimate endpoint of the medical intervention in the disease process (examples: pain relief at 4–6 hours after intervention, time from intervention to rescue analgesic dose, time to first mobilisation postoperatively, rate of postoperative nausea and vomiting). As intermediate outcomes are easier to measure and more likely to show changes over shorter periods of time, they are often measured and reported in clinical trials. Intermediate outcomes may or may not be important to the recipients of the interventions.
Surrogate outcome	A laboratory measurement or a physical sign used as a substitute for a clinically meaningful endpoint (examples: blood pressure or ECG changes versus incidence of postoperative myocardial infarction and mortality, reduced vital capacity versus incidence of postoperative pulmonary complications). To be useful a surrogate outcome should be a physiological variable; there should be a pathophysiological basis for believing that the surrogate outcome represents a direct link in the chain of events between the intervention and the clinically meaningful endpoint; and changes in the surrogate endpoint should predict changes in the clinically meaningful endpoint. Few surrogate outcomes meet all these requirements.
Patient-relevant outcome	An outcome that matters to the patient or their carers. These need to be outcomes that patients can experience (examples: a reduction in pain intensity that is valued as 'worthwhile' by the patient, improved quality of life, return to normal function).

Sources: Turner (1987), Temple (1999), NHMRC (2000) and Rathmell et al (2003).

CHAPTER 2

2.3.1 Outcome measures

Pain

Clinical management

Self-reports of pain intensity or pain relief (see above) are used to evaluate efficacy and adjust the analgesic management according to the individual patient's needs, until resolution of the pain or underlying illness. This outcome is of direct relevance to the patient.

Clinical trials

CHAPTER 2

The aim of many clinical trials is to determine whether a drug or intervention provides adequate pain relief for the majority of participants. This can be achieved by repeated single measures at fixed time points, which may encompass only a proportion of the total illness. When comparison is made with a placebo, a statistically significant result can be achieved with a relatively small number of patients (eg n=40) (Collins et al 2001). The primary outcome is chosen by the researcher and may not be of direct importance to the individual patient, particularly if it relates to only a proportion of the total time he/she was in pain. It is also important to consider that statistically significant differences in pain scores may not reflect clinically significant differences, although these are harder to define (see below).

Data derived from categorical and visual analogue scales of pain intensity or relief produce a range of summary outcomes that can be used to assess (Moore et al 2003):

- the degree of analgesic effect:
  - difference between the baseline and postintervention score of pain intensity or pain relief;
  - the area under the time-analgesic effect curve (see Table 2.3);
  - dose of rescue analgesic consumption required in a given time period;
- the time to analgesic effect:
  - the time to onset of analgesic effect;
  - mean time to maximum reduction in pain intensity or to peak relief;
- the duration of effect:
  - time for pain to return to at least 50% of baseline;
  - time for pain intensity to return to baseline or for pain relief to fall to zero;
  - time to remedication/rescue analgesia.

Table 2.3 Definitions of pain intensity and pain relief

Summed pain intensity difference (SPID)	The summed differences between initial pain intensity and pain intensity at a series of given time points after intervention. The reliability of SPID may be limited if groups differ with respect to the baseline pain severity
Visual analogue scale summed pain intensity difference (VASSPID)	The visual analogue equivalent of SPID
Total pain relief (TOTPAR)	The area under the curve for pain relief against time, usually for 4–6 hours after the intervention. As all patients have zero pain relief prior to intervention, results are more standardised than obtained with SPID
Visual analogue scale total pain relief (VASTOTPAR)	The visual analogue equivalent of TOTPAR

Source: Moore et al (2003).

Meta-analyses

In order to evaluate the overall efficacy of an intervention and adequately compare it with other treatments, a much larger group of patients is required and this information can be derived from a meta-analysis (Collins et al 2001).

A widely used method of describing the effectiveness of an analgesic intervention is the number-needed-to-treat (NNT). In this setting it is commonly defined as the number of patients that need to be treated to achieve at least 50% pain relief (eg at least 50% maximum TOTPAR) in one patient compared with a placebo over a 4–6 hour treatment period (Moore et al 2003). Analysis at other cut-off points (30–70% max TOTPAR) has shown the same relative efficacy of different treatments (McQuay et al 2003).

The validity of this approach as a true method of comparison may be questioned as there is no standardisation of the acute pain model or patient and only single doses of the analgesic agents are used. However, it may sometimes be reasonable to extrapolate estimates of analgesic efficacy from one pain model to another (Barden et al 2004, **Level I**).

Participant ratings of global improvement

Having measured the change in pain intensity attributable to a given intervention, the question arises as to whether the observed change is both statistically and clinically significant because a reduction in pain intensity does not inevitably lead to improved function and patient satisfaction (Svensson et al 2001, **Level IV**). A reduction in pain intensity by 30–35% has been rated as clinically meaningful by patients with postoperative pain (Cepeda et al 2003, **Level IV**; Jensen et al 2003, **Level IV**), acute pain in the emergency department (Lee et al 2003, **Level IV**), breakthrough cancer pain (Farrar et al 2000, **Level IV**) and chronic pain (Farrar et al 2001, **Level IV**).

Global ratings of efficacy or satisfaction allow patients to balance the unpleasantness or inconvenience of the intervention, the personal meaningfulness of any improvement in their pain and function, and the unpleasantness and meaning of any adverse events.

Global improvement scales usually incorporate a question-stem such as 'How effective do you think the treatment was?' with patient ratings scored on VAS or VNRS. Question-stems that address patient 'satisfaction' require the patient to compare their global improvement with their expectations.

Patients may report high levels of satisfaction even if they have moderate to severe acute pain (Svensson et al 2001, **Level IV**). Satisfaction may also be influenced by preoperative expectations of pain, effectiveness of pain relief, the patient-provider relationship (eg communication by medical and nursing staff), interference with function due to pain and number of opioid-related side effects (Svensson et al 2001, **Level IV**; Carlson et al 2003, **Level IV**; Jensen et al 2004, **Level IV**).

Notwithstanding these reservations, the evidence generally supports the validity of such measures in the study of acute and chronic pain (Chapman et al 1996, **Level IV**; Fischer et al 1999, **Level IV**; Collins et al 2001, **Level IV**; Katz 2002).

Physical functioning

Measures of physical functioning quantify many aspects of a patient's life including their ability to sleep, eat, think, deep breathe, cough, mobilise, perform activities of self-care and daily living, undertake their usual vocation, and to enjoy leisure activities and sport (Williams 1999). While not used commonly in single-dose analgesic trials, these measures may be useful in quantifying the functional outcome of multi-dose pharmacotherapy or non-pharmacological therapies for some acute pain states, in particular those affecting the musculoskeletal system and lasting weeks or months. Unidimensional measures of physical functioning include:

- lists of activities abandoned or performed in a limited manner due to pain;
- direct ratings of the degree to which pain interferes with given activities; and
- hours per week of given activities.

Global or multidimensional measures of function attempt to combine various abilities or disabilities to derive a summary measure. Scales that employ a large number of items might be comprehensive but risk patient exhaustion or error, while scales with fewer items might be patient-friendly but risk becoming insensitive to state or change (Williams 1999). These scales have been used in some studies of acute spinal pain and cancer-related pain:

- *disability scales* — generic scales include the Short Form 36 of Medical Outcomes Study (SF-36), the Sickness Impact Profile (SIP), and Roland & Morris Short SIP (Williams 1999); and
- *Quality of life (QOL) measures* — these measures are not widely used in pain studies other than for cancer-related pain (Higginson 1997).

Disease-specific measures quantify the impact of a specific pain problem on function and can be used to track changes after an intervention (eg ability to cough after thoracotomy, ability to lift a baby after caesarean section) (Garratt et al 2001). Generic measures facilitate comparisons among the functional limitations of different conditions and treatments, and may have advantages for audit of an acute pain service that includes patients with a range of conditions (Patrick & Deyo 1989).

Emotional functioning

Acute pain is an unpleasant sensory and emotional experience. The unpleasantness of the experience and its meaning for the individual may have short-term (anxiety, depression, irritability) and long-term consequences (lost confidence or self-efficacy or post-traumatic stress disorder) for the individual's emotional functioning.

Adverse symptoms and events

In trials of efficacy, adverse events are usually considered to be of secondary importance and inadequate reporting has been found in as many as half of randomised trials reviewed (Edwards et al 1999; Ioannidis & Lau 2001). If adverse events are sufficiently common (eg nausea with opioids) they may be quantifiable in trials of efficacy and specifically measured using dichotomous (present or absent), categorical (none, mild, moderate, severe) or interval scales (analogue or Likert). Analogous to NNTs, the number-needed-to-harm (NNH) may be used to describe the incidence of adverse effects.

Most efficacy trials will have inadequate power to detect rare adverse events and therefore they are also absent from systematic reviews. Large clinical trials specifically designed to detect adverse events are required (eg the VIGOR study investigated gastrointestinal toxicity and non-steroidal anti-inflammatory drugs [NSAIDs]) (Bombardier et al 2000). Spontaneous patient complaints and patient diaries (Edwards et al 1999) may detect unforeseeable adverse events. Case reports and post-marketing epidemiological research and surveillance (eg the Australian Adverse Drug Reactions Advisory Committee) remain important for detection of delayed events occurring after the initial trial period.

Besides the adverse outcomes attributed to acute pain management interventions, another area of interest is whether the adverse outcomes of trauma and surgery might be prevented by effective acute pain management. Outcomes such as mortality, morbidity due to derangements of the cardiovascular, respiratory, gastrointestinal and coagulation systems and progression to chronic pain have also been reported (Rathmell et al 2003).

Key message

The following tick box ☑ represents conclusions based on clinical experience and expert opinion.

☑ Multiple outcome measures are required to adequately capture the complexity of the pain experience and how it may be modified by pain management interventions.

CHAPTER 2

References

Aubrun F, Langeron O, Quesnel C et al (2003) Relationship between measurement of pain using visual analog score and morphine requirements during postoperative intravenous morphine titration. *Anesthesiology* 98: 1415–21.

Banos JE, Bosch F, Canellas M et al (1989) The acceptability of visual analogue scales in the clinical setting: a comparison with verbal rating scales in postoperative pain. *Methods Find Exp Clin Pharmacol* 11: 123–27.

Barden J, Edwards JE, McQuay HJ et al (2004) Pain and analgesic response after third molar extraction and other postsurgical pain. *Pain*107: 86–90.

Bennett M (2001) The LANSS Pain Scale: the Leeds assessment of neuropathic symptoms and signs. *Pain* 92: 147–57.

Bombardier C, Laine L, Reicin A et al (2000) Comparison of upper gastrointestinal toxicity of rofecoxib and naproxen in patients with rheumatoid arthritis. VIGOR Study Group. *New Engl J Med* 343: 1520–28.

Bouhassira D, Attal N, Fermanian J et al (2004) Development and validation of the Neuropathic Pain Symptom Inventory. *Pain* 108: 248–57.

Breivik EK, Bjornsson GA, Skovlund E (2000) A comparison of pain rating scales by sampling from clinical trial data. *Clin J Pain* 16: 22–28.

Campbell WI & Patterson CC (1998) Quantifying meaningful changes in pain. *Anaesthesia* 53: 121–25.

Carlson J, Youngblood R, Dalton JA et al (2003) Is patient satisfaction a legitimate outcome of pain management. *J Pain Symptom Manage* 25: 264-75.

Cepeda MS, Africano JM, Polo R et al (2003) What decline in pain intensity is meaningful to patients with acute pain. *Pain* 105: 151–57.

Chapman SL, Jamison RN, Sanders SH (1996) Treatment helpfulness questionnaire: a measure of patient satisfaction with treatment modalities provided in chronic pain management programs. *Pain* 68: 349–61.

Collins SL, Edwards J, Moore RA et al (2001) Seeking a simple measure of analgesia for mega-trials: is a single global assessment enough? *Pain* 91: 189–94.

Cook AK, Niven CA, Downs MG (1999) Assessing the pain of people with cognitive impairment. *Int J Geriatr Psych* 14: 421–25.

Daut RL, Cleeland CS, Flanery RC (1983) Development of the Wisconsin Brief Pain Questionnaire to assess pain in cancer and other diseases. *Pain* 17: 197–210.

DeLoach LJ, Higgins MS, Caplan AB et al (1998) The visual analog scale in the immediate postoperative period: intrasubject variability and correlation with a numeric scale. *Anesth Analg* 86: 102–06.

Edwards JE, McQuay HJ, Moore RA et al (1999) Reporting of adverse effects in clinical trials should be improved. Lessons from acute postoperative pain. *J Pain Sympt Manage* 18: 289–97.

Farrar JT, Portenoy RK, Berlin JA et al (2000) Defining the clinically important difference in pain outcome measures. *Pain* 88: 287–94.

Farrar JT, Young JP Jr, LaMoreaux L et al (2001) Clinical importance of changes in chronic pain intensity measured on an 11-point numerical pain rating scale. *Pain* 94: 149–58.

Fischer D, Stewart AL, Blich DA et al (1999) Capturing the patient's view of change as a clinical outcome measure. *JAMA* 282: 1157–62.

Galer BS & Jensen MP (1997) Development and preliminary validation of a pain measure specific to neuropathic pain: the Neuropathic Pain Scale. *Neurology* 48: 332–38.

Garratt AM, Maffett JK, Farrin AJ (2001) Responsiveness of generic and specific measures of health outcome in low back pain. *Spine* 26: 71–77.

Gould TH, Crosby DL, Harmer M et al (1992) Policy for controlling pain after surgery: effect of sequential changes in management. *BMJ* 305: 1187–93.

Higginson IJ (1997) Innovations in assessment: epidemiology and assessment of pain in advanced cancer. In: Jensen TS, Turner JA, Weisenfeld-Hallin Z (Eds). *Proceedings of the 8th World Congress on Pain, Progress in Pain Research and Management*. Volume 8. Seattle: IASP Press, pp 707–16.

Hobbs GJ & Hodgkinson V (2003) Assessment, measurement, history and examination. In: Rowbotham DJ & Macintyre PE (Eds) *Clinical Pain Management: Acute Pain*. London: Arnold Publishers.

Ioannidis JPA & Lau J (2001) Completeness of safety reporting in randomized trials: an evaluation of seven medical areas. *JAMA* 285: 437–43.

Jensen MP, Chen C, Brugger AM (2002) Postsurgical pain outcome assessment. *Pain* 99: 101–09.

Jensen MP, Chen C, Brugger AM (2003) Interpretation of visual analog scale ratings and change scores: a reanalysis of two clinical trials of postoperative pain. *J Pain* 4: 407–14.

Jensen MP, Mendoza T, Hanna D et al (2004) The analgesic effects that underlie patient satisfaction with treatment. *Pain* 110: 480–87.

JCAHO & NPC (2001) *Pain: Current Understanding of Assessment, Management and Treatments*. Joint Commission on Accreditation of Healthcare Organisations and the National Pharmaceutical Council, Inc. (www.jcaho.org/news+room/health+care+issues/pm+monographs.htm)

Katz J (2003) Timing of treatment and preemptive analgesia. In: Rowbotham DJ & Macintyre PE (Eds) *Clinical Pain Management: Acute Pain*. London: Arnold.

Katz N (2002) The impact of pain management on quality of life. *J Pain Sympt Manage* 24: S38–47.

Lee JS, Hobden E, Stiell IG et al (2003) Clinically important change in the visual analog scale after adequate pain control. *Acad Emerg Med* 10: 1128–30.

McQuay HJ, Barden J, Moore RA (2003) Clinically important changes – what's important and whose change is it anyway? *J Pain Symptom Manage* 25: 395–96.

Melzack R (1987) The short form McGill Pain Questionnaire. *Pain* 30: 191–97.

Moore A, Edwards J, Barden J et al (2003) *Bandolier's Little Book of Pain*. Oxford: Oxford University Press, pp14–18.

Murphy DF, McDonal A, Power C (1988) Measurement of pain: a comparison of the visual analogue scale with a nonvisual analogue scale. *Clin J Pain* 3: 197–99.

Myles PS, Troedel S, Boquest M et al (1999) The pain visual analog scale: is it linear or nonlinear? *Anesth Analg* 89: 1517–20.

NHMRC (2000) *How to use the Evidence: Assessment and Application of Scientific Evidence*. Handbook Series on Preparing Clinical Practice Guidelines. Canberra: National Health and Medical Research Council, pp24–29.

Patrick DL & Deyo RA (1989) Generic and disease-specific measures in assessing health status and quality of life. *Med Care* 27: S217–232.

Rathmell JP, Neal JM, Liu SS (2003) Outcome measures in acute pain management. In: Rowbotham DJ & Macintyre PE (Eds) *Clinical Pain Management: Acute Pain*. London: Arnold Publishers, pp163–81.

Svensson I, Sjostrom B, Halijamae H (2001) Influence of expectations and actual pain experience on satisfaction with postoperative pain management. *Eur J Pain* 5: 125–33.

Temple R (1999) Are surrogate markers adequate to assess cardiovascular disease drugs? *JAMA* 282: 790–95.

Turner GW (Ed) (1987) *The Australian Concise Oxford Dictionary*. Melbourne: Oxford University Press.

Williams AC de C (1999) Measures of function and psychology. In: Wall PD, Melzack R (Eds). *Textbook of Pain*. 4th Edition. Edinburgh: Churchill Livingstone, pp427–44.

Woolf C & Max M (2001) Mechanism-based pain diagnosis: issues for analgesic drug development. *Anaesthesiology* 95: 241–49.

3. PROVISION OF SAFE AND EFFECTIVE ACUTE PAIN MANAGEMENT

The safe and effective management of acute pain requires the appropriate education of all involved (ie medical, nursing and allied health staff and patients) and attention to the organisational aspects involved in the delivery of pain relief. These may include appropriate guidelines for drug prescription, monitoring of patients and recognition and treatment of any adverse effects of pain relief, and in some situations, the provision of an acute pain service. It is recognised that the need for and complexity of these requirements will vary according to the setting in which acute pain relief is delivered (eg hospital, general practice).

Successful acute pain management also requires close liaison with all personnel involved in the care of the patient including anaesthetists, pain specialists, surgeons, physicians, palliative care clinicians, general practitioners, specialists in addiction medicine, nurses, physiotherapists and psychologists (ANZCA &FPM 2000; RCA & Pain Society 2003; ASA 2004).

3.1 Education

3.1.1 Patients

Patient or carer education may take a number of forms — the most common methods are the use of booklets or short videos and specialist one-on-one education. The evidence for any benefit from preoperative education or the best educational technique is varied and inconsistent.

Patients may find that preoperative education is helpful (Shuldham 1999; Hodgkinson 2000) and it may increase patient or carer knowledge about pain and positive attitudes towards pain relief (Chambers et al 1997, **Level II**; Greenberg et al 1999, **Level II**; Knoerl et al 1999, **Level III-1**; Watkins 2001, **Level II**). However, pain relief is not always improved.

Some studies have shown no effect on postoperative pain or analgesic requirements (Griffin et al 1998, **Level II**; Greenberg et al 1999, **Level II**), including patient-controlled analgesia (PCA) (Chumbley et al 2004, **Level III-1**), although there may be an increase in patient satisfaction (Knoerl et al 1999, **Level III-1**; Watkins 2001, **Level II**; Sjoling et al 2003, **Level III-2**) and less preoperative anxiety (Sjoling et al 2003, **Level III-2**).

Others have suggested that, in general, structured preoperative patient education may improve patient outcome, including pain relief (Devine 1992, **Level III-2**; Guruge & Sidani 2002, **Level III-2**; Giraudet-Le Quintrec et al 2003, **Level II**).

In studies looking at specific types of surgery, there is no evidence that preoperative patient education has any effect on postoperative pain after:

- hip or knee replacement (McDonald & Green 2004, **Level I**);

- cardiac surgery in adults (Shuldham et al 2002, **Level II**; Watt-Watson et al 2004, **Level II**) or children (Huth et al 2003, **Level II**);
- gynaecological surgery (Lam et al 2001, **Level II**);
- gastric banding (Horchner & Tuinebreijer 1999, **Level III-1**); or
- spinal fusion in children and adolescents (Kotzer et al 1998, **Level III-3**).

Antenatal teaching about postnatal nipple pain and trauma results in reduced nipple pain and improved breast feeding (Duffy et al 1997, **Level II**).

3.1.2 Staff

Medical and nursing staff education may take a number of forms — the evidence for any benefit or the best educational technique is varied and inconsistent. Education may also include the provision of guidelines (see Section 3.2).

Improvements in nursing knowledge and ability to manage epidural analgesia followed the reintroduction of an epidural education program using an audit/ guideline/ problem-based teaching approach, accompanied by practical assessments (Richardson 2001, **Level III-3**). Pain documentation in surgical wards (Ravaud et al 2004, **Level III-1**) and intensive care units (Arbour 2003, **Level IV**; Erdek 2004, **Level III-3**) is also improved by education programs.

Improvements in postoperative pain relief, assessment of pain and prescribing practices can result from staff education as well as the introduction of medical and nursing guidelines (Harmer & Davies 1998, **Level III-3**; Gould et al 1992, **Level III-3**; MacDonald et al 2001, **Level IV**). Personalised feedback forms given to anaesthetists have been shown to increase the use of PCA, non-steroidal anti-inflammatory drugs (NSAIDs), epidural morphine and nerve blocks (Rose et al 1997, **Level III-3**). Education of residents in an emergency department can improve patient pain relief scores (Jones & Machen 2003, **Level III-3**).

However, education programs may not always be successful in improving nursing staff knowledge or attitudes (Dahlman et al 1999, **Level III-3**) or pain relief (Knoblauch & Wilson 1999, **Level IV**).

A number of studies have shown the benefits of education and/or guidelines on improved prescribing patterns both in general terms (Humphries 1997, **Level III-3**; Ury et al 2002, **Level III-3**) and specifically for NSAIDs (May et al 1999, **Level III-3**; Figueiras et al 2001, **Level I**; Ray et al 2001), paracetamol (Ripouteau et al 2000, **Level III-3**) and pethidine (Gordon et al 2000, **Level III-3**).

In rural and remote settings, distance and professional isolation could impact on the ability of health care staff to receive up-to-date education about pain relief. However, similarities between urban and rural nurses' knowledge and knowledge deficits relating to acute pain management have been reported (Kubecka et al 1996) and a tailored education program in a rural hospital improved the medical management of acute pain (Jones 1999, **Level III-3**).

3.2 Organisational requirements

More effective acute pain management will result from appropriate education and organisational structures for the delivery of pain relief rather than the analgesic techniques themselves (Wheatley & Madej 2003). Even simple methods of pain relief can be more effective if proper attention is given to education (see Section 3.1), analgesic drug orders, documentation, monitoring of patients and the provision of appropriate policies, protocols and guidelines (Gould et al 1992, **Level III-3**). In some institutions, acute pain services will assume responsibility for managing more advanced methods of pain relief such as PCA and epidural analgesia.

3.2.1 General requirements

Guidelines that aim to enhance patient outcomes and standardise analgesic techniques (eg drug and drug concentrations, dose, dose intervals, monitoring requirements, equipment and responses to inadequate or excessive analgesic doses and other complications) within or between institutions, may lead to consistency of practice, standardised educational programs for both staff and patients and potentially improved patient safety and analgesic efficacy (Wheatley & Madej 2003).

Marked improvements in conventional methods of pain relief have followed the introduction of guidelines for intramuscular opioid administration (Gould et al 1992, **Level III-3**; Humphries et al 1997, **Level III-3**). However, implementation of guidelines and not their development remains the greatest obstacle to their use. Compliance with available guidelines is highly variable and may be better in larger institutions (Carr et al 1998, **Level IV**). Resource availability, particularly staff with pain management expertise, and the existence of formal quality assurance programs to monitor pain management are positive predictors of compliance with guidelines (Jiang et al 2001, **Level IV**).

Professional bodies in a number of countries have issued guidelines for the management of acute pain (ANZCA &FPM 2000; ANZCA &FPM 2003; RCA & Pain Society 2003; ASA 2004).

3.2.2 Acute pain services

Many institutions would now say that they have an acute pain service. However, there is a very wide diversity of acute pain service structures (Powell et al 2004). Some are 'low-cost' nurse-based (Rawal 1997; Shapiro et al 2003), others are anaesthetist-led but there may not be daily clinical participation by an anaesthetist, relying primarily on acute pain service nurses (Harmer 2001; Nagi 2004; Powell et al 2004) and some are comprehensive and multidisciplinary services with acute pain service nursing staff, sometimes pharmacists or other staff and daily clinical input from and 24-hour cover by anaesthetists (Ready et al 1988; Macintyre et al 1990; Schug & Haridas 1993).

Some acute pain services supervise primarily 'high-tech' forms of pain relief while others have input into all forms of acute pain management in an institution and will work towards optimising traditional methods of pain relief so that all patients in that institution benefit (Macintyre & Ready 2001; Breivik 2002). There may also be inter-service variability in basic quality criteria (Stamer et al 2002).

Not surprisingly therefore, it is difficult to come up with a meaningful analysis of the benefits or otherwise of acute pain services. Individual publications have reported that the presence of an acute pain service reduced pain scores (Gould et al 1992, **Level III-3**; Miaskowski et al 1999, **Level IV**; Sartain & Barry 1999, **Level III-3**; Salomäki et al 2000, **Level III-3**; Bardiau et al 2003, **Level III-3**; Stadler et al 2004, **Level III-3**) and side effects (Schug & Torrie 1993, **Level IV**; Stacey et al 1997, **Level III-3**; Miaskowski et al 1999, **Level IV**).

A recent review of publications (primarily audits) looking at the effectiveness of acute pain services (all types) concluded that the implementation of an acute pain service is associated with a significant improvement in postoperative pain and a possible reduction in postoperative nausea and vomiting (Werner et al 2002, **Level IV**). The authors comment, however, that it is not possible to assess the contribution of factors such as an increased awareness of the importance of postoperative analgesia, the use of more effective analgesic regimens (eg epidural analgesia), the effects of acute pain service visits and better strategies for anti-emetic therapy.

Although systematic reviews have been attempted (McDonnell et al 2003; NICS 2003), the poor quality of the studies looking at the effectiveness or otherwise of acute pain services means that a proper meta-analysis cannot be performed and that the evidence for any benefit of acute pain services remains mixed.

Key messages

1. Preoperative education improves patient or carer knowledge of pain and encourages a more positive attitude towards pain relief (**Level II**).
2. Implementation of an acute pain service may improve pain relief and reduce the incidence of side effects (**Level III-3**).
3. Staff education and the use of guidelines improve pain assessment, pain relief and prescribing practices (**Level III-3**).
4. Even 'simple' techniques of pain relief can be more effective if attention is given to education, documentation, patient assessment and provision of appropriate guidelines and policies (**Level III-3**).

The following tick boxes ☑ represent conclusions based on clinical experience and expert opinion.

☑ Successful management of acute pain requires close liaison with all personnel involved in the care of the patient.

☑ More effective acute pain management will result from appropriate education and organisational structures for the delivery of pain relief rather than the analgesic techniques themselves.

References

ASA (2004) Practice guidelines for acute pain management in the perioperative setting. American Society of Anesthesiologists. *Anesthesiology* 100: 1573–81.

Arbour R (2003) A continuous quality improvement approach to improving clinical practice in the areas of sedation, analgesia, and neuromuscular blockade. *J Cont Ed Nursing* 34: 64–71.

ANZCA & FPM (2000) *Guidelines on Acute Pain Management*. ANZCA professional document PS41 2000. Australian and New Zealand College of Anaesthetists and Faculty of Pain Medicine. (www.anzca.edu.au/publications/profdocs/profstandards/PS41_2000.htm)

ANZCA & FPM (2003) *Guidelines for the Management of Major Regional Analgesia.* ANZCA professional document PS3 2003. Australian and New Zealand College of Anaesthetists and Faculty of Pain Medicine. (www.anzca.edu.au/publications/profdocs/profstandards/PS3_2003.htm)

Bardiau FM, Braeckman MM, Seidel L (1999) Effectiveness of an acute pain service inception in a general hospital. *J Clin Anesth* 11: 583–89.

Bardiau FM, Taviaux NF, Albert A et al (2003) An intervention study to enhance postoperative pain management. *Anesth Analg* 96: 179–85.

Breivik H (2002) How to implement an acute pain service. *Best Pract Res Clin Anaesthesiol* 16: 527–47.

Carr DB, Miaskowski C, Dedrick SC et al (1998) Management of perioperative pain in hospitalized patients: a national surgery. *J Clin Anesth* 10: 77–85.

Chambers CT, Reid GJ, McGrath PJ (1997) A randomized trial of a pain education booklet: effects on parents' attitudes and postoperative pain management. Presented at the meeting of the Canadian Psychological Association, Charlottetown, Prince Edward Island, June 1995. *Child Health Care* 26: 1–13.

Chumbley GM, Ward L, Hall GM et al (2004) Pre-operative information and patient-controlled analgesia: much ado about nothing. *Anaesthesia* 59: 354–58.

Dahlman G, Dykes A, Elander G (1999) Patients' evaluation of pain and nurses' management of analgesics after surgery. The effect of a study day on the subject of pain for nurses working at the thorax surgery department. *J Adv Nursing* 30: 866–74.

Devine EC (1992) Effects of psychoeducational care for adult surgical patients: a meta-analysis of 191 studies. *Patient Educ Couns* 19: 129–42.

Duffy EP, Percival P, Kershaw E (1997) Positive effects of an antenatal group teaching session on postnatal nipple pain, nipple trauma and breast feeding rates. *Midwifery* 13: 189–96.

Erdek M (2004) Improving assessment and treatment of pain in the critically ill. *Int J Qual Health Care* 16: 59–64.

Figueiras A, Sastre I, Tato F et al (2001) One-to-one versus group sessions to improve prescription in primary care: a pragmatic randomized controlled trial. *Med Care* 3: 158–67.

Giraudet-Le Quintrec JS, Coste J, Vastel L et al (2003) Positive effect of patient education for hip surgery: a randomized trial. *Clin Orthop* Sep: 112–20.

Gordon DB, Jones HD, Goshman LM et al (2000) A quality improvement approach to reducing use of meperidine. *Jt Comm J Qual Improv* 26: 686–99.

Gould TH, Crosby DL, Harmer M et al (1992) Policy for controlling pain after surgery; effect of sequential changes in management. *BMJ* 305: 1187–93.

Greenberg RS, Billett C, Zahurak M et al (1999) Videotape increases parental knowledge about pediatric pain management. *Anesth Analg* 89: 899–903.

Griffin MJ, Brennan L, McShane AJ (1998) Preoperative education and outcome of patient controlled analgesia. *Can J Anaesth* 45: 943–48.

Guruge S & Sidani S (2002) Effects of demographic characteristics on preoperative teaching outcomes: a meta-analysis. *Can J Nurs Res* 34: 25–33.

Harmer M & Davies KA (1998) The effect of education, assessment and a standardised prescription on postoperative pain management. The value of clinical audit in the establishment of acute pain services. *Anaesthesia* 53: 424–30.

Harmer M (2001) When is a standard not a standard? When it is a recommendation. *Anaesthesia* 56: 611–12.

Hodgkinson S (2000) Knowledge retention from pre-operative patient information. *Best Pract* 4: 1–6.

Horchner R & Tuinebreijer W (1999) Preoperative preparatory program has no effect on morbidly obese patients undergoing a Lap-Band operation. *Obes Surg* 9: 250–57.

Humphries C (1997) Audit of opioid prescribing: the effect of hospital guidelines. *Anaesthesia* 52: 745–49.

Huth MM, Broome ME, Mussatto KA et al (2003) A study of the effectiveness of a pain management education booklet for parents of children having cardiac surgery. *Pain Manage Nursing* 4: 31–39.

Jiang HJ, Lagasse RS, Ciccine K et al (2001) Factors influencing hospital implementation of acute pain management practice guidelines. *J Clin Anesth* 13: 268–76.

Jones JB (1999) Assessment of pain management skills in emergency medicine residents: the role of an education program. *J Emerg Med* 17: 349–54.

Jones GE & Machen I (2003) Pre-hospital pain management: the paramedics' perspective. *Accid Emerg Nursing* 11: 166–72.

Knoblauch SC & Wilson CJ (1999) Clinical outcomes of educating nurses about pediatric pain management. *Outcomes Manage Nurs Pract* 3: 87–89.

Knoerl DV, Faut-Callahan M, Paice J et al (1999) Preoperative PCA teaching program to manage postoperative pain. *Medsurg Nurs* 8: 25–33, 36.

Kotzer AM, Coy J, LeClaire AD (1998) The effectiveness of a standardized educational program for children using patient-controlled analgesia. *J Soc Ped Nurses* 3: 117–26.

Kubecka KE, Simon JM, Boettcher JH (1996) Pain management knowledge of hospital-based nurses in a rural Appalachian area. *J Adv Nurs* 23: 861–67.

Lam KK, Chan MT, Chen PP et al (2001) Structured preoperative patient education for patient-controlled analgesia. *J Clin Anesth* 13: 465–69.

Macintyre PE, Runciman WBR, Webb RK (1990) An acute pain service in an Australian teaching hospital: the first year. *Med J Aust* 153: 417–20.

Macintyre PE & Ready LB (2001) *Acute Pain Management: A Practical Guide*. 2nd Edition. London: WB Saunders.

May FW, Rowett DS, Gilbert AL et al (1999) Outcomes of an educational-outreach service for community medical practitioners: non-steroidal anti-inflammatory drugs. *Med J Aust* 170: 471–74.

McDonald DD, Freeland M, Thomas G et al (2001) Testing a preoperative pain management intervention for elders. *Res Nurs Health* 24: 402–09.

McDonald S, Hetrick S, Green S (2004) Pre-operative education for hip or knee replacement. *The Cochrane Database of Systematic Reviews 2004*, Issue 1. Art. No.: CD003526. DOI: 10.1002/14651858.CD003526.pub2.

McDonnell A, Nicholl J, Read SM (2003) Acute pain teams and the management of postoperative pain: a systematic review and meta-analysis. *J Adv Nurs* 41: 261–73.

Miaskowski C, Crews J, Ready B et al (1999) Anaesthesia-based pain services improve the quality of postoperative pain management. *Pain* 80: 23–29.

Nahi H (2004) Acute pain services in the United Kingdom. *Acute Pain* 5: 89–107.

NICS (2002) *Institutional Approaches to Pain Assessment and Management: A Systematic Literature Review*. Prepared by the Health Technology Assessment Unit, Department of Public Health, University of Adelaide. Melbourne: National Institute of Clinical Studies.

Powell AE, Davies HTO, Bannister J et al (2004) Rhetoric and reality on acute pain services in the UK: a national postal questionnaire survey. *Anaesthesia* 92: 689–92.

Ravaud P, Keita H, Porcher R et al (2004) Randomized clinical trial to assess the effect of an educational programme designed to improve nurses' assessment and recording of postoperative pain. *Br J Surg* 91: 692–98.

Rawal N (1997) Organization of acute pain services: a low cost model. *Acta Anaesthiol Scand* 111 (Supp): 188–90.

Ray WA, Stein CM, Byrd V et al (2001) Educational program for physicians to reduce use of non-steroidal anti-inflammatory drugs among community-dwelling elderly persons: a randomized controlled trial. *Med Care* 39: 425–35.

Ready LB, Oden R, Chadwick HS et al (1988) Development of an anesthesiology-based postoperative pain management service. *Anesthesiology* 68: 100–06.

Richardson J (2001) Post-operative epidural analgesia: introducing evidence-based guidelines through an education and assessment process. *J Clin Nursing* 10: 238–45.

Ripouteau C, Conort O, Lamas JP et al (2000) Quality improvement report: effect of multifaceted intervention promoting early switch from intravenous to oral acetaminophen for postoperative pain: controlled, prospective, before and after study. *BMJ* 321: 1460–63.

Rose DK, Cohen MM, Yee DA (1997) Changing the practice of pain management. *Anesth Analg* 84: 764–72.

Salomäki TE, Hokajärvi TM, Ranta P et al (2000) Improving the quality of postoperative pain relief. *Eur J Pain* 4: 367–72.

Sartain JB & Barry JJ (1999) The impact of an acute pain service on postoperative pain management. *Anaesth Intensive Care* 27: 375–80.

Schug SA & Haridas RP (1993) Development and organizational structure of an acute pain service in a major teaching hospital. *Aust N Z J Surg* 63: 8–13.

Schug SA & Torrie JJ (1993) Safety assessment of postoperative pain management by an acute pain service. *Pain* 55: 389–91.

Shapiro A, Zohar E, Kantor M et al (2003) Establishing a nurse-based anaesthesiologist-supervised inpatient acute pain service: experience of 4,617 patients. *J Clin Anesth* 16: 415–20.

Shuldham C (1999) A review of the impact of pre-operative education on recovery from surgery. *Int J Nurs Stud* 36: 171–77.

Shuldham CM, Fleming S, Goodman H (2002) The impact of pre-operative education on recovery following coronary artery bypass surgery. A randomized controlled clinical trial. *Eur Heart J* 23: 666–74.

Sjoling M, Nordahl G, Olofsson N et al (2003) The impact of preoperative information in state anxiety, postoperative pain and satisfaction with pain management. *Patient Ed Couns* 51: 169–76.

Stacey BR, Rudy TE, Nelhaus D (1997) Management of patient-controlled analgesia: a comparison of primary service and dedicated pain service. *Anesth Analg* 85: 130–34.

Stadler M, Schlander M, Braeckman M et al (2004) A cost-utility and cost-effectiveness analysis of an acute pain service. *J ClinAnesth* 16: 159–67.

Stamer UM, Mpasios N, Stüber F et al (2002) A survey of acute pain services in Germany and a discussion of international survey data. *Reg Anesth Pain Med* 27: 125–31.

RCA & Pain Society (2003) *Pain Management Services: Good Practice*. London: The Royal College of Anaesthetists, The British Pain Society.

Ury WA, Rahn M, Tolentino V et al (2002) Can a pain management and palliative care curriculum improve the opioid prescribing practices of medical residents? *J Gen Int Med* 17: 625–31.

Watkins GR (2001) *Effect of Pain Education on Postoperative Pain Management*. PhD thesis, University of Illinois at Chicago, Health Sciences Center.

Watt-Watson J, Stevens B, Katz J et al (2004) Impact of preoperative education on pain outcomes after coronary artery bypass graft surgery. *Pain* 109: 73–85.

Werner MU, Søholm L, Rotbøll-Nielsen et al (2002) Does an acute pain service improve postoperative outcome. *Anesth Analg* 95: 1361–72.

Wheatley RG & Madej TH (2003) Organization of an acute pain service. In: Rowbotham DJ & Macintyre PE (Eds) *Clinical Pain Management: Acute Pain*. London: Arnold Publishers.

4. SYSTEMICALLY ADMINISTERED ANALGESIC DRUGS

4.1 Opioids

Opioids remain the mainstay of systemic analgesia for the treatment of moderate to severe acute pain. Interpatient opioid requirements vary greatly (Lehmann et al 1990, **Level IV**; Macintyre & Jarvis 1996, **Level IV**) and opioid doses therefore need to be titrated to suit each patient. In adult patients, age rather than weight is the better predictor of opioid requirements (Macintyre & Jarvis 1996, **Level IV**).

4.1.1 Choice of opioids

All full opioid agonists given in equianalgesic doses produce the same analgesic effect (McQuay 1991); such equianalgesic doses are difficult to determine due to interindividual variabilities in kinetics and dynamics (Gammaitoni et al 2003).

Most available data do not suggest that any one opioid is superior to another, either in terms of better pain relief, differences in side effects or patient satisfaction (Sinatra et al 1989, **Level II**; Dunbar et al 1996, **Level III-2**; Rapp et al 1996, **Level II**; Stanley et al 1996, **Level II**; Woodhouse et al 1996, **Level II**; Silvasti et al 1998, **Level II**), but rather that some opioids may be better in some patients (Woodhouse et al 1999, **Level II**); although pethidine has been reported to have a higher incidence of nausea and vomiting compared with morphine (Ezri at al 2002, **Level II**; Silverman et al 2004, **Level III-3**).

While the data to support the concept of opioid rotation originate from cancer pain (Quigley 2004, **Level I**), it may be a useful strategy in the management of acute pain in patients with intolerable opioid-related side effects that are unresponsive to treatment.

4.1.2 Specific opioids

The efficacy of various opioids administered by the different routes used in the management of acute pain is discussed in detail in Chapter 6; the following section describes other relevant aspects of selected opioid agents including tramadol.

Codeine

Codeine is classified as a weak opioid but the molecule itself is devoid of analgesic activity. The principal metabolite of codeine is codeine-6-glucuronide, which has a similar potency to the parent drug and is renally excreted; metabolism to morphine (2–10% of dose given), the minor pathway, accounts for most of the analgesic effect of codeine (Mercadante & Arcuri 2004). The enzyme responsible for the conversion to morphine is cytochrome isoenzyme P450 (CYP) 2D6, which is lacking in 9% of Caucasians (Caraco et al 1996, **Level II**).

Given in doses of 60mg with paracetamol, codeine results in additional pain relief but may also increase the incidence of side effects (Moore et al 1998, **Level I**).

Dextropropoxyphene

Dextropropoxyphene (65mg) is a weak opioid with a number-needed-to-treat (NNT) of 7.7(Collins et al 1999b, **Level I**). It is often used in combination with paracetamol but this combination improves pain relief by only 7.3% compared with paracetamol alone and increases the incidence of dizziness (Li Wan Po & Zhang 1997, **Level I**).

The major metabolite of dextropropoxyphene is nordextropropoxyphene which is renally excreted; accumulation of nordextropropoxyphene can lead to central nervous system (CNS), respiratory and cardiac depression (Davies et al 1996).

Diamorphine

Diamorphine (diacetylmorphine, heroin) is rapidly hydrolysed to monoacetylmorphine (MAM) and morphine; diamorphine and MAM are more lipid soluble than morphine and penetrate the CNS more rapidly, although it is MAM and morphine that are thought to be responsible for the analgesic effects of diamorphine (Myoshi & Lackband, 2001). There is no difference between parenteral diamorphine and morphine in terms of analgesia and side effects (Kaiko et al 1981, **Level II**).

Dihydrocodeine

Dihydrocodeine is a semi-synthetic derivative of codeine, with an analgesic effect independent of its metabolism to dihydromorphine (Jurna et al 1997). Single doses of 30mg are ineffective in relieving postoperative pain (Edwards et al 2000b, **Level I**).

Fentanyl

Fentanyl is increasingly used in the treatment of acute pain because of its lack of active metabolites and fast onset of action (Peng & Sandler 1999).

Hydromorphone

Hydromorphone is a derivative of morphine that is approximately five times as potent as morphine. There is little difference between hydromorphone and other opioids in terms of analgesic efficacy or adverse effects (Quigley 2002, **Level I**). The main metabolite of hydromorphone is hydromorphone-3-glucuronide, a structural analogue of morphine-3-glucuronide (M3G), and like M3G (see below) it is dependent on the kidney for excretion, has no analgesic action and can lead to dose-dependent neurotoxic effects (Smith 2000; Wright et al 2001).

Methadone

Methadone is commonly used for the maintenance treatment of patients with an addiction to opioids because of its good oral bioavailability (60–95%), high potency and long duration of action. In addition, its lack of active metabolites, low cost and additional effects as an N-methyl-D-aspartate (NMDA) receptor antagonist and serotonin reuptake inhibitor have led to its increasing use in the treatment of cancer and chronic non-cancer pain (Bruera & Sweeney 2002). Its use in acute pain treatment is limited by its long and unpredictable duration of action and the risk of accumulation.

Morphine

Morphine remains the most widely used opioid for the management of pain and the standard against which other opioids are compared. Morphine-6-glucuronide (M6G) and M3G, the main metabolite of morphine, are formed by morphine glucuronidation, primarily in the liver. M6G is a mu opioid agonist, may be more potent than morphine and has morphine-like effects including analgesia; M3G has very low affinity for opioid receptors, has no analgesic activity, and animal studies have shown that it may antagonise the analgesic effects of morphine and be responsible for neurotoxic symptoms, such as hyperalgesia, allodynia and myoclonus, sometimes associated with high doses of morphine (Andersen et al 2003).

Both M6G and M3G are dependent on the kidney for excretion. Impaired renal function, the oral route of administration (first pass metabolism), higher doses and increased patient age are predictors of higher M3G and M6G concentrations (Faura et al 1998, **Level IV**; Klepstad et al 2003, **Level IV**).

Oxycodone

Oxycodone is a potent opioid agonist commonly used in acute pain management for patients able to take opioids by mouth (Macintyre & Ready 2001). It is effective in the treatment of postoperative pain (Edwards et al 2000c, **Level I**). Both its immediate-release (Macintyre & Ready 2001) and controlled-release (Ginsberg et al 2003, **Level IV**) formulations have also been used as 'step-down' analgesia following patient-controlled analgesia (PCA) with doses based on PCA opioid requirements.

Oxycodone is metabolised in the liver primarily to noroxycodone and oxymorphone; oxymorphone is weakly active but contributes minimally to any clinical effect (Mercadante & Arcuri 2004).

Pethidine

Pethidine is a synthetic opioid still widely used even though it has multiple disadvantages. Despite a common belief that it is the most effective opioid in the treatment of renal colic, it is no better than morphine (O'Connor et al 2000, **Level II**) or hydromorphone (Jasani et al 1994, **Level II**). Similarly, pethidine and morphine have similar effects on the sphincter of Oddi and biliary tract and there is no evidence that pethidine is better in the treatment of biliary colic (Latta et al 2002, **Level IV**).

Pethidine induces more nausea and vomiting than morphine when used parenterally in the emergency department (Silverman et al 2004, **Level III-3**) and after gynaecological surgery (Ezri at al 2002, **Level II**).

Accumulation of its active metabolite, norpethidine, is associated with neuroexcitatory effects that range from nervousness to tremors, twitches, multifocal myoclonus and seizures (Armstrong & Bersten 1986; Simopoulos et al 2002, **Level IV**). As impaired renal function increases the half-life of norpethidine, patients in renal failure are at increased risk of norpethidine toxicity. Naloxone does not reverse and may increase the problems related to norpethidine toxicity. Overall, the use of pethidine should be discouraged in favour of other opioids (Latta et al 2002).

Tramadol

Tramadol is commonly referred to as an atypical centrally-acting analgesic because of its combined effects as an opioid agonist (mainly its metabolite O-desmethyltramadol,

M1) and a serotonin and noradrenaline reuptake inhibitor (Raffa et al 1992), but it is listed as a weak opioid by the World Health Organization (WHO 1996).

Tramadol is an effective treatment of neuropathic pain with an NNT of 3.5 (Dühmke et al 2004, **Level I**).

Its adverse effect profile is different from other opioids. The risk of respiratory depression is significantly lower at equianalgesic doses (Tarkkila et al 1997, **Level II**; Tarkkila et al 1998, **Level II**; Mildh et al 1999, **Level II**) and it does not depress the hypoxic ventilatory response (Warren et al 2000, **Level II**). Significant respiratory depression has only been described in patients with severe renal failure, most likely due to accumulation of the metabolite M1, which has higher affinity for the opioid receptor (Barnung et al 1997).

In addition, tramadol has limited effects on gastrointestinal motor function (Wilder-Smith & Bettiga 1997, **Level II**), causes less constipation (Wilder-Smith et al 1999a, **Level II**) and has less effect on gastric emptying (Wilder-Smith et al 1999b, **Level II**) and postoperative bowel recovery (Lim & Schug 2001, **Level II**) than morphine. Nausea and vomiting are the most common adverse effects and occur at rates similar to other opioids (Radbruch et al 1996, **Level IV**). Tramadol does not increase the incidence of seizures compared with other analgesic agents (Gasse et al 2000, **Level III-2**).

4.1.3 Adverse effects of opioids

Common adverse effects of opioids are sedation, pruritus, nausea, vomiting, slowing of gastrointestinal function and urinary retention (Schug et al 1992). Clinically meaningful adverse effects of opioids are dose-related; once a threshold dose is reached, every 3–4mg increase of morphine-equivalent dose per day is associated with one additional adverse event or patient-day with such an event (Zhao et al 2004, **Level II**).

Opioid-related adverse effects in surgical patients increase length of stay in hospital and total hospital costs (Philips et al 2002, **Level III-2**; Oderda et al 2003, **Level IV**) and the use of opioid-sparing techniques can be cost-effective (Philips et al 2002, **Level III-2**).

Respiratory depression

Respiratory depression, the most feared side effect of opioids, can usually be avoided by careful titration of the dose against effect. A number of studies investigating hypoxia in the postoperative period, in patients receiving opioids for pain relief, have found that measurement of respiratory rate as an indicator of respiratory depression is of little value and that hypoxaemic episodes often occur in the absence of a low respiratory rate (Catley et al 1985, **Level IV**; Jones et al 1990; Wheatley et al 1990, **Level IV**; Kluger et al 1992, **Level IV**). As respiratory depression is almost always preceded by sedation, the best early clinical indicator is increasing sedation (Ready et al 1988; Leith et al 1994; Chaney 1995).

Supplemental oxygen in the first 48 hours following major surgery is beneficial (Rosenberg et al 1992, **Level II**), in particular in elderly and high risk patients because of the link between postoperative hypoxaemia, tachycardia (Stausholm et al 1995, **Level II**) and myocardial ischaemia (Rosenberg et al 1990).

Nausea and vomiting

Postoperative nausea and vomiting, is common and often related to opioid administration. The risk is significantly reduced by the use of droperidol, dexamethasone and ondansetron, which are equally effective (Tramèr et al 2001, **Level I**; Gan et al 2003; Apfel et al 2004, **Level II**); propofol and omission of nitrous oxide are less effective (Apfel et al 2004, **Level II**).

Pruritus

Naloxone, naltrexone, nalbuphine and droperidol are effective in the treatment of opioid-induced pruritus, although minimal effective doses remain unknown (Kjellberg & Tramèr 2001, **Level I**).

Key messages

1. Dextropropoxyphene has low analgesic efficacy (**Level I** [Cochrane Review]).
2. Tramadol is an effective treatment in neuropathic pain (**Level I** [Cochrane Review]).
3. Droperidol, dexamethasone and ondansetron are equally effective in prophylaxis of postoperative nausea and vomiting (**Level I**).
4. Naloxone, naltrexone, nalbuphine and droperidol are effective treatments for opioid-induced pruritus (**Level I**).
5. In the management of acute pain, one opioid is not superior over others but some opioids are better in some patients (**Level II**).
6. The incidence of clinically meaningful adverse effects of opioids is dose-related (**Level II**).
7. Tramadol has a lower risk of respiratory depression and impairs gastrointestinal motor function less than other opioids at equianalgesic doses (**Level II**).
8. Pethidine is not superior to morphine in treatment of pain of renal or biliary colic (**Level II**).
9. Supplemental oxygen in the postoperative period improves oxygen saturation and reduces tachycardia and myocardial ischaemia (**Level II**).
10. In adults, patient age rather than weight is a better predictor of opioid requirements, although there is a large interpatient variation (**Level IV**).
11. Impaired renal function and the oral route of administration result in higher concentrations of the morphine metabolites M3G and M6G (**Level IV**).

The following tick boxes ☑ represent conclusions based on clinical experience and expert opinion.

☑ Assessment of sedation level is a more reliable way of detecting early opioid-induced respiratory depression than a decreased respiratory rate.

☑ The use of pethidine should be discouraged in favour of other opioids.

4.2 PARACETAMOL, NSAIDs AND COX-2 SELECTIVE INHIBITORS

4.2.1 Paracetamol (acetaminophen)

Paracetamol is the remaining para-aminophenol used in clinical practice and is an effective analgesic (Barden 2004a, **Level I**) and antipyretic. It is absorbed rapidly and well from the small intestine after oral administration, can be given rectally, and parenteral preparations have recently been introduced into clinical practice (see Section 6) (Hernandez-Palazon et al 2001; Bannwarth & Pehourcq 2003; Van Aken et al 2004).

The mechanism of action of paracetamol remains unclear. In comparison with opioids, paracetamol has no known endogenous binding sites, and unlike non-steroidal anti-inflammatory drugs (NSAIDs), apparently does not inhibit peripheral cyclo-oxygenase activity. There is increasing evidence of a central antinociceptive effect. Potential mechanisms for this include inhibition of a COX-2 in the CNS, or inhibition of a putative central cyclo-oxygenase 'COX-3' (see below) that is selectively susceptible to paracetamol, and modulation of inhibitory descending serotonergic pathways (Warner & Mitchell 2002; Bonnefont et al 2003; Botting 2003). Paracetamol has also been shown to prevent prostaglandin production at the cellular transcriptional level, independent of cyclo-oxygenase activity (Mancini et al 2003).

Efficacy

Single doses of paracetamol are effective in the treatment of postoperative pain. The NNTs for at least 50% pain relief over 4–6 hours were: 325mg NNT 3.8 (2.2 to 13.3); 500mg NNT 3.5 (2.7 to 4.8); 600/650mg NNT 4.6 (3.9 to 5.5); 975/1,000mg NNT 3.8 (3.4 to 4.4); and 1,500mg NNT 3.7 (2.3 to 9.5) (Barden 2004a, **Level I**).

Paracetamol is also an effective adjunct to opioid analgesia, opioid requirements being reduced by 20–30% when combined with a regular regimen of oral or rectal paracetamol (Rømsing et al 2002, **Level I**). The use of oral paracetamol (1g every 4 hours) in addition to PCA morphine lowered pain scores, shortened the duration of PCA use and improved patient satisfaction (Schug et al 1998, **Level II**). The combination of paracetamol 1000mg plus codeine 60mg has a NNT of 2.2 (see Chapter 6 and Table 6.1). The addition of an NSAID to paracetamol further improves efficacy (Hyllested et al 2002, **Level I**; Rømsing et al 2002, **Level I**). In contrast, the commonly used lower dose of rectal paracetamol (1g every 6 hours) is insufficient for a maximal opioid-sparing benefit as it produces a sub-optimal plasma paracetamol concentration (Kvalsvik et al 2003, **Level II**).

Intravenous (IV) paracetamol is an effective analgesic after surgery (Hernandez-Palazon et al 2001, **Level II**), is as effective as ketorolac (Varrassi et al 1999, **Level II**; Zhou et al 2001, **Level II**), and is equivalent to morphine and better tolerated after dental surgery (Van Aken et al 2004, **Level II**), although there is evidence of a ceiling effect (Hahn et al 2003, **Level II**).

Adverse effects

Paracetamol has fewer side effects than NSAIDs and can be used when the latter are contraindicated (eg patients with a history of asthma or peptic ulcers). It should be used with caution or in reduced doses in patients with active liver disease, alcohol-related liver disease and glucose-6-phosphate dehydrogenase deficiency. In these situations, as well as in overdose, the rate of reactive metabolite production can result in centrilobular hepatocellular necrosis, occasionally with acute renal tubular necrosis (al-Swayeh et al 2000; Futter et al 2001; Moore & Marshall 2003; Romero-Sandoval et al 2003).

4.2.2 Non-steroidal anti-inflammatory drugs

NSAIDs have a spectrum of analgesic, anti-inflammatory and antipyretic effects and are effective analgesics in a variety of acute pain states. Unfortunately, significant contraindications and adverse effects limit the use of NSAIDs (RCA 1998), although some, including the renal effect, are being re-assessed (Lee et al 2003).

Many effects of NSAIDs can be explained by inhibition of prostaglandin synthesis in peripheral tissues, nerves, and the CNS (Botting 1999; Botting 2003). However, NSAIDs and aspirin may have other mechanisms of action independent of any effect on prostaglandins, including effects on basic cellular and neuronal processes (McCormack 1994). Prostaglandins are produced by the enzyme prostaglandin endoperoxide (PGH) synthase, which has both cyclo-oxygenase and hydroperoxidase sites. Two subtypes of cyclo-oxygenase enzyme have been identified — the 'constitutive' COX-1, and the 'inducible' COX-2, and now a COX-3 is being investigated (Seibert et al 1994; Botting 2003; Simmons 2003).

Prostaglandins have many physiological functions including gastric mucosal protection, renal tubular function and intrarenal vasodilation, bronchodilatation, production of endothelial prostacyclin that leads to vasodilation and prevents platelet adhesion, and platelet thromboxane that results in platelet aggregation and vessel spasm. Such physiological roles are mainly regulated by COX-1 and are the basis for many of the adverse effects associated with NSAID use. Tissue damage induces COX-2 production leading to synthesis of prostaglandins that result in pain and inflammation. COX-2 may be 'constitutive' in some tissues, including the kidney. NSAIDs are 'non-selective' cyclo-oxygenase inhibitors that inhibit both COX-1 and COX-2. Aspirin acetylates and inhibits cyclo-oxygenase irreversibly but NSAIDs are reversible inhibitors of the enzymes. The COX-2 inhibitors have been developed to inhibit selectively the inducible form (Kam & Power 2000).

Efficacy

Single doses of NSAIDs are effective in the treatment of pain after surgery (Gillis & Brogden 1997, **Level I**; Collins et al 1999a, **Level I**; Edwards et al 2000a, **Level I** ;Barden et al 2004b, **Level I**), low back pain (van Tulder et al 2000, **Level I**), and renal colic (Holdgate & Pollock 2004, **Level I**). The NNT of intramuscular (IM) ketorolac 10mg is 2.6, diclofenac 50mg 2.3, and ibuprofen 400mg 2.4. For comparison, the NNT of IM morphine 10mg is 2.9 and oral codeine 60mg 16.7 (see Chapter 6 and Table 6.1).

NSAIDs are inadequate as the sole analgesic agent in the treatment of severe postoperative pain although they are useful analgesic adjuncts; when given in combination with opioids after surgery, NSAIDs result in better analgesia and reduce opioid consumption (RCA 1998, **Level IV**). The addition of an oral NSAID to paracetamol also improves analgesia (Hyllested et al 2002, **Level I**; Rømsing et al 2002, **Level I**). NSAIDs are therefore integral components of multimodal analgesia (Kehlet 1997; Brodner et al 2001; Barratt et al 2002).

Opioid-sparing does not always result in a reduced incidence of adverse opioid-related effects but may have cost advantages compared with using opioid analgesics alone (RCA 1998, **Level IV**; Philips et al 2002, **Level III-2**).

Adverse effects

NSAID side effects are more common with long-term use — in the perioperative period the main concerns are renal impairment, interference with platelet function, peptic ulceration and bronchospasm in individuals who have aspirin-exacerbated respiratory disease (AERD). In general, the risk and severity of NSAID-associated side effects is increased in elderly people (RCA 1998, **Level IV**).

Renal function

Renal prostaglandins regulate tubular electrolyte handling, modulate the actions of renal hormones, and maintain renal blood flow and glomerular filtration rate in the presence of circulating vasoconstrictors. The adverse renal effects of chronic NSAID use are common and well-recognised. In some clinical conditions, including hypovolaemia and dehydration, high circulating concentrations of the vasoconstrictors angiotensin II, noradrenaline and vasopressin increase production of intrarenal vasodilators including prostacyclin — maintenance of renal function may then depend on prostaglandin synthesis and thus can be sensitive to brief NSAID administration.

Diclofenac has been shown to affect renal function in the immediate postoperative period after major surgery (Power et al 1992, **Level II**) and administration of other potential nephrotoxins, such as gentamicin, can increase the renal effects of ketorolac (Jaquenod et al 1998, **Level IV**). However, in clinical practice with careful patient selection and monitoring, the incidence of NSAID-induced renal impairment is low in the perioperative period (Lee et al 2003, **Level I**).

The risk of adverse renal effects of NSAIDs and COX-2 inhibitors is increased in the presence of factors such as pre-existing renal impairment, hypovolaemia, hypotension, use of other nephrotoxic agents and ACE inhibitors (RCA 1998, **Level IV**).

Platelet function

Single doses of NSAIDs such as ketorolac and diclofenac inhibit platelet function, but do not always significantly increase surgical blood loss (Power et al 1990, **Level II**; Power et al 1998, **Level II**; Møiniche et al 2003, **Level I**). However aspirin (Krishna et al 2003, **Level I**) and NSAIDs (number-needed-to-harm [NNH] 29–60) increased the risk of reoperation for post-tonsillectomy bleeding (Marret et al 2003, **Level I**; Møiniche et al 2003, **Level I**) (see also Sections 9.6.7 and10.1.5).

Nevertheless, NSAID use after tonsillectomy is associated with an increase in reoperation rate (Møiniche et al 2003, **Level I**) and more surgical blood loss (Rusy et al 1995, **Level II**) compared with paracetamol. In particular, aspirin, which irreversibly inhibits platelet aggregation, increases the risk of post-tonsillectomy haemorrhage (Krishna et al 2003, **Level I**). After gynaecological or breast surgery, NSAIDs cause more blood loss than the COX-2 inhibitor rofecoxib (Hegi et al 2004, **Level II**). Furthermore, the presence of a bleeding diathesis or administration of anticoagulants may increase the risk of significant surgical blood loss after NSAID administration (Schafer 1999).

Peptic ulceration

Acute gastroduodenal damage and bleeding can occur with short-term NSAID use — the risk is increased with higher doses, a history of peptic ulceration, use for more than 5 days and in elderly people (Strom et al 1996, **Level IV**). After 5 days of naproxen and ketorolac use in healthy elderly subjects, ulcers were found on gastroscopy in 20% and 31% of cases respectively (Harris et al 2001, **Level II**; Stoltz et al 2002, **Level II**; Goldstein et al 2003, **Level II**).

The gastric and duodenal epithelia have various protective mechanisms against acid and enzyme attack and many of these involve prostaglandin production. Chronic NSAID use is associated with peptic ulceration and bleeding and the latter may be exacerbated by the antiplatelet effect. It has been estimated that the relative risk of perforations, ulcers and bleeds associated with NSAIDs is 2.7 compared with people not consuming NSAIDs (Ofman et al 2002, **Level III-2**).

Aspirin-exacerbated respiratory disease

Precipitation of bronchospasm by aspirin is a recognised phenomenon in individuals with asthma, chronic rhinitis and nasal polyps. AERD affects 10–15% of people with asthma, can be severe and there is a cross-sensitivity with NSAIDs but not selective COX-2 inhibitors (Simon & Namazy 2003, **Level IV**; Szczeklik & Stevenson 2003, **Level IV**, West & Fernandez 2003, **Level I**). A history of AERD is a contraindication to NSAID use, although there is no reason to avoid NSAIDs in other people with asthma.

Bone healing

Prostaglandin production has been shown to be important in animal models of bone healing, but there is no good evidence of any clinically significant inhibitory effect of NSAIDs on bone healing (Harder & An 2003; Bandolier 2004).

4.2.3 Cyclo-oxygenase-2 selective inhibitors (COX-2 inhibitors)

New drugs have been developed that selectively inhibit the inducible cyclo-oxygenase enzyme, COX-2, and spare constitutive COX-1 (see above). The COX-2 inhibitors available at present include meloxicam, celecoxib, etoricoxib, valdecoxib and parecoxib, the injectable precursor of valdecoxib. By sparing physiological tissue prostaglandin production while inhibiting inflammatory prostaglandin release, COX-2 inhibitors offer the potential for effective analgesia with fewer side effects than NSAIDs.

Efficacy

COX-2 inhibitors are as effective as NSAIDs for postoperative pain (Rømsing & Møiniche 2004, **Level I**). NNTs are comparable with those for conventional NSAIDs for the treatment of moderate to severe acute pain: celecoxib 200mg, 4.5; parecoxib 20mg IV, 3.0; parecoxib 40mg IV, 2.2; valdecoxib 20mg, 1.7 (Ahuja et al 2003, **Level I**; Barden et al 2003a, **Level I**; Barden et al 2003b, **Level I**; Chavez & DeKorte 2003, **Level I**).

When given in combination with opioids after surgery, COX-2 inhibitors are opioid-sparing; as with traditional NSAIDs, opioid-sparing results in a reduced (Malan et al 2003, **Level II**; Gan et al 2004, **Level II**; Zhao et al 2004, **Level II**) or comparable (Hubbard et al 2003, **Level II**; Ng et al 2003; **Level II**; Reynolds et al 2003, **Level II**) incidence of adverse opioid-related effects.

Adverse effects

Renal function

COX-2 is constitutively expressed in the kidney and is highly regulated in response to alterations in intravascular volume. COX-2 has been implicated in maintenance of renal blood flow, mediation of renin release and regulation of sodium excretion (Cheng & Harris 2004, **Level IV**; Kramer et al 2004, **Level IV**). COX-2 inhibitors and NSAIDs have similar adverse effects on renal function (Curtis et al 2004, **Level I**).

Platelet function

Platelets produce only COX-1, not COX-2, and as a corollary COX-2 selective inhibitors do not impair platelet function. The use of COX-2 inhibitors reduces surgical blood loss in comparison with NSAIDs (Hegi et al 2004, **Level II**). The lack of antiplatelet effects may be an advantage for the patient with a bleeding diathesis, when anticoagulants are given, where central neuraxial blockade is performed, or where surgical blood loss is expected to be considerable or of particular relevance (orthopaedics, ear nose and throat [ENT], neurosurgery, plastic surgery).

The question has been raised whether COX-2 inhibitors can produce a tendency to thrombosis because they inhibit endothelial prostacyclin production but spare platelet thromboxane synthesis and aggregation. While the pharmacological evidence for a prothrombotic effect of COX-2 inhibitors is plausible, the published data on the clinical risk are conflicting (Clark et al 2004).

The VIGOR study, in which patients on low-dose aspirin were excluded, found an increased risk of myocardial infarction for patients given rofecoxib compared with naproxen (Bombardier 2002, **Level II**). Rofecoxib has recently been withdrawn from clinical practice because of further concerns about the risks of cardiovascular events including myocardial infarction and stroke (FDA 2004).

An increase in the incidence of cerebrovascular and cardiovascular events in patients given parecoxib, then valdecoxib after coronary artery bypass graft surgery has also been reported (Ott et al 2003, **Level II**; Nussmeier et al 2005, **Level II**). Therefore, their use is contraindicated after this type of surgery.

Gastrointestinal

Large outcome studies have demonstrated that COX-2 inhibitors produce less clinically significant peptic ulceration than NSAIDs (Hawkey & Skelly 2002, **Level IV**). Both rofecoxib and celecoxib have been associated with a substantial reduction in endoscopic ulcers compared with NSAID comparators (Bombardier 2000, **Level II**; Silverstein et al 2000, **Level II**). In the VIGOR study (Bombardier et al 2000, **Level II**) all upper GI events were reduced with rofecoxib compared with naproxen. In the CLASS study (Silverstein et al 2000, **Level II**) the incidence of ulcer complications was less with celecoxib compared with ibuprofen or diclofenac. While there is continuing discussion on the relevance of these findings with long-term use, short-term use of parecoxib as required to treat acute pain results in gastroscopic ulcer rates similar to placebo, even in elderly patients at increased risk (Harris et al 2001, **Level II**; Stoltz et al 2002, **Level II**; Goldstein et al 2003, **Level II**).

Aspirin-exacerbated respiratory disease

Investigation of patients with AERD has provided encouraging evidence that COX-2 selective inhibitors, administered at analgesic doses, do not produce bronchospasm in these patients (Martin-Garcia et al 2003, **Level II**; Szczeklik & Stevenson 2003, **Level IV**, West & Fernandez 2003, **Level I**).

Bone healing

At present the effect of COX-2 inhibitors on bone healing remains an effect demonstrated under laboratory conditions, but there is no good evidence of any clinically significant inhibitory effect of COX-2 inhibitors on bone healing (Gerstenfeld et al 2003; Harder & An 2003; Bandolier 2004).

Key messages

1. Paracetamol is an effective analgesic for acute pain (**Level I** [Cochrane Review]).
2. NSAIDs and COX-2 inhibitors are effective analgesics of similar efficacy for acute pain. (**Level I** [Cochrane Review]).
3. NSAIDs given in addition to paracetamol improve analgesia (**Level I**).
4. With careful patient selection and monitoring, the incidence of NSAID-induced perioperative renal impairment is low (**Level I** [Cochrane Review]).
5. Aspirin and some NSAIDs increase the risk of reoperation for post-tonsillectomy bleeding (**Level I**).
6. COX-2 inhibitors and NSAIDs have similar adverse effects on renal function (**Level I**).
7. COX-2 selective inhibitors do not appear to produce bronchospasm in individuals known to have aspirin-exacerbated respiratory disease (**Level I**).
8. Paracetamol, NSAIDs and COX-2 inhibitors are valuable components of multimodal analgesia (**Level II**).
9. COX-2 inhibitors do not impair platelet function (**Level II**).

10. Short-term use of COX-2 inhibitors results in gastric ulceration rates similar to placebo (**Level II**).

11. Use of parecoxib followed by valdecoxib after coronary artery bypass surgery increases the incidence of cardiovascular events (**Level II**).

The following tick boxes ☑ represent conclusions based on clinical experience and expert opinion.

☑ Adverse effects of NSAIDs are significant and may limit their use.

☑ The risk of adverse renal effects of NSAIDs and COX-2 inhibitors is increased in the presence of factors such as pre-existing renal impairment, hypovolaemia, hypotension, use of other nephrotoxic agents and ACE inhibitors.

☑ Serious cardiovascular complications have been reported with the use of COX-2 inhibitors in some settings and the use of these agents is currently being assessed; no recommendation about their use can be made until further evidence is available.

4.3 ADJUVANT DRUGS

4.3.1 Nitrous oxide

Nitrous oxide (N_2O) has been used since the inception of anaesthesia for its modest analgesic and sedative properties, with minimal respiratory and cardiovascular depression. N_2O in oxygen has some analgesic efficacy in labour (Rosen 2002, **Level I**) and is effective during painful procedures such as dental surgery, endoscopy, biopsy, burns dressing and venous cannulation (Harding & Gibson 2000, **Level II**; Castera et al 2001, **Level II**; Gerhardt et al 2001, **Level II**; Hee et al 2003, **Level II**). N_2O is at least as effective as topical local anaesthesia for IV cannulation in children (Murat et al 2003, **Level I**) and in relieving acute ischaemic chest pain, with a significant reduction in plasma beta-endorphin concentrations (O'Leary et al 1987, **Level II**).

N_2O diffuses more rapidly than nitrogen and can expand enclosed air-containing spaces within the body. Its use is therefore contraindicated in the presence of a pneumothorax, obstruction of middle ear and sinus cavities, recent vitreoretinal surgery, pneumocephalus, bowel obstruction and gas embolism (Shaw & Morgan 1998).

Toxicity

N_2O oxidises the cobalt ion in the vitamin B_{12}-dependent enzyme methionine synthetase (MS) resulting in the formation of hydroxyl radicals which are responsible for the inactivation and destruction of this enzyme and the subsequent depletion of vitamin B_{12} stores (Kondo et al 1981; Drummond & Matthews 1994; Riedel et al 1999). MS is required for the formation of: tetrahydrofolate, needed for deoxyribonucleic acid (DNA) synthesis and therefore the production of rapidly dividing tissues such as bone marrow and gastrointestinal mucosa (Nunn 1987); and methionine, necessary for the synthesis of myelin (Green & Kinsella 1995).

Bone marrow and neurological complications have been reported in patients exposed to N_2O (see below). It has also been reported in those who abuse the drug (Layzer 1978; Sahenk et al 1978; Stacy et al 1992). In critically ill individuals with increased metabolic demands or poor nutrition, the rate of inactivation of vitamin B_{12}-dependent enzymes may be greater, leading to increased morbidity (Amos et al 1982, **Level IV**).

N_2O-induced bone marrow toxicity is usually progressive but reversible. Early megaloblastic changes in the marrow with production of macrocytes and hypersegmented polymorphonuclear white blood cells may progress to thrombocytopenia, leucopoenia and anaemia (Nunn et al 1982; Blanco & Peters 1983; Skacel et al 1983). The bone marrow changes are almost completely prevented by administration of folinic acid (Amos et al 1984; Nunn et al 1986). Despite the lack of any good data assessing efficacy in humans, and even though the bone marrow changes are usually reversible, it may be reasonable to give patients repeatedly exposed to N_2O, vitamin B_{12} and folic or folinic acid supplements (Weimann 2001).

Neurotoxicity associated with N_2O use is rare but can be rapid and irreversible. Patients deficient in vitamin B_{12}, even without an associated anaemia (ie a subclinical deficiency) may develop a severe and progressive neuropathy even after brief exposure to N_2O (Schilling 1986; Berger et al 1988; Holloway & Alberico 1990; Flippo & Holder 1993; Kinsella & Green 1995; McMorrow et al 1995; Nestor & Stark 1996; Rosener & Dichgans 1996; Lee et al 1999; Sesso et al 1999; Marie et al 2000; McNeely et al 2000; Qaiyum & Sandrasegaran 2000). Those at risk of vitamin B_{12} deficiency include some vegetarians, the newborn of vegetarian mothers, patients with gastrointestinal pathology, elderly people or patients taking proton pump inhibitors and H_2 blockers (Schilling 1986; Berger et al 1988; Kinsella & Green 1995; Rosener & Dichgans 1996; Nilsson-Ehle 1998; Schenk et al 1999; Carmel 2000).

The neuropathy appears to be the result of decreased methionine and subsequent defective myelin formation (Scott 1981; Green & Kinsella 1995). The clinical picture is that of a vitamin B_{12} deficiency where subacute combined degeneration (SACD) of the spinal cord causes numbness, tingling, paresthesiae, ataxia and spasticity (Weimann 2001). Involvement of peripheral, autonomic and central nervous systems may also lead to incontinence, diplopia, confusion or impaired cognitive function (Weimann 2001). In patients with pernicious anaemia, SACD usually responds well to treatment with vitamin B_{12}, although it may take many months and response to treatment may be incomplete (Toh et al 1997).

In monkeys exposed continuously to N_2O, SACD is prevented by a diet supplemented with methionine (Scott 1981) and in cultured human fibroblasts, a methionine-rich media diminished the rate of MS activation (Christensen & Ueland 1993). Despite the lack of good data assessing efficacy in humans, it may be reasonable to give patients at risk of vitamin B_{12} deficiency and who are exposed to N_2O on a repeated basis, vitamin B_{12} and folic or folinic acid supplements (Weimann 2001) and additional methionine.

Another consequence of N_2O-induced inactivation of MS is elevation of plasma homocysteine, a known risk factor for coronary artery and cerebrovascular disease (Christensen et al 1994, **Level IV**; Badner et al 1998, **Level II**). The significance of this in respect to N_2O use in patients is unknown. Methionine given preoperatively to patients

CHAPTER 4

undergoing N_2O anaesthesia improved the rate of recovery of MS and prevented the prolonged postoperative rise in plasma homocysteine concentrations (Christensen et al 1994). Preoperative administration of oral B vitamins (folate, B_6 and B_{12}) also prevent the postoperative increase in homocysteine following N_2O anaesthesia (Badner et al 2001, **Level II**).

The information about the complications of N_2O comes from case reports only. There are no controlled studies that evaluate the safety of repeated intermittent exposure to N_2O in humans and no data to guide the appropriate maximum duration or number of times a patient can safely be exposed to N_2O. Nevertheless, the severity of the potential problems requires highlighting. The suggestions for the use of N_2O outlined below are extrapolations only from the information above.

Suggestions for the use of nitrous oxide as an analgesic

When N_2O is to be used *repeatedly* for painful short procedures, it may be reasonable to:

- exclude patients with a known vitamin B_{12} deficiency;
- screen patients at risk of B_{12} deficiency by examination of the blood picture and serum B_{12} concentrations before using nitrous oxide;
- exclude asymptomatic patients with macrocytic anaemia or hypersegmentation of neutrophils until it is established that vitamin B_{12} or folate deficiency is not the cause;
- exclude females who may be in the early stages of pregnancy, although this will depend on the relative harm of any alternative methods;
- limit exposure to N_2O to the briefest possible time — restricting the duration of exposure may require strict supervision and limited access to the gas;
- administer methionine, vitamin B_{12} and possibly folic or folinic acid to patients repeatedly exposed to N_2O. The doses that may prevent the complications of exposure to N_2O have not been established. Methionine and vitamin B_{12} are cheap and have a good safety profile; and
- monitor for clinical signs and symptoms of neuropathy on a regular basis.

See Section 10.1.4 for the use of nitrous oxide in children.

Key messages

1. Nitrous oxide has some analgesic efficacy and is safe during labour (**Level I**).
2. Nitrous oxide is an effective analgesic agent in a variety of other acute pain situations (**Level II**).

The following tick boxes ☑ represent conclusions based on clinical experience and expert opinion.

☑ Neuropathy and bone marrow suppression are rare but potentially serious complications of nitrous oxide use, particularly in at-risk patients.

CHAPTER 4

☑ The information about the complications of nitrous oxide comes from case reports only. There are no controlled studies that evaluate the safety of repeated intermittent exposure to nitrous oxide in humans and no data to guide the appropriate maximum duration or number of times a patient can safely be exposed to nitrous oxide. The suggestions for the use of nitrous oxide are extrapolations only from the information above. Consideration should be given to duration of exposure and supplementation with vitamin B_{12}, methionine, and folic or folinic acid.

☑ If nitrous oxide is used with other sedative or analgesic agents, appropriate clinical monitoring should be used.

4.3.2 N-methyl-D-aspartate receptor antagonists

N-methyl-D-aspartate (NMDA) receptors are sited peripherally and centrally (Petrenko et al 2003). Activation of NMDA receptors, via glutamate release from excitatory synapses (Carpenter & Dickenson 1999), augments the propagation of nociceptive information and is linked to learning and memory, neural development, neural plasticity, as well as acute and chronic pain states (Sikiennik & Kream 1995). At the spinal level, NMDA receptor activation results in the development of hyperalgesia and allodynia (Carpenter & Dickenson 1999).

The NMDA receptor antagonists ketamine and dextromethorphan are used clinically. In chronic pain states such as central pain, Complex Regional Pain Syndrome, fibromyalgia and ischaemic and neuropathic pain, there is moderate to weak evidence that ketamine, either as the sole agent or in combination with other analgesics, improves pain, allodynia and hyperalgesia and/or decreases the requirement for other analgesic agents (Hocking & Cousins 2003, **Level I**). Extrapolation into the acute pain setting would seem reasonable.

Ketamine may also reduce opioid requirements in opioid-tolerant patients (Bell 1999, **Level IV**; Eilers et al 2001, **Level IV**; Sator-Katzenschlager et al 2001, **Level IV**).

As an adjuvant to opioids for the treatment of postoperative pain, IV and epidural ketamine have an opioid-sparing effect (Subramaniam et al 2004, **Level I**). Best effects were seen when ketamine was given as a continuous IV infusion, while there was no evidence supporting the addition of ketamine to PCA morphine. Ketamine side effects were not apparent at the low doses used. In spite of an opioid-sparing effect, there was no reduction of opioid-related side effects.

In patients with severe pain that was incompletely relieved by morphine, the addition of ketamine to the morphine regimen provided rapid, effective and prolonged analgesia (Weinbroum 2003, **Level II**).

Individual studies of dextromethorphan have produced a wide range of contradictory results (Ilkjaer et al 1997, **Level II**; Gilron et al 2000, **Level II**; Ilkjaer et al 2000, **Level II**; Plesan et al 2000, **Level II**; Helmy & Bali 2001, **Level II**; Wadhwa et al 2001, **Level II**; Weinbroum et al 2001, **Level II**; Heiskanen et al 2002, **Level II**; Weinbroum 2002, **Level II**; Choi et al 2003, **Level II**; Weinbroum 2003, **Level II**).

NMDA receptor antagonist drugs may have preventive analgesic effects (McCartney et al 2004, **Level I**) (see Section 1.4).

Key messages

1 Ketamine has an opioid-sparing effect in postoperative pain although there is no concurrent reduction in opioid-related side effects (**Level I**).

2 NMDA receptor antagonist drugs show preventive analgesic effects (**Level I**).

3 Ketamine improves analgesia in patients with severe pain that is poorly responsive to opioids (**Level II**).

4. Ketamine may reduce opioid requirements in opioid-tolerant patients (**Level IV**).

The following tick box ☑ represents conclusions based on clinical experience and expert opinion.

☑ Ketamine may be a useful adjunct in conditions of allodynia, hyperalgesia and opioid tolerance.

CHAPTER 4

4.3.3 Antidepressant drugs

There are no published data on the use of antidepressants in the management of acute neuropathic pain. However, antidepressants are effective in the treatment of a variety of chronic neuropathic pain states (McQuay et al 1996, **Level I**; Sindrup & Jensen 1999, **Level I**; Collins et al 2000, **Level I**).

There is also good evidence for the effect of antidepressants in chronic headaches with an NNT of 3.2 (Tomkins et al 2001, **Level I**) and for pain relief, but not improved function, in chronic back pain (Salerno et al 2002, **Level I**).

Table 4.1 summarises NNTs and numbers-need-to-harm (NNH) for antidepressants used in the treatment of the two most commonly studied indications — diabetic neuropathy and postherpetic neuralgia.

Table 4.1 Antidepressants for the treatment of diabetic neuropathy and postherpetic neuralgia (placebo-controlled trials)

Efficacy	**NNT (95% CI)**
Diabetic neuropathy	
TCAs	2.4 (2.0–3.0)
SSRIs	6.7 (3.4–435)
Postherpetic neuralgia	
TCAs	2.1 (1.7–3.0)
Minor adverse effects	**NNH (95% CI)**
Pooled diagnoses	
TCAs	2.8 (2.0–4.7)
SSRIs	no dichotomous data available
Major adverse effects	**NNH (95% CI)**
Pooled diagnoses	
TCAs	17.0 (10–43)
SSRIs	not different from placebo

Note: CI = confidence interval; TCA = tricyclic antidepressants; SSRI = selective serotonin re-uptake inhibitors

Source: Adapted from Collins et al (2000) and McQuay (2002).

Currently the use of antidepressants for acute neuropathic pain is mainly based on extrapolation of the above data. However, amitriptyline (Kalso et al 1996, **Level II**) and venlafaxine (Tasmuth et al 2002, **Level II**) are effective in the treatment of established neuropathic pain following breast surgery. In addition there is a possible preventive effect — given before and continued after surgery, venlafaxine significantly reduced the incidence of chronic pain at 6 months (Reuben et al 2004, **Level II**), and amitriptyline given to patients with acute herpes zoster reduced the incidence of postherpetic neuralgia at 6 months (Bowsher 1997, **Level II**).

Clinical experience in chronic pain suggests that tricyclic antidepressants (TCAs) should be started at low doses (eg amitriptyline 5–10mg at night) and subsequent doses increased slowly if needed, in order to minimise the incidence of adverse effects.

There are very limited data on the use of TCAs in acute nociceptive pain. Desipramine given prior to dental surgery increased and prolonged the analgesic effect of a single dose of morphine but had no analgesic effect in the absence of morphine (Levine et al 1986, **Level II**). However, when used in experimental pain, desipramine had no effect on pain or hyperalgesia (Wallace et al 2002, **Level II**). Amitriptyline given prior to dental surgery (Levine et al 1986, **Level II**) or after orthopaedic surgery (Kerrick et al 1993, **Level II**) did not improve morphine analgesia.

Key messages

1. Tricyclic antidepressants are effective in the treatment of chronic neuropathic pain states, chronic headaches and chronic back pain (**Level I**).
2. In neuropathic pain, tricyclic antidepressants are more effective than selective serotonergic re-uptake inhibitors (**Level I**).
3. Antidepressants reduce the incidence of chronic neuropathic pain after acute zoster and breast surgery (**Level II**).

The following tick boxes ☑ represent conclusions based on clinical experience and expert opinion.

☑ Based on the experience in chronic neuropathic pain states, it would seem reasonable to use tricyclic antidepressants in the management of acute neuropathic pain.

☑ To minimise adverse effects, particularly in elderly people, it is advisable to initiate treatment with low doses.

4.3.4 Anticonvulsant drugs

There are only limited data on the treatment of acute neuropathic pain with anticonvulsant medications. However, anticonvulsants have been used to treat chronic neuropathic pain and various systematic reviews have shown their efficacy in a variety of neuropathic pain states. (McQuay et al 1995, **Level I**; Sindrup & Jensen 1999, **Level I**; Collins et al 2000, **Level I**; Wiffen et al 2000, **Level I** ;Jensen 2002, **Level I**; McQuay 2002, **Level I**).

Table 4.2 shows a summary of NNTs and NNHs for all anticonvulsants used in the treatment of the two most commonly studied indications — diabetic neuropathy and postherpetic neuralgia.

Table 4.2 Anticonvulsants for the treatment of diabetic neuropathy and postherpetic neuralgia (placebo-controlled trials)

Efficacy	**NNT (95% CI)**
Diabetic neuropathy	2.7 (2.2–3.8)
Postherpetic neuralgia	3.2 (2.4–5.0)
Minor adverse effects	**NNH (95% CI)**
Pooled diagnoses	2.7 (2.2–3.4)
Major adverse effects	**NNH (95% CI)**
Pooled diagnoses	Not different from placebo

Source: Adapted from McQuay (2002).

Currently the use of anticonvulsants for acute neuropathic pain can only be based on extrapolation of the above data.

In acute nociceptive pain after surgery, sodium valproate is of no benefit (Martin et al 1988, **Level II**). Perioperative gabapentin leads to substantial reductions in both postoperative analgesic requirements and pain (Dahl et al 2004, **Level I**).

CHAPTER 4

Specific anticonvulsant agents used in the treatment of chronic neuropathic pain

Carbamazepine

In a systematic review, carbamazepine was found to have an NNT of 2.6 in trigeminal neuralgia and 3.3 in diabetic neuropathy (Backonja 2002, **Level I**). The NNH was 3.4 for minor adverse effects and 24 for severe adverse effects.

Gabapentin

In the same review the NNTs for gabapentin ranged between 3.2 and 3.8 in the treatment of chronic neuropathic pain states (Backonja 2002, **Level I**). The NNH for a minor adverse effect compared with a placebo was 2.6 (2.1 to 3.3) (Collins et al 2000, **Level I**). Gabapentin is also effective in the treatment of postamputation phantom pain (Bone et al 2002, **Level I**).

Lamotrigine

The NNT of lamotrigine, based on a limited number of studies in trigeminal neuralgia, is 2.1 (1.3–6.1) (Backonja 2002, **Level I**).

Sodium valproate

Sodium valproate has an NNT of 3.5 for at least a 50% reduction in migraine frequency (Moore et al 2003, **Level I**). The NNHs for nausea, tremor, dizziness and drowsiness were 3.3, 6.2, 6.5 and 6.3 respectively. The NNH for withdrawals due to adverse effects with sodium valproate was 9.4.

Key messages

1. Anticonvulsants are effective in the treatment of chronic neuropathic pain states (**Level I**).
2. Perioperative gabapentin reduces postoperative pain and opioid requirements (**Level I**).

The following tick box ☑ represents conclusions based on clinical experience and expert opinion.

☑ Based on the experience in chronic neuropathic pain states, it would seem reasonable to use anticonvulsants in the management of acute neuropathic pain.

4.3.5 Membrane stabilisers

There are only limited data on the treatment of acute pain with membrane stabilisers. A lignocaine (lidocaine) infusion started before abdominal incision and stopped 1 hour after surgery resulted in less pain on movement and lower morphine requirements in the first 72 hours after major abdominal surgery (Koppert et al 2004 **Level II**). This is possibly a preventive effect (see Section 1.4).

IV lignocaine infusions are effective in reducing pain and allodynia in chronic neuropathic pain conditions (Kalso et al 1998, **Level I**; Baranowski et al 1999, **Level II**). Overall, the strongest evidence is for use of membrane stabilisers in pain due to peripheral nerve trauma (Kalso et al 1998, **Level I**).

Oral mexiletine showed limited efficacy with an NNT of 10 for diabetic neuropathy (Kalso et al 1998, **Level I**).

Currently, the use of membrane stabilisers for acute neuropathic pain can only be based on extrapolation of the above data.

Key messages

1. Membrane stabilisers are effective in the treatment of chronic neuropathic pain states, particularly after peripheral nerve trauma (**Level I**).
2. Perioperative intravenous lignocaine (lidocaine) reduces pain on movement and morphine requirements following major abdominal surgery (**Level II**).

The following tick boxes ☑ represent conclusions based on clinical experience and expert opinion.

☑ Based on the experience in chronic neuropathic pain states, it would seem reasonable to use membrane stabilisers in the management of acute neuropathic pain.

☑ Lignocaine (lidocaine) (intravenous or subcutaneous) may be a useful agent to treat acute neuropathic pain.

4.3.6 Alpha-2 agonists

Systemic administration (oral, intramuscular [IM], IV) of single doses of the alpha-2 agonists clonidine and dexmedetomidine decreases perioperative opioid requirements in surgical patients (Aho et al 1991, **Level II**; Bernard et al 1991, **Level II**; De Kock et al 1992, **Level II**; Park et al 1996, **Level II**; Jalonen et al 1997, **Level II**; Arian et al 2004, **Level II**).

Higher doses of clonidine result in a significant reduction in opioid requirements but a greater degree of sedation and hypotension (Marinangeli et al 2002, **Level II**).

In the intensive care setting, IV dexmedetomidine infusions used for sedation of ventilated patients resulted in a 50% reduction in morphine requirements (Venn et al 1999, **Level II**).

Few controlled studies have been performed on the systemic administration of alpha-2 agonists for chronic pain. In a comparison of epidural and IV clonidine the routine use of systemic clonidine does not appear to be of benefit (Carroll et al 1993, **Level II**).

CHAPTER 4

Key message

1. The use of systemic alpha-2-agonists consistently improves perioperative opioid analgesia, but frequency and severity of side effects may limit their clinical usefulness (**Level II**).

4.3.7 Calcitonin

Vertebral fractures due to osteoporosis can result in significant acute pain. Calcitonin, given parenterally, intransally or rectally, has been shown to have analgesic efficacy in this setting (Blau & Hoehns 2003, **Level I**).

Key message

1. Calcitonin is effective in the treatment of acute pain after osteoporosis-related vertebral fractures (**Level I**).

4.3.8 Cannabinoids

Cannabinoids are a diverse group of substances derived from natural (plant and animal) and synthetic sources that affect cannabinoid receptors. Although over 60 cannabinoids have been identified in products of the cannabis plants (Ashton 1999), the most potent psychoactive agent is delta^9-tetrahydrocannabinol (delta^9-THC). Potentially useful actions of cannabis include mood elevation, appetite stimulation, an anti-emetic effect and antinociception. The clinical use of naturally occurring cannabis is unfortunately limited due to a wide range of side effects, which include dysphoria, sedation, impaired psychomotor performance and withdrawal symptoms (Ashton 1999).

A number of expert committees have examined the scientific evidence assessing the efficacy and safety of cannabinoids in clinical practice (House of Lords Committee on Science and Technology 1998; Joy et al 1999; Working Party on the Use of Cannabis for Medicinal Purposes 2000). Insufficient rigorous scientific evidence was found to support the use of cannabinoids in clinical practice.

In 2001 a qualitative systematic review examined the evidence for cannabinoids as analgesics (Campbell et al 2001, **Level I**) and found no evidence for clinically relevant effectiveness, but significant side effects.

A more recent study found no benefit with 5mg of oral THC in acute postoperative pain (Buggy et al 2003, **Level II**).

It should be noted that all clinical studies to date have only used non-selective highly lipophilic cannabinoid compounds. The possible benefits from more selective agonists have yet to be investigated in the clinical setting.

Key message

1. **Current evidence does not support the use of cannabinoids in acute pain management (Level I).**

4.3.9 Complementary and alternative medicines

Herbal, traditional Chinese and homeopathic medicines may be described as complementary or alternative medicines (CAMs) because their use lies outside the dominant, 'orthodox' health system of Western industrialised society (Belgrade 2003). In other cultures these therapies may be mainstream.

CAMs include:

- *herbal medicine* — plant substances such as roots and leaves;
- *traditional Chinese medicine* — herbal medicines, animal and mineral substances;
- *homeopathy* — ultra-diluted substances; and
- *others* — vitamins, minerals, animal substances, metals and chelation agents.

A drug is any substance or product that is used or intended to be used to modify or explore physiological systems or pathological states (WHO 1966). While the use of CAM therapies is commonplace, their efficacy in many areas, including in the management of acute pain, has not yet been subject to adequate scientific evaluation.

There are limited data on the use of CAMs in the management of acute pain. In dysmenorrhoea, vitamin B_1 (Proctor & Murphy 2001, **Level I**) and fennel (Namavar Jahromi et al 2003, **Level III-2**) are effective. Willow bark extract is more effective than placebo in relieving acute low back pain (Chrubasik et al 2000, **Level II**) and as effective as rofecoxib (Chrubasik et al 2001, **Level II**).

CAMs are effective in the treatment of a variety of chronic pain states. Peppermint oil has an NNT of 3.1 for improvement of pain in irritable bowel syndrome over 2–4 weeks (Pittler & Ernst 1998, **Level I**). In osteoarthritis, willow bark (Schmid et al 2000, **Level II**), devil's claw (Soeken 2004, **Level I**), chondroitin sulphate (Leeb et al 2000, **Level I**), glucosamine (Towheed et al 2000, **Level I**) and avocado-soybean unsaponifiables (Little et al 2000, **Level I**) reduce pain. Fish oil reduces tenderness and pain in rheumatoid arthritis (Fortin et al 1995, **Level I**). Phytodolor (a standardised herbal preparation of aspen, ash and golden rod) is superior to placebo and similar to indomethacin (indometacin) and diclofenac in the treatment of pain associated with arthritic and rheumatoid diseases (Ernst 1999, **Level I**).

There is no evidence of benefit of homeopathy in the treatment of pain of osteoarthritis (Long & Ernst 2001, **Level I**) or of homeopathic arnica in treating a variety of pain states (Ernst & Pittler 1998, **Level I**). Homeopathic arnica was ineffective for pain relief after hand surgery (Stevinson et al 2003, **Level II**) and abdominal hysterectomy (Hart et al 1997, **Level II**).

Adverse effects and interactions with other medications have been described with CAMs and must be considered before their use. For details see:

- herb side effects and drug interactions — www.asahq.org/patientEducation/herbPhysician.pdf; and/or
- herb-opioid interactions — www.clinicaltrials.gov/show/NCT00027014.

CHAPTER 4

REFERENCES

Aho MS, Erkola OA, Scheinin H et al (1991) Effect of intravenously administered dexmedetomidine on pain after laparoscopic tubal ligation. *Anesth Analg* 73: 112–18.

Ahuja N, Singh A, Singh B (2003) Rofecoxib: an update on physicochemical, ISSN pharmaceutical, pharmacodynamic and pharmacokinetic aspects. *J Pharm Pharmacol* 55: 859–94.

al-Swayeh OA, Futter LE, Clifford RH et al (2000) Nitroparacetamol exhibits anti-inflammatory and anti- nociceptive activity. *Br J Pharmacol* 130: 1453–56.

Amos RJ, Amess JA, Hinds CJ et al (1982) Incidence and pathogenesis of acute megaloblastic bone-marrow change in patients receiving intensive care. *Lancet* 2: 835–38.

Amos RJ, Amess JA, Nancekievill DG et al (1984) Prevention of nitrous oxide-induced megaloblastic changes in bone marrow using folinic acid. *Br J Anaesth* 56: 103–07.

Andersen G, Christrup L, Sjogren P (2003) Relationships among morphine metabolism, pain and side effects during long-term treatment: an update. *J Pain Symptom Manage* 25: 74–91.

Apfel CC, Korttila K, Abdalla M et al (2004) A factorial trial of six interventions for the prevention of postoperative nausea and vomiting. *N Engl J Med* 350: 2441–51.

Arian SR, Ruehlow RM, Uhrich TD et al (2004) The efficacy of dexmedetomidine versus morphine for postoperative analgesia after major impatient surgery. *Anesth Analg* 98: 153–58.

Armstrong PJ & Bersten A (1986) Normeperidine toxicity. *Anesth Analg* 65: 536–38.

Ashton CH (1999) Adverse effects of cannabis and cannabinoids. *Br J Anaesth* 83: 637–49.

Backonja MM (2002) Use of anticonvulsants for treatment of neuropathic pain. *Neurology* 59: S14–S17.

Badner NH, Drader K, Freeman D et al (1998) The use of intraoperative nitrous oxide leads to postoperative increases in plasma homocysteine. *Anesth Analg* 87: 711–13.

Badner NH, Freeman D, Spence JD (2001) Preoperative oral B vitamins prevent nitrous oxide-induced postoperative plasma homocysteine increases. *Anesth Analg* 93: 1507–10.

Bandolier (2004) NSAIDs, coxibs, smoking and bone. *Bandolier Extra*: www.ebandolier.com. (www.jr2.ox.ac.uk/bandolier/booth/painpag/wisdom/NSB.pdf)

Bannwarth B & Pehourcq F (2003) Pharmacological rationale for the clinical use of paracetamol: Pharmacokinetic and pharmacodynamic issues. *Drugs* 63: 5–13.

Baranowski AP, de Courcey J, Bonello E (1999) A trial of intravenous lidocaine on the pain and allodynia of postherpetic neuralgia. *J Pain Sympt Manage* 17: 429–33.

Barden J, Edwards JE, McQuay HJ et al (2003a) Oral valdecoxib and injected parecoxib for acute postoperative pain: a quantitative systematic review. *BMC Anesthesiol* 3: 1. (www.biomedcentral.com/1471-2253/3/1)

Barden J, Edwards JE, McQuay HJ, Moore RA (2003b) Single dose oral celecoxib for postoperative pain. *The Cochrane Database of Systematic Reviews*, Issue 1. Art. No.: CD004233. DOI: 10.1002/14651858.CD004233.

Barden J, Edwards J, Moore A, McQuay H (2004a) Single dose oral paracetamol (acetaminophen) for postoperative pain. *The Cochrane Database of Systematic Reviews*, Issue 1. Art. No.: CD004602. DOI: 10.1002/14651858.CD004602.

Barden J, Edwards J, Moore RA, McQuay HJ (2004b) Single dose oral diclofenac for postoperative pain. *The Cochrane Database of Systematic Reviews*, Issue 2. Art. No.: CD004768. DOI: 10.1002/14651858.CD004768.

Barnung S K, Treschow M, Borgbjerg FM (1997) Respiratory depression following oral tramadol in a patient with impaired renal function. *Pain* 71: 111–12.

Barratt S M, Smith RC, Kee A J et al (2002) Multimodal analgesia and intravenous nutrition preserves total body protein following major upper gastrointestinal surgery. *Reg Anesth Pain Med* 27: 15–22.

Belgrade MJ (2003) Alternative and complementary therapies. In: Jensen TS, Wilson PR, Rice ASC (Eds) *Clinical Pain Management; Chronic Pain.* London: Arnold.

Bell RF (1999) Low-dose subcutaneous ketamine infusion and morphine tolerance. *Pain* 83: 101–03.

Berger JJ, Modell JH, Sypert GW (1988) Megaloblastic anemia and brief exposure to nitrous oxide--a causal relationship. *Anesth Analg* 67: 197–98.

Bernard JM, Hommeril JL Passuti N et al (1991) Postoperative analgesia by intravenous clonidine. *Anesthesiology* 75: 577–82.

Blanco G & Peters HA (1983) Myeloneuropathy and macrocytosis associated with nitrous oxide abuse. *Arch Neurol* 40: 416–18.

Blau LA &Hoehns JD (2003) Analgesic efficacy of calcitonin for vertebral fracture pain. *Ann Pharmacother* 37: 564–70.

Bombardier C, Laine L, Reicin A et al (2000) Comparison of upper gastrointestinal toxicity of rofecoxib and naproxen in patients with rheumatoid arthritis. VIGOR Study Group. *New Engl J Med* 343: 1520–28.

Bone M, Critchlet P, Buggy DJ (2002) Gabapentin in postamputation phantom limb pain: a randomized, double-blind, placebo-controlled, cross-over study. *Reg Anesth Pain Med* 27: 481–86.

Bonnefont J, Courade JP, Alloui A et al (2003) Mechanism of the antinociceptive effect of paracetamol. *Drugs* 63: 1–4.

Botting JH (1999) Nonsteroidal antiinflammatory agents. *Drugs Today (Barc)* 35: 225–35.

Botting R (2003) COX-1 and COX-3 inhibitors. *Thromb Res* 110: 269–22.

Bowsher D (1997) The effects of preemptive treatment of postherpetic neuralgia with amitriptyline: a randomised double-blind placebo-controlled trial. *J Pain Sympt Manage* 13: 327–31.

Brodner G, Van Aken H, Hertle L et al (2001) Multimodal perioperative management — combining thoracic epidural analgesia, forced mobilization, and oral nutrition — reduces hormonal and metabolic stress and improves convalescence after major urologic surgery. *Anesth Analg* 92: 1594–1600.

Bruera E & Sweeney C (2002) Methadone use in cancer patients with pain: a review. *J Palliat Med* 5: 127–38.

Buggy DJ, Toogood L, Maric S et al (2003) Lack of analgesic efficacy or oral d-9-tetrahydrocannabinol in postoperative pain. *Pain* 106: 169–72.

Campbell F A, Tamer M R, Carroll D et al (2001) Are cannabinoids an effective and safe treatment option in the management of pain? A qualitative systematic review. *BMJ* 323: 1–6.

Caraco Y, Sheller J, Wood AJJ (1996) Pharmacogenetic determination of the effects of codeine and prediction of drug interactions. *J Pharmacol Exp Ther* 278: 1165–74.

Carmel R (2000) Current concepts in cobalamin deficiency. *Annu Rev Med* 51: 357–75.

Catley DM, Thornton C, Jordan C et al (1985) Pronounced, episodic oxygen desaturation in the postoperative period: Its association with ventilatory pattern and analgesic regimen. *Anesthesiology* 63: 20–28.

Carpenter KJ & Dickenson AH (1999) NMDA receptors and pain — hopes for novel analgesics. *Reg Anaesth Pain Med* 24: 506–08.

Carroll D, Jadad A, King V et al (1993) Single dose, randomised, double blind, double dummy cross over comparison of extradural and iv clonidine in chronic pain. *Br J Anaesth* 71: 665–69.

Castera L, Negre I, Samii K et al (2001) Patient-administered nitrous oxide/oxygen inhalation provides safe and effective analgesia for percutaneous liver biopsy: a randomized placebo-controlled trial. *Am J Gastroenterol* 96: 1553–57.

Catley DM, Thornton C, Jordan C et al (1985) Pronounced, episodic oxygen desaturation in the postoperative period: its association with ventilatory pattern and analgesic regimen. *Anesthesiology* 63: 20–28.

Chaney MA (1995) Side effects of intrathecal and epidural opioids. *Can J Anaesthesiol* 42: 891–903.

Chavez ML & DeKorte CJ (2003) Valdecoxib: A review. *Clin Ther* 25: 817–51.

Cheng HF & Harris RC (2004) Cyclooxygenases, the kidney, and hypertension. *Hypertension* 43: 525–30.

Choi DMA, Kliffer AP, Douglas MJ (2003) Dextromethorphan and intrathecal morphine for analgesia after Caesarean section under spinal anaesthesia. *Br J Anaesth* 90: 653–58.

Christensen B & Ueland PM (1993) Methionine synthase inactivation by nitrous oxide during methionine loading of normal human fibroblasts. Homocysteine remethylation as determinant of enzyme inactivation and homocysteine export. *J Pharmacol Exp Ther* 267: 1298–303.

Christensen B, Guttormsen AB, Schneede J et al (1994) Preoperative methionine loading enhances restoration of the cobalamin-dependent enzyme methionine synthase after nitrous oxide anesthesia. *Anesthesiology* 80: 1046–56.

Chrubasik S, Eisenberg E, Balan E et al (2000) Treatment of low back pain exacerbations with willow bark extract: a randomized double-blind study. *Am J Med* 109: 9–14.

Chrubasik S, Kunzel O, Model A et al (2001) Treatment of low back pain with a herbal or synthetic anti-rheumatic: a randomised controlled study. Willow bark extract for low back pain. *Rheumatology* 40: 1388–93.

Clark DWJ, Layton D, Shakir SAW (2004) Do some inhibitors of COX-2 increase the risk of thromboembolic events? Linking pharmacology with pharmacoepidemiology. *Drug Safety* 27: 427–56.

Collins SL, Moore RA, McQuay HJ et al (2000) Antidepressants and anticonvulsants for diabetic neuropathy and postherpetic neuralgia: a quantitative systematic review. *J Pain Symptom Manage* 20: 449–58.

Collins SL, Moore RA, McQuay HJ, Wiffen PJ, Edwards JE (1999a) Single dose oral ibuprofen and diclofenac for postoperative pain. *The Cochrane Database of Systematic Reviews*, Issue 1. Art. No.: CD001548. DOI: 10.1002/14651858.CD001548.

Collins SL, Edwards JE, Moore RA, McQuay HJ (1999b) Single dose dextropropoxyphene, alone and with paracetamol (acetaminophen), for postoperative pain. *The Cochrane Database of Systematic Reviews*, Issue 1. Art. No.: CD001440. DOI: 10.1002/14651858.CD001440.

Curtis SP, Ng J, Yu QF et al (2004) Renal effects of etoricoxib and comparator nonsteroidal anti-inflammatory drugs in controlled clinical trials. *Clin Ther* 26: 70–83.

Dahl B, Mathiesen O, Moniche S (2004) A review of gabapentin and pregabalin in the treatment of postoperative pain. *Acta Anaesthesiol Scand* 48: 1130–36.

Davies G, Kingswood C, Street M (1996) Pharmacokinetics of opioids in renal dysfunction. *Clin Pharmacokin* 31: 410–22.

De Kock MF, Pichon G, Scholtes JL (1992) Intraoperative clonidine enhances postoperative morphine patient-controlled analgesia. *Can J Anaesth* 39: 537–44.

Drummond JT & Matthews RG (1994) Nitrous oxide inactivation of cobalamin-dependent methionine synthase from Escherichia coli: characterization of the damage to the enzyme and prosthetic group. *Biochemistry* 33: 3742–50.

Dühmke RM, Cornblath DD, Hollingshead JRF (2004) Tramadol for neuropathic pain. *The Cochrane Database of Systematic Reviews*, Issue 2. Art. No.: CD003726. DOI: 10.1002/14651858.CD003726.pub2.

Dunbar PJ, Chapman CR, Buckley FP et al (1996) Clinical analgesia equivalence for morphine and hydromorphone with prolonged PCA. *Pain* 68 : 265–70.

Edwards JE, Loke YK, Moore RA, McQuay HJ (2000a) Single dose piroxicam for acute postoperative pain. *The Cochrane Database of Systematic Reviews*, Issue 2. Art. No.: CD002762. DOI: 10.1002/14651858.CD002762.

Edwards JE, McQuay HJ, Moore RA (2000b) Single dose dihydrocodeine for acute postoperative pain. *The Cochrane Database of Systematic Reviews*, Issue 2. Art. No.: CD002760. DOI: 10.1002/14651858.CD002760.

Edwards JE, Moore RA, McQuay HJ (2000c) Single dose oxycodone and oxycodone plus paracetamol (acetominophen) for acute postoperative pain. *The Cochrane Database of Systematic Reviews*, Issue 2. Art. No.: CD002763. DOI: 10.1002/14651858.CD002763.

Eilers H, Philip LA, Bickler PE et al (2001) The reversal of fentanyl-induced tolerance by administration of 'small-dose' ketamine. *Anesth Analg* 93: 213–14.

Ernst E & Pittler MH (1998) Efficacy of homeopathic arnica: a systematic review of placebo controlled clinical trials. *Arch Surg* 133: 1187–90.

Ernst E (1999) The efficacy of Phytodolor for the treatment of musculoskeletal pain — a systematic review of randomised clinical trials. *Nat Med J* 2: 14–17.

Ezri T, Lurie S, Stein A et al (2002). Postoperative nausea and vomiting: comparison of the effect of meperidine or morphine in gynecologic surgery patients. *J Clin Anaesth* 14: 262–66.

Faura CC, Collins SL, Moore RA et al (1998) Systematic review of factors affecting the ratios of morphine and its major metabolites. *Pain* 74: 43–53.

FDA (2004) *FDA Public Health Advisory: Safety of Vioxx*. US Food and Drug Administration. (www.fda.gov/cder/drug/infopage/vioxx/PHA_ioxx.htm).

Flippo TS & Holder WD Jr (1993) Neurologic degeneration associated with nitrous oxide anesthesia in patients with vitamin B12 deficiency. *Arch Surg* 128: 1391–95.

Fortin PR, Lew RA, Liang MH et al (1995) Validation of a meta-analysis: the effects of fish oil in rheumatoid arthritis. *J Clin Epidemiol* 48: 1379–90.

Futter LE, al-Swayeh OA, Moore PK (2001) A comparison of the effect of nitroparacetamol and paracetamol on liver injury. *Br J Pharmacol* 132: 10–12.

Gammaitoni AR, Fine P, Alvarez N et al (2003) Clinical application of opioid equianalgesic data. *Clin J Pain* 19: 286–297.

Gan TJ, Meyer T, Apfel C et al (2003) Consensus guidelines for managing postoperative nausea and vomiting. *Anesth Analag* 97: 62–71.

Gan TJ, Joshi GP, Zhao SZ et al (2004) Presurgical intravenous parecoxib sodium and follow-up valdcoxib for pain management after laparoscopic cholecystectomy surgery reduces opioid requirements and opioid-related adverse effects. *Acta Anaesthesiol Scand* 48: 1194–207.

Gasse C, Derby L, Vasilakis-Scaramozza C et al (2000) Incidence of first-time idiopathic seizures in users of tramodol. *Pharmacotherapy* 20: 629–34.

Gerhardt RT, King KM, Wiegert RS (2001) Inhaled nitrous oxide versus placebo as an analgesic and anxiolytic adjunct to peripheral intravenous cannulation. *Am J Emerg Med* 19: 492–94.

Gerstenfeld LC, Thiede M, Seibert K et al (2003) Differential inhibition of fracture healing by non-selective and cyclooxygenase-2 selective non-steroidal anti-inflammatory drugs. *J Orthop Res* 21: 670–75.

Gillis JC & Brogden RN (1997) Ketorolac. A reappraisal of its pharmacodynamic and pharmacokinetic properties and therapeutic use in pain management. *Drugs* 53:139–88.

Gilron I, Booher SL, Rowan MS et al (2000) A randomized, controlled trial of high-dose dextromethorphan in facial neuralgias. *Neurology* 55: 964–71.

Ginsberg B, Sinatra RS, Adler LJ et al (2003) Conversion to oral controlled-release oxycodone from intravenous opioid analgesic in the postoperative setting. *Pain Med* 4: 31–38.

Goldstein JL, Kivitz AJ, Verburg KM et al (2003) A comparison of the upper gastrointestinal mucosal effects of valdecoxib, naproxen and placebo in healthy elderly subjects. *Aliment Pharmacol Ther* 18: 125–32.

Green R & Kinsella J (1995) Current concepts in the diagnosis of cobalamin deficiency. *Neurology* 45: 1435–40.

Hahn TW, Mogensen T, Lund C et al (2003) Analgesic effect of i.v. paracetamol: possible ceiling effect of paracetamol in postoperative pain. *Acta Anaesthesiol Scand* 47: 138–45.

Harder AT & An YHH (2003) The mechanisms of the inhibitory effects of nonsteroidal anti-inflammatory drugs on bone healing: A concise review. *J Clin Pharmacol* 43: 807–15.

Harding TA & Gibson JA (2000) The use of inhaled nitrous oxide for flexible sigmoidoscopy: a placebo-controlled trial. *Endoscopy* 32: 457–60.

Harris SI, Kuss M, Hubbard RC et al (2001) Upper gastrointestinal safety evaluation of parecoxib sodium, a new parenteral cyclooxygenase-2-specific inhibitor, compared with ketorolac, naproxen, and placebo. *Clin Ther* 23: 1422–28.

Hart O, Mullee MA, Lewith G et al (1997) Double-blind, placebo-controlled, randomized clinical trial of homeopathic arnica C30 for pain and infection after total abdominal hysterectomy *J R Soc Med* 90: 73–78.

Hawkey CJ & Skelly MM (2002) Gastrointestinal safety of selective COX-2 inhibitors. *Curr Pharm Des* 8: 1077–89.

Hee HI, Goy RW, Ng AS (2003) Effective reduction of anxiety and pain during venous cannulation in children: a comparison of analgesic efficacy conferred by nitrous oxide, EMLA and combination. *Paediatr Anaesth* 13: 210–16.

Hegi TR, Bombeli T, Seifert B et al (2004) Effect of rofecoxib on platelet aggregation and blood loss in gynaecological and breast surgery compared with diclofenac. *Br J Anaesth* 92: 523–31.

Heiskanen T, Härtel B, Dahl ML et al (2002) Analgesic effects of dextromethorphan and morphine in patients with chronic pain. *Pain* 96: 261–67.

Helmy SAK & Bali A (2001) The effect of the preemptive use of the NMDA receptor antagonist dextromethorphan on postoperative analgesic requirements. *Anesth Analg* 92: 739–44.

Hernandez-Palazon J, Tortosa JA, Martinez-Lage JF et al (2001) Intravenous administration of propacetamol reduces morphine consumption after spinal fusion surgery. *Anesth Analg* 92: 1473–76.

Hocking G & Cousins MJ (2003) Ketamine in chronic pain management: an evidence-based review. *Anesth Analg* 97: 1730–39.

Holdgate A, Pollock T (2004) Nonsteroidal anti-inflammatory drugs (NSAIDs) versus opioids for acute renal colic. *The Cochrane Database of Systematic Reviews*, Issue 1. Art. No.: CD004137. DOI: 10.1002/14651858.CD004137.pub2

Holloway KL & Alberico AM (1990) Postoperative myeloneuropathy: a preventable complication in patients with B12 deficiency. *J Neurosurg* 72: 732–36.

House of Lords Committee on Science and Technology (1998) *Cannabis: The Scientific and Medical Evidence*. Science and Technology — 9th Report. London: The United Kingdom Parliament.

Hubbard RC, Naumann TM, TraylorL et al (2003) Parecoxib sodium has opioid-sparing effects in patients undergoing total knee arthroplasty under spinal anaesthesia. *Br J Anaesth* 90: 166–72.

Hyllested M, Jones S, Pedersen J L et al (2002) Comparative effect of paracetamol, NSAIDs or their combination in postoperative pain management: a qualitative review. *Br J Anaesth* 88: 199–214.

Ilkjaer S, Dirks J, Brennum J et al (1997) Effect of systemic N-methyl-D-aspartate receptor antagonist (dextromethorphan) on primary and secondary hyperalgesia in humans. *Br J Anaesth* 79: 600–05.

Ilkjaer S, Bach LF, Nielsen PA et al (2000) Effect of preoperative oral dextromethorphan on immediate and late postoperative pain and hyperalgesia after total abdominal hysterectomy. *Pain* 86: 19–24.

Jalonen J, Hynynen M, Kuitunen A et al (1997) Dexmedetomidine as an anaesthetic adjunct in coronary bypass grafting. *Anesthesiology* 86: 331–45.

Jaquenod M, Ronnedh C, Cousins M J et al (1998) Factors influencing ketorolac-associated perioperative renal dysfunction. *Anesth Analg* 86: 1090–97.

Jasani NB, O'Conner RE, Bouzoukis JK (1994) Comparison of hydromorphone and meperidine for ureteral colic. *Acad Emerg Med* 1: 539–43.

Jensen TS (2002) Anticonvulsants in neuropathic pain: rationale and clinical evidence. *Eur J Pain* 6 (Suppl A): 61–68.

Jones JG, Sapsford DJ, Wheatley RG (1990) Postoperative hypoxaemia: mechanisms and time course. *Anaesthesia* 45: 566–73.

Joy J E, Watson SJ, Benson JA (1999) *Marijuana and Medicine: Assessing the Science Base.* Washington DC: National Academy Press.

Jurna I, Komen W, Baldauf J et al (1997) Analgesia by dihydrocodeine is not due to formation of dihydromorphine: evidence from nociceptive activity in rat thalamus. *J Pharmacol Exp Ther* 281: 1164–70.

Kaiko RF, Wallenstein SL, Rogers AG, et al (1981) Analgesic and mood effects of heroin and morphine in cancer patients with postoperative pain. *N Engl J Med* 304: 1501–05.

Kalso E, Tasmuth T, Neuvonen PJ (1996) Amitriptyline effectively relieves neuropathic pain following treatment of breast cancer. *Pain* 64: 2293–302.

Kalso E, Tramèr MR, McQuay HJ et al (1998) Systemic local-anaesthetic-type drugs in chronic pain: a systematic review. *Eur J Pain* 2: 3–14.

Kam PC & Power I (2000) New selective cox-2 inhibitors. *Pain Rev* 7: 3–13.

Kehlet H (1997) Multimodal approach to control postoperative pathophysiology and rehabilitation. *Br J Anaesth* 78: 606–17.

Kerrick JM, Fine PG, Lipman AG et al (1993) Low-dose amitriptyline as an adjunct to opioids for postoperative orthopedic pain: a placebo-controlled trial. *Pain* 52: 325–30.

Kinsella LJ & Green R (1995) Anesthesia paresthetica: nitrous oxide-induced cobalamin deficiency. *Neurology* 45: 1608–10.

Kjellberg F & Tramer MR (2001) Pharmacological control of opioid-induced pruritus: a quantitative systematic review of randomized trials. *Eur J Anaesthesiol* 18: 346–57.

Klepstad P, Dale O, Kaasa S et al (2003) Influences on serum concentrations of morphine, M6G and M3G during routine clinical drug monitoring: a prospective survey in 300 adult cancer patients. *Acta Anaesthesiol Scand* 47: 725–31.

Kluger MT, Owen H, Watson D et al (1992) Oxyhaemoglobin saturation following elective abdominal surgery in patients receiving continuous intravenous infusion or intramuscular morphine analgesia. *Anaesthesia* 47: 256–60.

Kondo H, Osborne ML, Kolhouse JF et al (1981) Nitrous oxide has multiple deleterious effects on cobalamin metabolism and causes decreases in activities of both mammalian cobalamin-dependent enzymes in rats. *J Clin Invest* 67: 1270–83.

Koppert W, Weigand M, Nuemann F et al (2004) Perioperative intravenous lidocaine has preventive effects on postoperative pain and morphine consumption after major abdominal surgery. *Anesth Analg* 98: 1050–55.

Kramer BK, Kammerl MC, Komhoff M (2004) Renal cyclooxygenase-2 (Cox-2) — physiological, pathophysiological, and clinical implications. *Kidney Blood Press Res* 27: 43–62.

Krishna S, Hughes LF, Lin SY (2003) Postoperative hemorrhage with nonsteroidal anti-inflammatory drug use after tonsillectomy: a meta-analysis. *Arch Otolaryngol Head Neck Surg* 129: 1086–89.

Kvalsvik O, Borchgrevink P C, Hagen L et al (2003) Randomized, double-blind, placebo-controlled study of the effect of rectal paracetamol on morphine consumption after abdominal hysterectomy. *Acta Anaesthesiol Scand* 47: 451–56.

Latta K S, Ginsberg B, Barkin RL (2002) Meperidine: a critical review. *Am J Ther* 9: 53–68.

Layzer RB (1978) Myeloneuropathy after prolonged exposure to nitrous oxide. *Lancet* 2: 1227–30.

Lee A, Cooper MC, Craig JC, Knight JF, Keneally JP (2003) Effects of nonsteroidal anti-inflammatory drugs on postoperative renal function in adults with normal renal function. *The Cochrane Database of Systematic Reviews*, Issue 3. Art. No.: CD002765. DOI: 10.1002/14651858.CD002765.pub2.

Lee P, Smith I, Piesowicz A et al (1999) Spastic paraparesis after anaesthesia. *Lancet* 353: 554.

Leeb BF, Schweitzer H, Montag K et al (2000) A metaanalysis of chondroitin sulfate in the treatment of osteoarthritis. *J Rheumatol* 27: 205–11.

Lehmann KA, Ribbert N, Horrichs-Haermeyer G (1990) Postoperative patient-controlled analgesia with alfentanil: Analgesic efficacy and minimum effective concentrations. *J Pain Symptom Manage* 5: 249–58.

Leith S, Wheatley RG, Jackson IJB et al (1994) Extradural infusion analgesia for postoperative pain relief. *Br J Anaesth* 73: 552–58.

Levine JD, Gordon NC, Smith R et al (1986) Desipramine enhances opiate postoperative analgesia. *Pain* 27: 45–49.

Li Wan Po A & Zhang WY (1997) Systematic overview of co-proxamol to assess analgesic effects of addition of dextropropoxyphene to paracetamol. *BMJ* 315: 1565–71.

Lim AW & Schug SA (2001) Tramadol versus morphine as oral step-down analgesia after postoperative epidural analgesia. *Reg Anesth Pain Med* 26: S133.

Little CV, Parsons T, Logan S (2000) Herbal therapy for treating osteoarthritis. *The Cochrane Database of Systematic Reviews*, Issue 4. Art. No.: CD002947. DOI: 10.1002/14651858.CD002947.

Long L & Ernst E (2001) Homeopathic remedies for the treatment of osteoarthritis: a systematic review. *Br Homeopath J* 90: 175–76.

Macintyre PE & Jarvis DA (1996) Age is the best predictor of postoperative morphine requirements. *Pain* 64: 357–64.

Macintyre PE & Ready LB (2001) *Acute Pain Management: A Practical Guide*. 2nd Edition. London: WB Saunders.

Malan TP, Marsh G, Hakki SI (2003) Parecoxib sodium, a parenteral cyclooxygenase 2 selective inhibitor, improves morphine analgesia and is opioid-sparing following total hip arthroplasty. *Anesthesiology* 98: 590–96.

Mancini F, Landolfi C, Muzio M et al (2003) Acetaminophen down-regulates interleukin-1 beta-induced nuclear factor-kappa B nuclear translocation in a human astrocytic cell line. *Neurosci Lett* 353: 79–82.

Marret E, Flahault A, Samama CM et al (2003) Effects of postoperative, nonsteroidal, antiinflammatory drugs on bleeding risk after tonsillectomy: meta-analysis of randomized, controlled trials. *Anesthesiology* 98: 1497–502.

Marie RM, Le Biez E, Busson P (2000) Nitrous oxide anesthesia-associated myelopathy. *Arch Neurol* 57: 380–82.

Marinangeli F, Ciccizzi A, Donatelli F et al (2002) Clonidine for treatment of postoperative pain: a dose-finding study. *Eur J Pain* 6: 35–42.

Martin C, Martin A, Rud C et al (1988) Comparative study of sodium valproate and ketoprofen in the treatment of postoperative pain. *Ann Fr Anesth Reanim* 7: 387–92.

Martin-Garcia C, Hinojosa M, Berges P et al (2003) Celecoxib, a highly selective COX 2 inhibitor, is safe in aspirin-induced asthma patients. *J Investig Allergol Clin Immunol* 13: 20–25.

McCartney CJ, Sinha A, Katz J (2004) A qualitative systematic review of the role of N-methyl-D-aspartate receptor antagonists in preventive analgesia. *Anesth Analg* 98: 1385–400.

McCormack K (1994) Non-steroidal anti-inflammatory drugs and spinal nociceptive processing. *Pain* 59: 9–43.

McMorrow AM, Adams RJ, Rubenstein MN (1995) Combined system disease after nitrous oxide anesthesia: A case report. *Neurology* 45: 1224–25.

McNeely JK, Buczulinski B, Rosner DR (2000) Severe neurological impairment in an infant after nitrous oxide. *Anesth Anesth* 93: 1549–50.

McQuay HJ (1991) Opioid clinical pharmacology and routes of administration. *Br Med Bull* 47: 703–17.

McQuay H, Carroll D, Jadad AJ et al (1995) Anticonvulsant drugs for management of pain: a systematic review. *BMJ* 311: 1047–53.

McQuay HJ, Tramèr M, Nye BA et al (1996) A systematic review of antidepressants in neuropathic pain. *Pain* 68: 217–27.

McQuay HJ (2002) Neuropathic pain: evidence matters. *Eur J Pain* 6(A): 11–18.

Mercadante S & Arcuri E (2004) Opioids and renal function. *J Pain* 5: 2–19.

Mildh LH, Leino KA, Kirvela OA (1999) Effects of tramadol and meperidine on respiration, plasma catecholamine concentrations, and hemodynamics. *J Clin Anesth* 11: 310–16.

Miyoshi RH, Lackband SG (2001) Systemic Opioid Analgesics. Bonica's Management of Pain. 3rd edition (Ed J Loeser). Lippincott Williams & Wilkins.

Møiniche S, Rømsing J, Dahl J B et al (2003) Nonsteroidal antiinflammatory drugs and the risk of operative site bleeding after tonsillectomy: a quantitative systematic review. *Anesth Analg* 96: 68–77.

Moore A, Collins S, Carroll D, McQuay H, Edwards J (1998) Single dose paracetamol (acetaminophen), with and without codeine, for postoperative pain. *The Cochrane Database of Systematic Reviews*, Issue 4. Art. No.: CD001547. DOI: 10.1002/14651858.CD001547.

Moore A, Edwards J, Barden J et al (2003) *Bandolier's Little Book of Pain*. Oxford: Oxford University Press.

Moore PK & Marshall M (2003) Nitric oxide releasing acetaminophen (nitroacetaminophen). *Dig Liver Dis* 35: S49–S60.

Murat I, Gall O, Tourniaire B (2003) Procedural pain in children: evidence-based best practice and guidelines. *Reg Anesth Pain Med* 28: 561–72.

Namavar Jahromi B, Tartifizadeh A, Khabnadideh S (2003) Comparison of fennel and mefenamic acid for the treatment of primary dysmenorrhoea. *Int J Gynaecol Obstet* 80: 153–57.

Nestor PJ & Stark RJ (1996) Vitamin B12 myeloneuropathy precipitated by nitrous oxide anaesthesia. *Med J Aust* 165: 174.

Ng A, Smith G, Davidson AC (2003) Analgesic effects of parecoxib following total abdominal hysterectomy. *Br J Anaesth* 90: 746–49.

Nilsson-Ehle H (1998) Age-related changes in cobalamin (vitamin B12) handling. Implications for therapy. *Drugs Aging* 12: 277–92.

Nunn JF, Sharer NM, Gorchein A et al (1982) Megaloblastic haemopoiesis after multiple short-term exposure to nitrous oxide. *Lancet* 1: 1379–81.

Nunn JF, Chanarin I, Tanner AG et al (1986) Megaloblastic bone marrow changes after repeated nitrous oxide anaesthesia. *Br J Anaesth* 58: 1469–70.

Nunn JF (1987) Clinical aspects of the interaction between nitrous oxide and vitamin B12. *Br J Anaesth* 59: 3–13.

Nussmeier NA, Whelton AA, Brown MT et al (2005)Complications of the COX-2 inhibitors parecoxib and valdecoxib after cardiac surgery. *New Engl J Med* 352: 1081–91.

O'Connor A, Schug SA, Cardwell HJ (2000) A comparison of the efficacy and safety of morphine and pethidine as analgesia for suspected renal colic in the emergency setting. *J Accid Emerg Med* 17: 261–64.

Oderda GM, Evans RS, Lloyd J (2003) Costs of opioid-related adverse events in surgical patients. *J Pain Symptom Manage* 25: 276–83.

Ofman JJ, MacLean CH, Straus WL et al (2002) A metaanalysis of severe upper gastrointestinal complications of nonsteroidal antiinflammatory drugs. *J Rheumatol* 29: 804–12.

O'Leary U, Puglia C, Friehling TD et al (1987) Nitrous oxide anesthesia in patients with ischemic chest discomfort: effect on beta-endorphins. *J Clin Pharmacol* 27: 957–61.

Ott E, Nussmeier NA, Duke PC et al (2003) Efficacy and safety of the cyclooxygenase 2 inhibitors parecoxib and valdecoxib in patients undergoing coronary artery bypass surgery. *J Thorac Cardiovasc Surg* 125: 1481–92.

Park J, Forrest J, Kolesar R et al (1992) Oral clonidine reduces postoperative PCA morphine requirements. *Can J Anaesth* 43: 900–06.

Peng PW & Sandler AN (1999) A review of the use of fentanyl analgesia in the management of acute pain in adults. *Anesthesiology* 90: 576–99.

Petrenko AB, Yamakura T, Baba H et al (2003) The role of N-methyl-D-aspartate receptors in pain: A review. *Anaesth Analg* 97: 1108–16.

Pittler MH & Ernst E (1998) Peppermint oil for irritable bowel syndrome; a critical review and metaanalysis. *Am J Gastroenterol* 93: 1131–35.

Philip BK, Reese PR, Burch SP (2002) The economic impact of opioids on postoperative pain management. *J Clin Anesth* 14: 354–64.

Plesan A, Sollevi A, Segerdahl M (2000) The N-methyl-D-aspartate-receptor antagonist dextromethorphan lacks analgesic effect in a human experimental ischaemic pain model. *Acta Anaesthesiol Scand* 44: 924–28.

Power I, Chambers WA, Greer I A et al (1990) Platelet function after intramuscular diclofenac. *Anaesthesia* 45: 916–19.

Power I, Cumming AD, Pugh GC (1992) Effect of diclofenac on renal function and prostacyclin generation after surgery. *Br J Anaesth* 69: 451–56.

Power I, Noble DW, Winter A et al (1998) Effects of ketorolac and dextran-70 alone and in combination on haemostasis. *Acta Anaesthesiol Scand* 42: 982–86.

Proctor ML, Murphy PA (2001). Herbal and dietary therapies for primary and secondary dysmenorrhoea. *The Cochrane Database of Systematic Reviews*, Issue 2. Art. No.: CD002124. DOI: 10.1002/14651858.CD002124.

Qaiyum M & Sandrasegaran K (2000) Post-operative paraesthesia. *Br J Radiol* 73: 791–92.

Quigley C (2002). Hydromorphone for acute and chronic pain. *The Cochrane Database of Systematic Reviews*, Issue 1. Art. No.: CD003447. DOI: 10.1002/14651858.CD003447.

Quigley C. Opioid switching to improve pain relief and drug tolerability. *The Cochrane Database of Systematic Reviews* 2004, Issue 3. Art. No.: CD004847. DOI: 10.1002/14651858.CD004847.

Radbruch L, Grond S, Lehmann KA (1996) A risk-benefit assessment of tramadol in the management of pain. *Drug Safety* 15: 8–29.

Raffa R B, Friderichs E, Reimann W et al (1992) Opioid and nonopioid components independently contribute to the mechanism of action of tramadol, an 'atypical' opioid analgesic. *J Pharmacol Exp Ther* 260: 275–85.

Rapp SE, Egan KJ, Ross BK et al (1996) A multidimensional comparison of morphine and hydromorphone patient-controlled analgesia. *Anesth Analg* 82: 1043–48.

RCA (1998) *Guidelines for the Use of Non-steroidal Anti-inflammatory Drugs in the Perioperative Period.* Oxford: Royal College of Anaesthetists (UK).

Ready LB, Oden R, Chadwick HS et al (1988) Development of an Anesthesiology-based postoperative pain management service. *Anesthesiology* 68: 100–06.

Reuben SS, Makari-Judson G, Lurie SD (2004) Evaluation of the efficacy of the perioperative administration of venlafaxine SR in the prevention of postmastectomy pain syndrome. *J Pain Sympt Manage* 27: 133–39.

Reynolds LW, Hoo RK, Brill RJ et al (2003) The COX-2 specific inhibitor, valdecoxib, is an effective, opioid-sparing analgesic in patients undergoing total knee arthroplasty. *J Pain Symptom Manage* 25: 133–41.

Riedel B, Fiskerstrand T, Refsum H et al (1999) Co-ordinate variations in methylmalonyl-CoA mutase and methionine synthase, and the cobalamin cofactors in human glioma cells during nitrous oxide exposure and the subsequent recovery phase. *Biochem J* 341: 133–38.

Romero-Sandoval EA, Del Soldato P, Herrero JF (2003) The effects of sham and full spinalization on the antinociceptive effects of NCX-701 (nitroparacetamol) in monoarthritic rats. *Neuropharmacol* 45: 412–19.

Rømsing J, Møiniche S, Dahl JB (2002) Rectal and parenteral paracetamol, and paracetamol in combination with NSAIDs, for postoperative analgesia. *Br J Anaesth* 88: 215–26.

Rømsing J, Møiniche S (2004) A systematic review of COX-2 inhibitors compared with traditional NSAIDs, or different COX-2 inhibitors for postoperative pain. *Acta Anaesthesiol Scand* 48: 525–46.

Rosen MA (2002) Nitrous oxide for relief of labor pain: a systematic review. *Am J Obstet Gynecol* 186: S110–26.

Rosenberg J, Rasmussen V, Von Jessen F et al (1990) Late postoperative episodic and constant hypoxaemia and associated ECG abnormalities. *Br J Anaesth* 65: 684–91.

Rosenberg J, Pedersen MH, Gebuhr P et al (1992) Effect of oxygen therapy on late postoperative episodic and constant hypoxaemia. *Br J Anaesth* 68: 18–22.

Rosener M & Dichgans J (1996) Severe combined degeneration of the spinal cord after nitrous oxide anaesthesia in a vegetarian. *J Neurol Neurosurg Psych* 60: 354.

Rusy LM, Houck CS, Sullivan L et al (1995) A double-blind evaluation of ketorolac tromethamine versus acetaminophen in pediatric tonsillectomy: analgesia and bleeding. *Anesth Analg* 80: 226–29.

Salerno SM, Browning R, Jackson JL (2002) The effect of antidepressant treatment on chronic back pain. *Arch Intern Med* 162: 19–24.

Sahenk Z, Mendell JR, Couri D et al (1978) Polyneuropathy from inhalation of N2O cartridges through a whipped-cream dispenser. *Neurology* 28: 485–87.

Sator-Katzenschlager S, Deusch E, Maier P et al (2001) The long-term antinociceptive effect of intrathecal S(+)-ketamine in a patient with established morphine tolerance. *Anesth Analg* 93: 1032–34.

Schafer AI (1999) Effects of nonsteroidal anti-inflammatory therapy on platelets. *Am J Med* 106: 25S–36S.

Schenk BE, Kuipers EJ, Klinkenberg-Knol EC et al (1999) Atrophic gastritis during long-term omeprazole therapy affects serum vitamin B12 levels. *Aliment Pharmacol Ther* 13: 1343–46.

Schilling RF (1986) Is nitrous oxide a dangerous anesthetic for vitamin B12-deficient subjects? *JAMA* 255: 1605–06.

Schmid B, Ludtke R, Selbmann HK et al (2000) [Effectiveness and tolerance of standardized willow bark extract in arthrosis patients. Randomised, placebo controlled double-blind study.] *Z Rheumatol* 49: 314–20.

Schug SA, Zech D, Grond S (1992) Adverse effects of systemic opioid analgesics. *Drug Safety* 7: 200–13.

Schug SA, Sidebotham DA, Mcguinnety M et al (1998) Acetaminophen as an adjunct to morphine by patient-controlled analgesia in the management of acute postoperative pain. *Anesth Analg* 87: 368–72.

Scott JM, Dinn JJ, Wilson P et al (1981) Pathogenesis of subacute combined degeneration: a result of methyl group deficiency. *Lancet* 2: 334–37.

Seibert K, Zhang Y, Leahy K et al (1994) Pharmacological and biochemical demonstration of the role of cyclooxygenase 2 in inflammation and pain. *Proc Natl Acad Sci* 91: 12013–17.

Sesso RM, Iunes Y, Melo AC (1999) Myeloneuropathy following nitrous oxide anesthaesia in a patient with macrocytic anaemia. *Neuroradiol* 41: 588–90.

Shaw AD & Morgan M (1998) Nitrous oxide: time to stop laughing? *Anaesthesia* 53: 213–15.

Sikiennik AW & Kream RM (1995) N-methyl-D-aspartate receptors and pain. *Curr Op Anaesthesiol* 8: 445–49.

Silvasti M, Rosenberg P, Seppala T et al (1998) Comparison of analgesic efficacy of oxycodone and morphine in postoperative intravenous patient-controlled analgesia. *Acta Anaesthesiol Scand* 42: 576–80.

Silverman M. Shih R, Allegra J (2004) Morphine indices less nausea than meperidine when administered parenterally. *J Emerg Med* 27: 241–43.

Silverstein FE, Faich G, Goldstein JL et al (2000) Gastrointestinal toxicity with celecoxib vs nonsteroidal anti-inflammatory drugs for osteoarthritis and rheumatoid arthritis — The CLASS study: a randomized controlled trial. *JAMA* 284: 1247–55.

Simopoulos TT, Smith HS, Peeters-Asdourian C et al (2002) Use of meperidine in patient-controlled analgesia and the development of a normeperidine toxic reaction. *Arch Surg* 137: 84–88.

Simmons DL (2003) Variants of cyclooxygenase-1 and their roles in medicine. *Thromb Res* 110: 265–68.

Simon RA & Namazy J (2003) Adverse reactions to aspirin and nonsteroidal anti inflammatory drugs (NSAIDs). *Clin Rev Allergy Immunol* 24: 239–51.

Sinatra RS, Lodge K, Sibert K et al (1989) A comparison of morphine, meperidine and oxymorphone as utilized in patient-controlled analgesia following Cesarean delivery. *Anesthesiology* 70: 585–90.

Sindrup S H & Jensen TS (1999) Efficacy of pharmacological treatments of neuropathic pain, an update and effect related to mechanism of drug action. *Pain* 83: 389–400.

Skacel PO, Hewlett AM, Lewis JD et al (1983) Studies on the haemopoietic toxicity of nitrous oxide in man. *Br J Haematol* 53: 189–200.

Smith MT (2000) Neuroexcitatory effects of morphine and hydromorphone: evidence implicating the 3-glucuronide metabolites. *Clin Exp Pharmacol Physiol* 27: 524–28.

Soeken KL (2004) Selected CAM therapies for arthritis-related pain: the evidence from systematic reviews. *Clin J Pain* 20: 13–18.

Stacy CB, Di Rocco A, Gould RJ (1992) Methionine in the treatment of nitrous-oxide-induced neuropathy and myeloneuropathy. *J Neurol* 239: 401–03.

Stanley G, Appadu B, Mead M et al (1996) Dose requirements, efficacy and side effects of morphine and pethidine delivered by patient-controlled analgesia after gynaecological surgery. *Br J Anaesth* 76: 484–86.

Stausholm K, Kehlet H, Rosenberg J (1995) Oxygen therapy reduces postoperative tachycardia. *Anaesthesia* 50: 737–39.

Stevinson C, Devaraj VS, Fountain-Barber A et al (2003) Homeopathic arnica for prevention of pain and bruising: a randomized placebo-controlled trial in hand surgery. *J R Soc Med* 90: 60–65.

Stoltz RR, Harris SI, Kuss ME et al (2002) Upper GI mucosal effects of parecoxib sodium in healthy elderly subjects. *Am J Gastroenterol* 97: 65–71.

Strom BL, Berlin JA, Kinman JL et al (1996) Parenteral ketorolac and risk of gastrointestinal and operative site bleeding. A postmarketing surveillance study. *JAMA* 275: 376–82.

Subramaniam K, Sibramaniam B, Steinbrook RA (2004) Ketamine as adjuvant analgesic to opioids: a quantitative and qualitative systematic review. *Anesth Analg* 99: 482–95.

Szczeklik A & Stevenson DD (2003) Aspirin-induced asthma: Advances in pathogenesis, diagnosis, and management. *J Allergy Clin Immunol* 111: 913–21.

Tarkkila P, Tuominen M, Lindgren L (1997) Comparison of respiratory effects of tramadol and oxycodone. *J Clin Anesth* 9: 582–85.

Tarkkila P, Tuominen M, Lindgren L (1998) Comparison of respiratory effects of tramadol and pethidine. *Eur J Anaesthesiol* 15: 64–68.

Tasmuth T, Hartel B, Kalso E (2002) Venlafaxine in neuropathic pain following treatment of breast cancer. *Eur J Pain* 6: 17–24.

Toh B-H, van Driel IR, Gleeson PA (1997) Pernicious anemia. *N Engl J Med* 337: 1441–48.

Tomkins GE, Jackson JL, O'Malley PG et al (2001) Treatment of chronic headache with antidepressants: A meta-analysis. *Am J Med* 111: 54–63.

Towheed TE, Anastassiades TP, Shea B, Houpt J, Welch V, Hochberg MC (2000) Glucosamine therapy for treating osteoarthritis. The Cochrane Database of Systematic Reviews, Issue 2. Art. No.: CD002946. DOI: 10.1002/14651858.CD002946.

Tramèr M (2001) A rational approach to the control of postoperative nausea and vomiting: evidence from systematic reviews. Part II. Recommendations for prevention and treatment, and research agenda. *Acta Anaesthesiol Scand* 45: 14–19.

Van Aken H, Thys L, Veekman L et al (2004) Assessing analgesia in single and repeated administrations of propacetamol for postoperative pain: Comparison with morphine after dental surgery. *Anesth Analg* 98: 159–65.

van Tulder MW, Scholten RJPM, Koes BW, Deyo RA (2000). Non-steroidal anti-inflammatory drugs for low-back pain. *The Cochrane Database of Systematic Reviews*, Issue 2. Art. No.: CD000396. DOI: 10.1002/14651858.CD000396.

Varrassi G, Marinangeli F, Agro F et al (1999) A double-blinded evaluation of propacetamol versus ketorolac in combination with patient-controlled analgesia morphine: analgesic efficacy and tolerability after gynecologic surgery. *Anesth Analg* 88: 611–16.

Venn RM, Bradshaw CJ, Spencer R et al (1999) Preliminary UK experience of dexmedetomidine, a novel agent for postoperative sedation in the intensive care unit. *Anaesthesia* 54: 1136–42.

Wadhwa A, Clarke D, Goodchild CS et al (2001) Large-dose oral dextromethorphan as an adjunct to patient-controlled analgesia with morphine after knee surgery. *Anaesth Analg* 92: 448–54.

Wallace MS, Berger D, Schulteis G (2002) The effect of oral desipramine on capsaicin-induced allodynia and hyperalgesia: a double-blinded. placebo-controlled, crossover study. *Anesth Analg* 95: 973–78.

Warner TD & Mitchell JA (2002) Cyclooxygenase-3 (COX-3): Filling in the gaps toward a COX continuum? *Proc Natl Acad Sci* 99: 13371–73.

Warren PM, Taylor JH, Nicholson KE et al (2000) Influence of tramadol on the ventilatory response to hypoxia in humans. *Br J Anaesth* 85: 211–16.

Weimann J (2001) Toxicity of nitrous oxide. *Best Pract Res Clin Anaesthesiol* 15: 47–61.

Weinbroum AA, Lalayev G, Yashar T et al (2001) Combined pre-incision oral dextromethorphan and epidural lidocaine for postoperative pain reduction and morphine sparing: a randomized double-blind study on day-surgery patients. *Anaesthesia* 56: 616–22.

Weinbroum AA (2002) Dextromethorphan reduces immediate and late postoperative analgesic requirements and improves patients' subjective scorings after epidural lidocaine and general anesthesia. *Anesth Analg* 94: 1547–52.

Weinbroum AA (2003) A single small dose of postoperative ketamine provides rapid and sustained improvement in morphine analgesia in the presence of morphine-resistance pain. *Anaesth Analg* 96: 789–95.

West PM & Fernadnez C (2003) Safety of COX-2 inhibitors in asthma patients with aspirin hypersensitivity. *Ann Pharmacother* 37: 1497–501.

Wheatley RG, Somerville ID, Sapsford DJ et al (1990) Postoperative hypoxaemia: comparison of extradural, IM and patient-controlled opioid analgesia. *Br J Anaesth* 64: 267–75.

WHO (1966) World Health Organization Tech Rep Ser 1966; 341:7. In: Laurence DR & Bennett PN (Eds) *Clinical Pharmacology.* 5th ed. Edinburgh: Christchurch Livingstone.

WHO (1996) Cancer Pain Relief: with a Guide to Opioid Availability. Geneva: World Health Organisation.

Wilder-Smith C H, Bettiga A (1997) The analgesic tramadol has minimal effect on gastrointestinal motor function. *Br J Clin Pharmacol* 43: 71–75.

Wilder-Smith CH, Hill L, Osler W et al (1999a) Effect of tramadol and morphine on pain and gastro-intestinal motor function in patients with chronic pancreatitis. *Dig Dis Sci* 44: 1107–16.

Wilder-Smith CH, Hill L, Wilkins J et al (1999b) Effects of morphine and tramadol on somatic and visceral sensory function and gastrointestinal motility after abdominal surgery. *Anesthesiology* 91: 639–47.

Wiffen P, Collins S, McQuay H, Carroll D et al (2000) Anticonvulsant drugs for acute and chronic pain. *The Cochrane Database of Systematic Reviews*, Issue 3. Art. No.: CD001133. DOI: 10.1002/14651858.CD001133.

Woodhouse A, Hobbes AFT, Mather LE et al (1996) A comparison of morphine, pethidine and fentanyl in the postsurgical patient-controlled analgesia (PCA) environment. *Pain* 64: 115–21.

Woodhouse A, Ward M, Mather L (1999) Inter-subject variability in post-operative patient-controlled analgesia (PCA): Is the patient equally satisfied with morphine, pethidine and fentanyl? *Pain* 80: 545–53.

Working Party on the Use of Cannabis for Medical Purposes (2000) *The Use of Cannabis for Medical Purposes.* Sydney: NSW Government.

Wright AW, Mather LE, Smith MT (2001) Hydromorphone-3-glucuronide: a more potent neuro-excitant than its structural analogue, morphine-3-glucuronide. *Life Sci* 69: 409–20.

Zhao SZ, Chung F, Hanna DB et al (2004) Dose-response relationship between opioid use and adverse effects after ambulatory surgery. *J Pain Symptom Manage* 28: 35–46.

Zhou TJ, Tang J, White PF (2001) Propacetamol versus ketorolac for treatment of acute postoperative pain after total hip or knee replacement. *Anesth Analg* 92: 1569–75.

5. REGIONALLY AND LOCALLY ADMINISTERED ANALGESIC DRUGS

5.1 LOCAL ANAESTHETICS

Local anaesthetics exert their effect as analgesics by the blockade of sodium channels and hence impeding neuronal excitation and/or conduction.

5.1.1 Short duration local anaesthetics

Lignocaine (lidocaine) is the most widely used short duration local anaesthetic in acute pain management. Although the plasma half-life is approximately 90 minutes, the duration of local anaesthetic effect depends very much on site of administration, dose administered and the presence or absence of vasoconstrictors. Although lignocaine is hydrophilic it is delivered in high concentrations and therefore usually diffuses well into nerve bundles, resulting in little separation of sensory and motor blocking actions (Covino & Wildsmith 1998).

The use of lignocaine (lidocaine) in ongoing acute pain management is usually restricted to the short-term re-establishment of a local anaesthetic infusion block; it is unsuited to long-term (ie days) use because of the development of tachyphylaxis or acute tolerance (Mogensen 1995). For example, 24-hour continuous perineural infusions of lignocaine result in less effective analgesia and more motor block than infusions of the long-acting local anaesthetic agent ropivacaine (Casati et al 2003a, **Level II**).

5.1.2 Long duration local anaesthetics

The three commonly used long duration local anaesthetic agents, bupivacaine, levobupivacaine and ropivacaine, are structurally related (Markham & Faulds 1996; McLeod & Burke 2001). Whereas bupivacaine is a racemic mixture of S- and R-enantiomers, levobupivacaine is the S (or *levo*) enantiomer of bupivacaine; ropivacaine is likewise an S enantiomer.

There are consistent laboratory data showing that the S-enantiomers of these local anaesthetics exhibit less central nervous system (CNS) or cardiac toxicity than the R-enantiomers or the racemic mixtures for doses resulting in equivalent sensory nerve conduction block. It is difficult to define relative toxicities for these agents because it depends on the parameters measured.

In blinded human volunteer studies, CNS symptoms were detected at intravenous (IV) doses and plasma levels that were 25% higher for ropivacaine compared with bupivacaine (Scott et al 1989, **Level II**) and 16% higher for levobupivacaine than bupivacaine (Bardsley et al 1998, **Level II**). Although these data show that CNS toxicity might occur less frequently or be less severe with the S-enantiomers, all local anaesthetics are toxic. A rapid IV bolus of any of these agents may overwhelm any of the more subtle differences found at lower plasma concentrations.

Severe myocardial depression and refractory ventricular fibrillation have been described as the hallmark of accidental IV administration of moderately large doses of bupivacaine. This has been attributed to the slow dissociation of bupivacaine from the myocardial sodium channel, which is less marked with levobupivacaine and ropivacaine (Mather & Chang 2001). Animal studies confirm that higher systemic doses of ropivacaine and levobupivacaine are required to induce ventricular arrhythmias, circulatory collapse or asystole (Ohmura et al 2001), with the ranking of toxicity risk being bupivacaine > levobupivacaine > ropivacaine (Groban & Dolinski 2001).

Controlled human studies are only possible when looking at surrogate endpoints such as electrocardiogram (ECG) changes or myocardial depression and suggest a similar ranking of effect (Scott et al 1989, **Level II**; Knudsen et al 1997, **Level II**; Bardsley et al 1998, **Level II**; Mather & Chang 2001, **Level II**), with bupivacaine being the most toxic and levobupivacaine being less toxic and similar to ropivacaine (Stewart et al 2003, **Level II**).

Resuscitation from a massive overdose is of greater relevance to toxicity in clinical practice. A canine study investigating resuscitation and survival following local anaesthetic-induced circulatory collapse showed survivals of 50%, 70% and 90% with bupivacaine, levobupivacaine and ropivacaine respectively (Groban et al 2001).

Case reports of accidental toxic overdosage with ropivacaine and bupivacaine suggest that outcomes are more favourable and resuscitation more straightforward (in particular requiring less cardiovascular support) with ropivacaine (Pham-Dang et al 2000; Chazalon et al 2003; Huet et al 2003; Klein et al 2003; Soltesz et al 2003). However, toxicity data are of little use if the relative potencies of these agents are not known.

The issue with relative potency emerges with lower doses and concentrations of local anaesthetic. When doses are carefully titrated, a minimum local anaesthetic concentration (MLAC) can be found at which 50% of patients will achieve a satisfactory analgesic block. In obstetric epidural analgesia, two separate studies found the MLAC of bupivacaine was 0.6 times that of ropivacaine (Capogna et al 1999, **Level II**; Polley et al 1999, **Level II**). The motor-blocking potency showed a similar ratio of 0.66 (Lacassie et al 2002, **Level II**).

When comparing bupivacaine with levobupivacaine, the 'percentage' bupivacaine solution is by weight of bupivacaine HCl, whereas % levobupivacaine solution is for the active molecule alone. This means that the molar dose of equal 'percentage concentration' is13% higher for levobupivacaine (Schug 2001). The sensory MLAC potency ratio of levobupivacaine to bupivacaine is 0.98, although if correction is made for molar concentrations this falls to 0.87 (neither value being different from unity) (Lyons et al 1998, **Level II**). Levobupivacaine has been shown to have slightly less motor blocking capacity than bupivacaine with a levobupivacaine / bupivacaine potency ratio for epidural motor blockade of 0.87 (95% CI, 0.77-0.98) (Lacassie & Columb 2003, **Level II**). Another labour epidural analgesia study has found no difference in MLAC between levobupivacaine and ropivacaine with a ropivacaine:levobupivacaine potency ratio of 0.98 (95% CI, 0.80-1.20) (Polley et al 2003, **Level II**).

For postoperative epidural infusions, dose-ranging studies established that 0.2% ropivacaine was a suitable concentration (Scott et al 1995, **Level II**; Schug et al 1996,

Level II). Therefore, most investigators compare infusions of bupivacaine or levobupivacaine at 0.1% or 0.125% with ropivacaine 0.2% which removes any imbalance in comparative potency.

The majority of studies find similar analgesic outcomes with postoperative epidural infusions based on these strengths (Jorgensen et al 2000, **Level II**; Macias et al 2002, **Level II**; Casati et al 2003b, **Level II**), although others have found bupivacaine to be superior to ropivacaine (Muldoon et al 1998, **Level II**). The quality of pain relief from low-dose epidural infusions of plain local anaesthetic consistently benefits from the addition of adjuvants such as opioids (Crews et al 1999, **Level II**; Scott et al 1999, **Level II**; Hubler et al 2001, **Level II**; Senard et al 2002, **Level II**) or alpha-2 adrenoceptor agonists (Milligan et al 2000, **Level II**; Niemi & Breivik 2002, **Level II**).

Motor block is of clinical relevance in low thoracic or lumbar epidural infusions and has been reported to be less intense with epidural ropivacaine than with bupivacaine (Zaric et al 1996, **Level II**; Muldoon et al 1998, **Level II**; Merson 2001, **Level II**). However, this finding has not been supported by other authors (Casati et al 2003b, **Level II**).

The effect of motor block in labour analgesic infusions has been studied specifically because of the implications for prolonged labour or instrumental delivery. In a recent large trial comparing 0.08% ropivacaine to 0.08% bupivacaine (both with fentanyl 2 microgram/mL), no differences were found in labour analgesia, outcomes or delivery (Halpern et al 2003, **Level II**). A subsequent meta-analysis concluded that both ropivacaine and bupivacaine provide excellent labour analgesia and there was no difference in maternal satisfaction or neonatal outcomes (Halpern & Walsh 2003, **Level I**). The effects on motor block were inconsistent.

At concentrations of 0.5% or greater, there are no significant differences in onset time, intensity or duration of sensory blockade between bupivacaine, levobupivacaine or ropivacaine in epidural (Cheng et al 2002, **Level II**; Casati et al 2003b, **Level II**), sciatic (Casati et al 2002, **Level II**), interscalene (Casati et al 2003c, **Level II**) or axillary brachial plexus blocks (McGlade et al 1998, **Level II**). The intensity and duration of motor block is frequently less with ropivacaine compared with bupivacaine or levobupivacaine, but this has little effect on the quality of block for surgery (McGlade et al 1998, **Level II**; Casati et al 2003c, **Level II**).

Total plasma levels of local anaesthetic tend to rise during the first 48 hours of postoperative infusion, although free levels remain relatively low (Emanuelsson et al 1995; Scott et al 1997). Thus in normal circumstances toxicity due to systemic absorption from epidural or perineural infusions is not a problem. However, the risk of accidental absolute overdose with postoperative infusions suggests that the less toxic agents should be used in preference.

Key messages

1. Continuous perineural infusions of lignocaine (lidocaine) result in less effective analgesia and more motor block than long-acting local anaesthetic agents (**Level II**).
2. There are no consistent differences between ropivacaine, levobupivacaine and bupivacaine when given in low doses for regional analgesia in terms of quality of analgesia or motor blockade (**Level II**).
3. Cardiovascular and central nervous system toxicity of the stereospecific isomers ropivacaine and levobupivacaine is less severe than with racemic bupivacaine (**Level II**).

The following tick box ☑ represents conclusions based on clinical experience and expert opinion.

☑ Case reports following accidental overdose with ropivacaine and bupivacaine suggest that resuscitation is likely to be more successful with ropivacaine.

5.2 Opioids

CHAPTER 5

5.2.1 Neuraxial opioids

Opioid receptors were described in the spinal cord of the rat in 1976 (Pert et al 1976) and the same year a potent analgesic effect of directly applied intrathecal morphine was reported in these animals (Yaksh & Rudy 1976). Opioid analgesia is spinally mediated via presynaptic and postsynaptic receptors in the substantia gelatinosa in the dorsal horn (Yaksh 1981). In addition to this a local anaesthetic action has been described for pethidine (meperidine) that may contribute to the clinical effect when administered intrathecally (Jaffe & Rowe 1996). The first clinical use of intrathecal morphine was for analgesia for cancer patients (Wang et al 1979).

Intrathecal opioids

The lipid solubility of opioids largely determines the speed of onset and duration of intrathecal analgesia; hydrophilic drugs (eg morphine) have a slower onset of action and longer half-lives in cerebrospinal fluid with greater cephalad migration compared with lipophilic opioids (eg fentanyl) (Bernards 2004).

Safety studies and widespread clinical experience with morphine, fentanyl and sufentanil have shown no neurotoxicity or behavioural changes at normal clinical intrathecal doses (Hodgson et al 1999, **Level IV**). Other opioid agonists or partial agonists do not have animal or human safety data.

Although early clinical studies used very high intrathecal morphine doses (ie 1mg or more), adequate postoperative analgesia with fewer adverse effects may be obtained with less morphine (see Section 7.3). For patients undergoing caesarean section with spinal anaesthesia, intrathecal morphine provided better reductions in postoperative pain and analgesic consumption compared with fentanyl (Dahl et al 1999, **Level I**).

Epidural opioids

The behaviour of epidural opioids is also governed largely by their lipid solubility. The greater sequestration of lipid soluble opioids into epidural fat and slow re-release back into the epidural space means that elimination from the epidural space is prolonged, resulting in relatively smaller fractions of drug reaching the cerebrospinal fluid (Bernards 2004). Lipophilic opioids (eg fentanyl) have a faster onset but shorter duration of action compared with hydrophilic drugs (eg morphine) (de-Leon Casasola & Lema 1996).

Morphine is the least lipid soluble of the opioids administered epidurally; it has the slowest onset and offset of action (Cousins & Mather 1984). As it has a prolonged analgesic effect it can be given by intermittent bolus dose or infusion; the risk of respiratory depression may be higher and analgesia less effective with bolus dose regimens (de-Leon Casasola & Lema 1996).

Pethidine (meperidine) is effective when administered epidurally by bolus dose, continuous infusion and by epidural patient-controlled analgesia. It is more lipid soluble than morphine (but less than fentanyl and its analogues), thus its onset and offset of epidural analgesic action is more rapid than morphine (Ngan Kee 1998, **Level IV**). The analgesic effect of smaller doses appears to be spinally mediated but systemic effects are likely after larger doses; in the smaller doses it is not known whether the local anaesthetic properties of pethidine contribute significantly to pain relief (Ngan Kee 1998, **Level IV**). Epidural pethidine has been used predominantly in the obstetric setting. After caesarean section epidural pethidine resulted in better pain relief and less sedation than IV pethidine(Paech 1994, **Level II**) but inferior analgesia compared with intrathecal morphine, albeit with less pruritus, nausea and drowsiness (Paech 2000, **Level II**).

Diamorphine (diacetylmorphine, heroin) is rapidly hydrolysed to monoacetylmorphine (MAM) and morphine. Diamorphine and MAM are more lipid soluble than morphine and penetrate the CNS more rapidly, although it is MAM and morphine that are thought to be responsible for the analgesic effects of diamorphine (Myoshi & Lackband, 2001). Epidural administration of diamorphine is common in the United Kingdom and is effective administered by intermittent bolus dose or infusion (McLeod et al 2005).

The quality of epidural analgesia with hydromorphone is similar to morphine (Chaplan et al 1992, **Level II**). In a comparison of epidural and IV hydromorphone, patients required twice as much IV hydromorphone to obtain the same degree of analgesia (Liu et al 1995, **Level II**).

The evidence that epidural fentanyl acts via a spinal rather than systemic effect is conflicting and it has been suggested that any benefit when comparing epidural with systemic fentanyl alone is marginal (Wheatley et al 2001; Bernards 2002). However, the conflicting results may be due to differing modes of administration. An infusion of epidural fentanyl appears to produce analgesia by uptake into the systemic circulation, whereas a bolus dose of fentanyl produces analgesia by a selective spinal mechanism (Ginosar et al 2003, **Level IV**). There is no evidence of benefit of epidural versus systemic administration of alfentanil or sufentanil (Bernards 2002).

Neuraxial opioids may cause respiratory depression, sedation, nausea, vomiting, pruritus, urinary retention and decreased gastrointestinal motility. Depending on type and dose of the opioid, a combination of spinal and systemic mechanisms may be responsible for these adverse effects. Many of these effects are more frequent with morphine and are to some extent dose related (Dahl et al 1999, **Level I**; Cole 2000, **Level I**). Late onset respiratory depression, which is believed to be a result of the cephalad spread of opioids within the cerebrospinal fluid, is also seen more commonly with hydrophilic opioids such as morphine (Cousins & Mather 1984).

Local anaesthetic/opioid combinations

Most studies show that the combination of an opioid with an epidural local anaesthetic improves analgesic efficacy and reduces the dose requirements of both drugs (Walker et al 2002, **Level I**). Potential benefits are more obvious for local anaesthetic side effects (hypotension and motor block) than for opioid-related side effects (Walker et al 2002, **Level I**).

5.2.2 Peripheral opioids

CHAPTER 5

Opioid receptors on sensory unmyelinated C nerve fibres mediate anti-nociceptive effects in animal studies (Stein et al 1990). In the presence of inflammation, opioid receptors are transported to the periphery and increased amounts of endogenous opioid peptides are present in infiltrating immune cells (Stein 1995; Schafer 1999). An experimental model of inflammatory hyperalgesia caused by ultra violet light showed that analgesia mediated via peripheral opioid mechanisms could also occur in humans (Koppert et al 1999, **Level II**).

In clinical practice, morphine injected as a single dose into the knee intra-articular space produces analgesia which may last up to 24 hours, but evidence for a peripheral rather than a systemic effect is not conclusive (Gupta et al 2001, **Level I**; Kalso et al 2002, **Level I**) Confounding variables that hinder analysis included the pre-existing degree of inflammation, type of surgery, the baseline pain severity and the overall relatively weak clinical effect (Gupta et al 2001, **Level I**) (see also Section 7.5).

There is no evidence for analgesic efficacy of peripheral opioids at non intra-articular sites, including with perineural blockade (Picard et al 1997, **Level I**). However a later study showed that, after iliac bone graft, morphine compared with local infiltration of saline or intramuscular (IM) morphine resulted in less local pain, both in the postoperative period and at 1 year after surgery, and lower postoperative morphine requirements (Reuben et al 2001, **Level II**).

Key messages

1. Intrathecal morphine produces better postoperative analgesia than intrathecal fentanyl after caesarean section (**Level I**).

2. The combination of an opioid with an epidural local anaesthetic improves analgesic efficacy and reduces the dose requirements of both drugs (**Level I**).

3. Morphine injected as a single dose into the intra-articular space produces analgesia that lasts up to 24 hours (**Level I**).

4. Evidence for a clinically relevant peripheral opioid effect at non-articular sites, including perineural, is inconclusive (**Level I**).

5. Epidural pethidine produces better pain relief and less sedation than IV pethidine after caesarean section (**Level II**).

The following tick boxes ☑ represent conclusions based on clinical experience and expert opinion.

☑ No neurotoxicity has been shown at normal clinical intrathecal doses of morphine, fentanyl and sufentanil.

☑ Neuraxial administration of bolus doses of hydrophilic opioids carries an increased risk of delayed sedation and respiratory depression compared with lipophilic opioids.

5.3 ADJUVANT DRUGS

5.3.1 Clonidine

Spinal

Clonidine is an alpha-2 adrenoceptor agonist that acts as an analgesic at the level of the spinal cord. There is no human or animal evidence of neurotoxicity when preservative-free clonidine is administered intrathecally (Hodgson et al 1999).

Epidural clonidine is approved by the United States Food and Drug Administration for relief of chronic cancer pain. Other neuraxial use of alpha-2 agonists is not endorsed by regulatory authorities, and no clinical trials of the use of newer drugs such as dexmedetomidine as analgesics have been published.

There is inconsistent evidence that the addition of clonidine to an epidural or intrathecal opioid is more effective than clonidine or the opioid alone (Walker et al 2002, **Level I**).

Intrathecal clonidine in combination with local anaesthetics may prolong the duration of spinal block, but the evidence is inconsistent (Racle et al 1987, **Level II**; Bonnet et al 1990, **Level II**; Dobrydnjov & Samarutel 1999, **Level II**; Slappendal et al 1999, **Level II**; Dobrydnjov et al 2003, **Level II**). The addition of intrathecal clonidine to bupivacaine and fentanyl for combined spinal-epidural analgesia during labour failed to increase duration of analgesia (Paech et al 2002, **Level II**). The combination of subarachnoid bupivacaine, fentanyl, morphine and clonidine significantly prolonged pain relief following caesarean section, but with increased sedation (Paech et al 2004, **Level II**).

Clonidine also prolongs the analgesic effect of epidural local anaesthetics (Eisenach et al 1996, **Level II**). The addition of clonidine to levobupivacaine has been shown to significantly reduce postoperative morphine requirements compared with either drug alone (Milligan et al 2000, **Level II**).

Plexus blocks

There is evidence of analgesic benefit with the addition of clonidine to local anaesthetics for brachial plexus blocks (Murphy et al 2000, **Level I**) but many of the studies have methodological limitations. Later reports show both lack of postoperative analgesic benefit from the addition of clonidine to bupivacaine for interscalene (Culebras et al 2001, **Level II**) and levobupivacaine for axillary brachial plexus block (Duma et al 2005, **Level II**), and prolongation of analgesia when clonidine is added to ropivacaine for axillary brachial plexus block (El Saied et al 2000, **Level II**).

5.3.2 Adrenaline (epinephrine)

Spinal

In thoracic epidural infusions used after surgery the addition of adrenaline (epinephrine) to fentanyl and ropivacaine or bupivacaine improved analgesia (Sakaguchi et al 2000, **Level II**; Niemi & Breivnik 2002, **Level II**; Niemi & Breivnik 2003, **Level II**). This was not demonstrated in lumbar epidural infusion (Forster et al 2003, **Level II**).

The addition of adrenaline (epinephrine) (0.2mg) to intrathecal bupivacaine prolongs motor block and some sensory block modalities (Moore et al 1998, **Level II**).

5.3.3 Other adjuvants

Midazolam

Midazolam, the preservative-free preparation, has been proposed as a potential spinal analgesic due to its action on $GABA_A$ receptors. It is not approved for this indication and efficacy and safety issues remain unclear.

Limited reports of intrathecal midazolam administration have appeared in the literature for many years, despite concerns regarding potential neurotoxicity (Yaksh & Allen 2004). Recent clinical series (Tucker 2004a and 2004b, **Level III-2**) and laboratory investigations (Johansen et al 2004) suggest a low risk of toxicity — neurotoxic damage was not seen in sheep and pigs given continuous intrathecal midazolam (Johansen et al 2004) and a 1-month questionnaire follow-up of patients who had received intrathecal midazolam failed to show any evidence of neurologic or urologic complications (Tucker et al 2004a, **Level III-2**).

The addition of subarachnoid midazolam for labour pain produced no effect on its own, but potentiated the analgesic effect of intrathecal fentanyl (Tucker et al 2004b, **Level II**). The addition of intrathecal midazolam to a mixture of bupivacaine and buprenorphine also prolonged the time to first analgesia (Shah et al 2003, **Level II**).

Midazolam added to bupivacaine for epidural infusion improved analgesia but increased sedation (Nishiyama et al 2002).

Neostigmine

Neostigmine acts as a spinal analgesic by potentiation of muscarinic cholinergic activity. In a literature review of animal and human studies there is no evidence of neurotoxicity with spinal neostigmine (Hodgson et al 1999).

The addition of intrathecal neostigmine to local anaesthetic reduces postoperative analgesic requirements (Liu et al 1999, **Level II**; Walker et al 2002, **Level I**; Almeida et al 2003, **Level II**; Yegin et al 2003, **Level II**) but increases the incidence of nausea and vomiting (Walker et al 2002, **Level I**; Almeida et al 2003, **Level II**) unless given in low doses.

Epidural neostigmine combined with an opioid reduces the dose of epidural opioid that is required for analgesia but there may not be any decrease in side effects compared with the opioid alone (Walker et al 2002, **Level I**).

Ketamine

Some commercially available preparations of ketamine contain an untested preservative (benzethonium chloride) and a low pH (pH 3.5 to 5.5), and so cannot be recommended for intrathecal use in humans (Hodgson et al 1999).

The addition of intrathecal ketamine to bupivacaine does not prolong postoperative analgesia or reduce analgesic requirements, but may lead to significantly more side effects of nausea and vomiting, sedation, dizziness, nystagmus and 'strange feelings' (Kathirvel et al 2000, **Level II**).

Combination of ketamine with opioid-based (+/- local anaesthetic) solutions for epidural analgesia improves pain relief (Subramaniam et al 2004, **Level I**) and may reduce overall opioid requirements (Walker et al 2002, **Level I**) without increasing the incidence of adverse effects (Walker et al 2002, **Level I**; Subramaniam et al 2004, **Level I**).

Key messages

1. Evidence that the addition of clonidine to an epidural or intrathecal opioid is more effective than clonidine or the opioid alone is weak and inconsistent (**Level I**).
2. Epidural ketamine (without preservative) added to opioid-based epidural analgesia regimens improves pain relief without reducing side effects (**Level I**).
3. Epidural neostigmine combined with an opioid reduces the dose of epidural opioid that is required for analgesia (**Level I**).
4. Intrathecal neostigmine prolongs the analgesic effect of intrathecal morphine and bupivacaine but increases the incidence of nausea and vomiting unless given in low doses (**Level I**).
5. Epidural and intrathecal clonidine prolong the effects of local anaesthetics (**Level II**).
6. Epidural adrenaline (epinephrine) in combination with a local anaesthetic improves the quality of postoperative thoracic epidural analgesia (**Level II**).

The following tick box ☑ represents conclusions based on clinical experience and expert opinion.

☑ There is conflicting evidence of analgesic efficacy for the addition of clonidine to brachial plexus blocks.

REFERENCES

Almeida RA, Lauretti GR, Mattos AL (2003) Antinociceptive effect of low-dose intrathecal neostigmine combined with intrathecal morphine following gynecologic surgery. *Anesthesiology* 98: 495–98.

Bardsley H, Gristwood R, Baker H et al (1998) A comparison of the cardiovascular effects of levobupivacaine and rac-bupivacaine following intravenous administration to healthy volunteers. *Br J Clin Pharmacol* 46: 245–49.

Bernards CM (2002) Understanding the physiology and pharmacology of epidural and intrathecal opioids. *Best Pract Res Clin Anaesthesiol* 16: 489–505.

Bernards CM (2004) Recent insights into the pharmacokinetics of spinal opioids and the relevance to opioid selection. *Curr Opin Anaesthesiol* 17: 441–47.

Bonnet F, Buisson VB, Francois Y et al (1990) Effects of oral and subarachnoid clonidine on spinal anesthesia with bupivacaine. *Reg Anesth* 15: 211–14.

Capogna G, Celleno D, Fusco P (1999) Relative potencies of bupivacaine and ropivacaine for analgesia in labour. *Br J Anaesthesia* 82: 371–73.

Casati A, Borghi B, Fanelli G et al (2002) A double-blinded, randomized comparison of either 0.5% levobupivacaine or 0.5% ropivacaine for sciatic nerve block. *Anesth Analg* 94: 987–90.

Casati A, Vinciguerra F, Scarioni M et al (2003a) Lidocaine versus ropivacaine for continuous interscalene brachial plexus block after open shoulder surgery. *Acta Anaesthesiol Scand* 47: 355–60.

Casati A, Santorsola R, Aldegheri G et al (2003b) Intraoperative epidural anesthesia and postoperative analgesia with levobupivacaine for major orthopedic surgery: a double-blind, randomized comparison of racemic bupivacaine and ropivacaine. *J Clin Anesth* 15: 126–31.

Casati A, Borghi B, Fanelli G et al (2003c) Interscalene brachial plexus anesthesia and analgesia for open shoulder surgery: a randomized, double-blinded comparison between levobupivacaine and ropivacaine. *Anesth Analg* 96: 253–59.

Chaplan SR, Duncan SR, Brodsky JB et al (1992) Morphine and hydromorphone epidural analgesia. *Anesthesiology* 77: 1090–94.

Chazalon P, Tourtier JP, Villevielle T et al (2003) Ropivacaine-induced cardiac arrest after peripheral nerve block: successful resuscitation. *Anesthesiology* 99: 1449–51.

Cheng CR, Su TH, Hung YC et al (2002) A comparative study of the safety and efficacy of 0.5% levobupivacaine and 0.5% bupivacaine for epidural anesthesia in subjects undergoing elective caesarean section. *Acta Anaesthesiol Sin* 40: 13–20.

Cole PJ, Craske DA, Wheatley RG (2000) Efficacy and respiratory effects of low-dose spinal morphine for postoperative analgesia following knee arthroplasty. *Br J Anaesth* 85: 233–37.

Cousins MJ & Mather LE (1984) Intrathecal and epidural administration of opioids. *Anesthesiology* 61: 276–310.

Covino BG & Wildsmith JA (1998) Clinical pharmacology of local anaesthetic agents. In: Cousins MJ & Bridenbough *Neural Blockade*. 3rd Edition Philadelphia: Lippincott-Raven.

Crews JC, Hord AH, Denson DD et al (1999) A comparison of the analgesic efficacy of 0.25% levobupivacaine combined with 0.005% morphine, 0.25% levobupivacaine alone, or 0.005% morphine alone for the management of postoperative pain in patients undergoing major abdominal surgery. *Anesth Analg* 89: 1504–09.

CHAPTER 5

Culebras X, Van Gessel E, Hoffmeyer P et al (2001) Clonidine combined with a long acting local anesthetic does not prolong postoperative analgesia after brachial plexus block but does induce hemodynamic changes. *Anesth Analg* 92: 199–204.

Dahl JB, Jeppsen IS, Jorgensen H et al (1999) Intraoperative and postoperative analgesic efficacy and adverse effects of intrathecal opioids in patients undergoing cesarean section with spinal anesthesia: a qualitative and quantitative systematic review of randomised controlled clinical trials. *Anesthesiology* 91: 1919–27.

De Leon-Casasola OA, Lema MJ (1996) Postoperative epidural opioid analgesia: what are the choices? *Anesth Analg* 83: 867–75.

Dobrydnjov I & Samarutel J (1999) Enhancement of intrathecal lidocaine by addition of local and systemic clonidine. *Acta Anaesthesiol Scand* 43: 556–62.

Dobrydnjov I, Axelsson K, Thorn SE et al (2003) Clonidine combined with small-dose bupivacaine during spinal anesthesia for inguinal herniorrhaphy: a randomized double-blinded study. *Anesth Analg* 96: 1496–503.

Duma A, Urbanek B, Sitzwol C et al (2005) Clonidine as an adjuvant to local anaesthetic axillary brachial plexus block: a randomized, controlled study *Br J Anaesth* 94: 112–16.

Eisenach JC, De Kock M, Klimscha W (1996) Alpha 2 adrenergic gonists for regional anesthesia: a clinical review of clonidine (1984–1995). *Anesthesiol* 85: 655–74.

El Saied AH, Steyn MP, Ansermino JM (2000) Clonidine prolongs the effect of ropivacaine for axillary brachial plexus blockade. *Can J Anaesth* 47: 962–67.

Emanuelsson BM, Zaric D, Nydahl PA et al (1995) Pharmacokinetics of ropivacaine and bupivacaine during 21 hours of continuous epidural infusion in healthy male volunteers. *Anesth Analg* 81: 1163–68.

Forster JG, Niemi TT, Aromaa U et al (2003) Epinephrine added to a lumbar epidural infusion of a small-dose ropivacaine-fentanyl mixture after arterial bypass surgery of the lower extremities. *Acta Anaesthesiol Scand* 47: 1106–13.

Ginoras Y, Riley ET, Angst MS (2003) The site of epidural fentanyl in humans: the difference between infusion and bolus administration. *Anesth Analg* 97: 1428–36.

Groban L & Dolinski S (2001) Differences in cardiac toxicity among ropivacaine, levobupivacaine, bupivacaine and lidocaine. *Tech Reg Anesth Pain Manage* 5: 48–55.

Groban L, Deal DD, Vernon JC et al (2001) Cardiac resuscitation after incremental overdosage with lidocaine, bupivacaine, levobupivacaine, and ropivacaine in anesthetized dogs. *Anesth Analg* 92: 37–43.

Gupta A, Bodin L, Holmstrom B et al (2001) A systematic review of the peripheral analgesic effects of intra-articular morphine. *Anesth Analg* 93: 761–70.

Gwirtz K, Young J, Byers R et al (1999) The safety and efficacy of intrathecal opioid analgesia for acute postoperative pain: Seven years experience with 5969 surgical patients at Indiana University Hospital. *Anesth Analg* 88: 599–604.

Halpern SH & Walsh V (2003) Epidural ropivacaine versus bupivacaine for labor: a meta-analysis. *Anesth Analg* 96: 1473–79.

Halpern SH, Breen TW, Campbell DC et al (2003) A multicenter, randomized, controlled trial comparing bupivacaine with ropivacaine for labor analgesia. *Anesthesiology* 98: 1431–35.

Hodgson PS, Neal JM, Pollock JE et al (1999) The neurotoxicity of drugs given intrathecally (spinal). *Anesth Analg* 88: 797–809.

Hubler M, Litz RJ, Sengebusch KH et al (2001) A comparison of five solutions of local anaesthetics and/or sufentanil for continuous, postoperative epidural analgesia after major urological surgery. *Eur J Anaesthesiol* 18: 450–57.

Huet O, Eyrolle LJ, Mazoit JX et al (2003) Cardiac arrest after injection of ropivacaine for posterior lumbar plexus blockade. *Anesthesiology* 99: 1451–53.

Jaffe RA & Rowe MA (1996) A comparison of the local anesthetic effects of meperidine, fentanyl and sufentanil on dorsal root axons. *Anesth Analg* 83: 776–81.

Johansen MJ, Gradert TL, Satterfield WC et al (2004) Safety of continuous intrathecal midazolam infusion in the sheep model. *Anesth Analg* 98: 1528–35.

Jorgensen H, Fomsgaard JS, Dirks J et al (2000) Effect of continuous epidural 0.2% ropivacaine vs 0.2% bupivacaine on postoperative pain, motor block and gastrointestinal function after abdominal hysterectomy. *Br J Anaesth* 84: 144–50.

Kalso E, Smith L, McQuay HJ et al (2002) No pain, no gain: clinical excellence and scientific rigour — lessons learned from IA morphine. *Pain* 98: 269–75.

Kathirvel S, Sadhasivam S, Saxena A et al (2000) Effects of intrathecal ketamine added to bupivacaine for spinal anaesthesia. *Anaesthesia* 55: 899–904.

Klein SM, Pierce T, Rubin Y et al (2003) Successful resuscitation after ropivacaine-induced ventricular fibrillation. *Anesth Analg* 97: 901–03.

Knudsen K, Beckman Suurkula M, Blomberg S et al (1997) Central nervous and cardiovascular effects of i.v. infusions of ropivacaine, bupivacaine and placebo in volunteers. *Br J Anaesth* 78: 507–14.

Koppert W, Likar R, Geisslinger G et al (1999) Peripheral antihyperalgesic effect of morphine to heat but not mechanical stimulation in healthy volunteers after ultraviolet-B irradiation. *Anesth Analg* 88: 117–22.

Lacassie HJ, Columb MO, Lacassie HP et al (2002) The relative motor blocking potencies of epidural bupivacaine and ropivacaine in labor. *Anesth Analg* 95: 204–08.

Lacassie HJ & Columb MO (2003) The relative motor blocking potencies of bupivacaine and levobupivacaine in labor. *Anesth Analg* 97: 1509–13.

Liu SS, Carpenter RL Mulroy MF et al (1994) Intravenous versus epidural administration of hydromorphone. Effects on analgesia and recovery after radical retropubic prostatectomy. *Anes Analg* 82: 682–88.

Liu SS, Hodgson PS, Moore JM et al (1999) Dose response effects of spinal neostigmine added to bupivacaine spinal anaesthesia in volunteers. *Anesthesiology* 90: 710–17.

Lyons G, Columb M, Wilson RC et al (1998) Epidural pain relief in labour: potencies of levobupivacaine and racemic bupivacaine. *Br J Anaesth* 81: 899–901.

Macias A, Monedero P, Adame M et al (2002) A randomized, double-blinded comparison of thoracic epidural ropivacaine, ropivacaine/fentanyl, or bupivacaine/fentanyl for postthoracotomy analgesia. *Anesth Analg* 95: 1344–50.

Markham A & Faulds D (1996) Ropivacaine. A review of its pharmacology and therapeutic use in regional anaesthesia. *Drugs* 52: 429–49.

Mather LE & Chang DH (2001) Cardiotoxicity with modern local anaesthetics: is there a safer choice? *Drugs* 61: 333–42.

McGlade DP, Kalpokas MV, Mooney PH et al (1998) A comparison of 0.5% ropivacaine and 0.5% bupivacaine for axillary brachial plexus anaesthesia. *Anaesth Int Care* 26: 515–20.

McLeod GA & Burke D (2001) Levobupivacaine. *Anaesthesia* 56: 331–41.

McLeod GA, Munishankar B, Columb MO (2005) Is the clinical efficacy of epidural morphine concentration-dependent when used as analgesia for labour? *Br J Anaesth* 94: 229–33.

Merson N (2001) A comparison of motor block between ropivacaine and bupivacaine for continuous labor epidural analgesia. *AANA J* 69: 54–58.

Milligan KR, Convery PN, Weir P et al (2000) The efficacy and safety of epidural infusions of levobupivacaine with and without clonidine for postoperative pain relief in patients undergoing total hip replacement. *Anesth Analg* 91: 393–97.

Miyoshi RH & Lackband SG (2001) Systemic opioid analgesics. In: Loeser J (Ed) *Bonica's Management of Pain.* 3rd edition. Lippincott Williams & Wilkins.

Mogensen T (1995) Tachyphylaxis to epidural local anaesthetics. *Dan Med Bull* 42: 141–46.

Moore JM, Liu SS, Pollock JE et al (1998) The effect of epinephrine on small-dose hyperbaric bupivacaine spinal anesthesia: clinical implications for ambulatory surgery. *Anesth Analg* 86: 973–77.

Muldoon T, Milligan K, Quinn P et al (1998) Comparison between extradural infusion of ropivacaine or bupivacaine for the prevention of postoperative pain after total knee arthroplasty. *Br J Anaesth* 80: 680–81.

Murphy DB, McCartney CJ, Chan VW (2000) Novel analgesic adjuncts for brachial plexus block: a systematic review. *Anesth Analg* 90:1122–28.

Ngan Kee WD (1998) Epidural pethidine: pharmacology and clinical experience. *Anaesth Intensive Care* 26: 247–55.

Niemi G & Breivik H (2002) Epinephrine markedly improves thoracic epidural analgesia produced by a small-dose infusion of ropivacaine, fentanyl, and epinephrine after major thoracic or abdominal surgery: a randomized, double-blinded crossover study with and without epinephrine. *Anesth Analg* 94: 1598–605.

Niemi G & Breivik H (2003) The minimally effective concentration of adrenaline in a low-concentration thoracic epidural analgesic infusion of bupivacaine, fentanyl and adrenaline after major surgery. A randomized, double-blind, dose-finding study. *Acta Anaesthesiol Scand* 47: 439–50.

Nishiyama T, Matsukawa T, Hanaoka K (2002) Effects of adding midazolam on the postoperative epidural analgesia with two different doses of bupivacaine. *J Clin Anesth* 14: 92–97.

Ohmura S, Kawada M, Ohta T et al (2001) Systemic toxicity and resuscitation in bupivacaine-, levobupivacaine-, or ropivacaine-infused rats. *Anesth Analg* 93: 743–48.

Paech MJ, Moore JS, Evans SF (1994 Meperidine for patient-controlled analgesia after cesarean section. Intravenous versus epidural administration. *Anesthesiology* 80: 1268–76.

Paech MJ, Pavy TJ, Orlikowski CE et al (2000) Postoperative intraspinal opioid analgesia after caesarean section; a randomised comparison of subarachnoid morphine and epidural pethidine. *Int J Obstet Anesth* 9: 238–45.

Paech MJ, Banks SL, Gurrin LC et al (2002) A randomized, double-blinded trial of subarachnoid bupivacaine and fentanyl, with or without clonidine, for combined spinal/epidural analgesia during labor. *Anesth Analg* 95: 1396–401.

Paech MJ,Pavy TJG, Orlikowski CEP et al (2004) Postcesarean analgesia with spinal morphine, clonidine, or their combination. *Anesth Analg* 98: 1460–66.

Pert CB, Kuhar MJ, Snyder SH. et al (1976) Opioid receptor: autoradiographic localization in rat brain. *Proc Natl Acad Sci* 73: 3729–33.

Pham-Dang C, Beaumont S, Floch H et al (2000) Acute toxic accident following lumbar plexus block with bupivacaine. *Ann Fr Anesth Reanim* 19: 356–59.

Picard PR, Tramèr MR, McQuay HJ et al (1997) Analgesic efficacy of peripheral opioids (all except intra-articular): a qualitative systematic review of randomised controlled trials. *Pain* 72: 309–18.

Polley LS, Columb MO, Naughton NN et al (1999) Relative analgesic potencies of ropivacaine and bupivacaine for epidural analgesia in labor: implications for therapeutic indexes. *Anesthesiology* 90: 944–50.

Polley LS, Columb MO, Naughton NN et al (2003) Relative analgesic potencies of levobupivacaine and ropivacaine for epidural analgesia in labor. *Anesthesiology* 99: 1354–58.

Racle JP, Benkhadra A, Poy JY et al (1987) Prolongation of isobaric bupivacaine spinal anesthesia with epinephrine and clonidine for hip surgery in the elderly. *Anesth Analg* 66: 442–46.

Reuben SS, Vieria P, Faruqi S et al (2001) Local administration of morphine for analgesia after iliac bone graft harvest. *Anesthesiology* 95: 390–94.

Sakaguchi Y, Sakura S, Shinzawa M et al (2000) Does adrenaline improve bupivacaine and fentanyl analgesia after abdominal surgery. *Anesth Int Care* 28: 522–26.

Schafer M (1999) Peripheral opioid analgesia: from experimental to clinical studies. *Curr Opin Anaesthesiol* 12: 603–07.

Schug SS, Scott DA, Payne J et al (1996) Postoperative analgesia by continuous extradural infusion of ropivacaine after upper abdominal surgery. *Br J Anaesth* 76: 487–91.

Schug SA (2001) Correction factor for comparisons between levobupivacaine and racemic bupivacaine. *Reg Anesth Pain Med* 26: 91.

Scott DA, Chamley DM, Mooney PH et al (1995) Epidural ropivacaine infusion for postoperative analgesia after major lower abdominal surgery--a dose finding study. *Anesth Analg* 81: 982–86.

Scott DA, Emanuelsson BM, Mooney PH et al (1997) Pharmacokinetics and efficacy of long-term epidural ropivacaine infusion for postoperative analgesia. *Anesth Analg* 85: 1322–30.

Scott DA, Blake D, Buckland M et al (1999) A comparison of epidural ropivacaine infusion alone and in combination with 1, 2, and 4 microg/mL fentanyl for seventy-two hours of postoperative analgesia after major abdominal surgery. *Anesth Analg* 88: 857–64.

Scott DB, Lee A, Fagan D et al (1989) Acute toxicity of ropivacaine compared with that of bupivacaine. *Anesth Analg* 69: 563–69.

Senard M, Joris JL, Ledoux D et al (2002) A comparison of 0.1% and 0.2% ropivacaine and bupivacaine combined with morphine for postoperative patient-controlled epidural analgesia after major abdominal surgery. *Anesth Analg* 95: 444–49.

Shah FR, Halbe AR, Panchal ID et al (2003) Improvement in postoperative pain relief by the addition of midazolam to an intrathecal injection of buprenorphine and bupivacaine. *Eur J Anaesthesiol* 20: 904–10.

Slappendel R, Weber E, Dirksen R et al (1999) Optimization of the dose of intrathecal morphine in total hip surgery: a dose finding study. *Anesth Analg* 88: 822–26.

Soltesz EG, van Pelt F, Byrne JG (2003) Emergent cardiopulmonary bypass for bupivacaine cardiotoxicity. *J Cardiothorac Vasc Anesth* 17: 357–58.

Stein C, Hassan AH, Przewlocki R et al (1990) Opioids from immunocytes interact with receptors on sensory nerves to inhibit nociception in inflammation. *Proc Natl Acad Sci* 87: 5935–39.

Stein C (1995) Mechanisms of disease: The control of pain in peripheral tissue by opioids. *New Engl J Med* 332: 1685–90.

Stewart J, Kellett N, Castro D et al (2003) The central nervous system and cardiovascular effects of levobupivacaine and ropivacaine in healthy volunteers. *Anesth Analg* 97: 412–16.

Subramaniam K, Subramaniam B, Steinbrook RA (2004) Ketamine as adjuvant analgesic to opioids: a quantitative and qualitative systematic review. *Anesth Analg* 99: 482–95.

Tan CNH, Guha A, Scawn NDA et al (2004) Optimal concentration of epidural fentanyl in bupivacaine 0.1% after thoracotomy. *Br J Anaesth* 92: 670–74.

Tucker AP, Lai C, Nadeson R et al (2004a) Intrathecal midazolam i: a cohort study investigating safety. *Anesth Analg* 98: 1512–20.

Tucker AP, Mezzatesta J, Nadeson R et al (2004b) Intrathecal midazolam ii: combination with intrathecal fentanyl for labor pain. *Anesth Analg* 98:1521–27.

Walker SM, Goudas LC, Cousins MJ et al (2002) Combination spinal analgesic chemotherapy: a systematic review *Anesth Analg* 95: 674–715.

Wang JK, Nauss LA, Thomas JE (1979) Pain relief by intrathecally applied morphine in man. *Anesthesiology*: 149–51.

Wheatley RG, Schug SA, Watson D. et al (2001) Safety and efficacy of postoperative epidural analgesia. *Br J Anaesth* 87: 47–61.

Yaksh TL & Rudy TA (1976) Analgesia mediated by a direct spinal action of narcotics. *Science* 192: 1357–58.

Yaksh TL (1981) Spinal opiateopioid analgesia: characteristics and principles of action. *Pain* 11: 293–346.

Yaksh TL & Allen JW (2004) preclinical insights into the implementation of intrathecal midazolam: a cautionary tale. *Anesth Analg* 98: 1509–11.

Yegin A, Yilmaz M, Karsli B et al (2003) Analgesic effects of intrathecal neostigmine in perianal surgery. *Eur J Anaesthesiol* 20: 404–08.

Zaric D, Nydahl PA, Adel SO et al (1996) The effect of continuous epidural infusion of ropivacaine (0.1%, 0.2% and 0.3%) on nerve conduction velocity and postural control in volunteers. *Acta Anaesthesiol Scand* 40: 342–49.

6. ROUTES OF SYSTEMIC DRUG ADMINISTRATION

Opioid and non-opioid analgesic drugs can be administered systemically by a number of different routes. The choice of route may be determined by various factors, including the aetiology, severity, location and type of pain, the patient's overall condition and the characteristics of the chosen administration technique. Additional factors to consider with any route of administration are ease of use, accessibility, speed of analgesic onset, reliability of effect, duration of action, patient acceptability and cost.

The principles of individualisation of dose and dosing intervals apply to the administration of all analgesic agents, particularly opioids, by any route. A lack of flexibility in dose schedules has often meant that intermittent and 'prn' (as needed) methods of pain relief have been ineffective when the routes of administration discussed below have been used (Bandolier 2003). Frequent assessment of the patient's pain and their response to treatment (including the occurrence of any side effects) rather than strict adherence to a given dosing regimen is required if adequate analgesia is to be obtained.

6.1 Oral route

Oral administration of analgesic agents is simple, non-invasive, has good efficacy in most settings and high patient acceptability. Other than in the treatment of severe acute pain and providing there are no contraindications to its use, it is the route of choice for the administration of most analgesic drugs.

Limitations to the oral route include vomiting or delayed gastric emptying, when absorption is likely to be impaired. If multiple doses of an oral analgesic drug are given before return of normal gastric motility, accumulated doses may enter the small intestine at the same time once emptying resumes ('dumping effect'). This would result in an unexpectedly large systemic uptake of the drug and an increased risk of adverse effects.

Rates of absorption will vary according to the formulation of the oral analgesic agent (eg tablet, suspension, controlled-release preparation). Bioavailability will also vary between drugs because of the effects of first-pass hepatic metabolism following uptake into the portal circulation. Titration of pain relief with oral analgesic drugs is slower compared with some of the other routes of administration discussed below.

Direct comparisons between oral opioid and non-opioid analgesics, or between oral and other routes of administration, are limited. Indirect comparisons, where the individual drugs have been compared with a placebo, have been used to generate a 'league table' of analgesic efficacy (see Table 6.1). This table is based on randomised, double-blind, single-dose studies in patients with *moderate to severe pain* and shows the number of patients that need to be given the active drug (number-needed-to-treat or NNT) to achieve at least 50% pain relief in one patient compared with a placebo over a 4–6 hour treatment period (Moore et al 2003).

The validity of this approach as a true method of comparison of drugs may be questioned as there is no standardisation of the acute pain model or patient and only single doses of the analgesic agents are used. However, it may be reasonable to extrapolate estimates of analgesic efficacy from one pain model to another (Barden et al 2004a, **Level I**).

Table 6.1 The Oxford league table of analgesic efficacy (commonly used analgesic doses)

Analgesic	Number of patients in comparison	At least 50% pain relief (%)	NNT	Lower confidence interval	Higher confidence interval
Valdecoxib 40	473	73	1.6	1.4	1.8
Valdecoxib 20	204	68	1.7	1.4	2.0
Diclofenac 100	411	67	1.9	1.6	2.2
Paracetamol 1000 + Codeine 60	197	57	2.2	1.7	2.9
Parecoxib 40 (intravenous)	349	63	2.2	1.8	2.7
Diclofenac 50	738	63	2.3	2.0	2.7
Naproxen 440	257	50	2.3	2.0	2.9
Ibuprofen 600	203	79	2.4	2.0	4.2
Ibuprofen 400	4,703	56	2.4	2.3	2.6
Naproxen 550	500	50	2.6	2.2	3.2
Ketorolac 10	790	50	2.6	2.3	3.1
Ibuprofen 200	1,414	45	2.7	2.5	3.1
Piroxicam 20	280	63	2.7	2.1	3.8
Diclofenac 25	204	54	2.8	2.1	4.3
Pethidine 100 (intramuscular)	364	54	2.9	2.3	3.9
Morphine 10 (intramuscular)	946	50	2.9	2.6	3.6
Parecoxib 20 (intravenous)	346	50	3.0	2.3	4.1
Naproxen 220/250	183	58	3.1	2.2	5.2
Ketorolac 30 (intramuscular)	359	53	3.4	2.5	4.9
Paracetamol 500	561	61	3.5	2.2	13.3
Paracetamol 1000	2,759	46	3.8	3.4	4.4
Paracetamol 600/650 + Codeine 60	1,123	42	4.2	3.4	5.3

Analgesic	Number of patients in comparison	At least 50% pain relief (%)	NNT	Lower confidence interval	Higher confidence interval
Paracetamol 650 + Dextropropoxyphene (65mg hydrochloride or 100mg napsylate)	963	38	4.4	3.5	5.6
Aspirin 600/650	5,061	38	4.4	4.0	4.9
Paracetamol 600/650	1,886	38	4.6	3.9	5.5
Tramadol 100	882	30	4.8	3.8	6.1
Tramadol 75	563	32	5.3	3.9	8.2
Aspirin 650 + Codeine 60	598	25	5.3	4.1	7.4
Paracetamol 300 + Codeine 30	379	26	5.7	4.0	9.8
Tramadol 50	770	19	8.3	6.0	13.0
Codeine 60	1,305	15	16.7	11.0	48.0

Source: Bandolier (www.jr2.ox.ac.uk/bandolier/). Reproduced with permission.

6.1.1 Opioids and tramadol

Oral opioids can be as effective in the treatment of acute pain as opioids given by other more invasive routes if equianalgesic doses are administered. Both immediate-release (IR) and controlled-release (CR) formulations have been used.

Effectiveness of individual oral opioids and tramadol

- *Codeine* in a single dose of 60mg is not an effective analgesic agent (Moore & McQuay 1997, **Level I**); it is effective when combined with 600/650mg paracetamol (Barden et al 2004b, **Level I**; Moore et al 1998b, **Level I**).
- *Dextropropoxyphene* 65mg is not an effective analgesic agent; it is effective when combined with 650mg paracetamol (Collins et al 1999a, **Level I**).
- *Dihydrocodeine* in a single dose of 30mg is no more effective than placebo; 60mg is less effective than non-steroidal anti-inflammatory drugs (Edwards et al 2000a, **Level I**).
- *Oxycodone* (IR), in a single dose of 5mg shows no benefit over placebo for the treatment of moderate to severe acute pain; doses of 15mg, 10mg plus paracetamol and 5mg plus paracetamol are effective (Edwards et al 2000b, **Level I**).
- *Tramadol* is an effective analgesic agent (Moore & McQuay 1997, **Level I**). The combination of tramadol 75mg or 112.5mg with paracetamol (acetaminophen) 560mg or 975mg is more effective than either of its two components administered alone (McQuay & Edwards 2003, **Level I**).
- *Morphine (IR, oral)* is effective in the treatment of acute pain. Following pre-loading with intravenous (IV) morphine, morphine liquid 20mg (initial dose 20mg; subsequent doses increased by 5mg if breakthrough doses needed) every 4 hours with additional 10mg doses as needed has been shown to provide better pain relief after

CHAPTER 6

hip surgery than intramuscular (IM) morphine 5–10mg prn (McCormack et al 1993, **Level II**).

The NNTs of each of these drugs is listed in Table 6.1.

IR oral opioids such as oxycodone, morphine and tramadol have also been used as 'step down' analgesia after patient-controlled analgesia (PCA), with doses based on prior PCA requirements (Macintyre & Ready 2001) and after epidural analgesia (Lim & Schug 2001, **Level II**).

Controlled-release formulations

CR formulations, also referred to as slow-release (SR) or prolonged-release, may take 3–4 hours or more to reach peak effect. In contrast and in most cases, the analgesic effect of the IR opioid preparations will be seen within about 45–60 minutes. This means that rapid titration to effect is easier and safer with IR formulations.

CR oral oxycodone comprises an IR component as well as the delayed-release compound and therefore has a more rapid onset of action than other CR agents. CR oxycodone may be effective in the immediate management of acute pain (Sunshine et al 1996, **Level II**; Reuben et al 2002, **Level II**; Kampe et al 2004, **Level II**) and may be more effective than either fixed-dose or 'prn' IR oxycodone regimens (Reuben et al 1999, **Level II**).

CR opioid preparations should only be used at set time intervals and IR opioids should be used for acute and breakthrough pain, and for titration of CR opioids. The use of CR opioid preparations as the sole agents for the early management of acute pain is discouraged because of difficulties in short-term dose adjustments needed for titration.

CR oral oxycodone was found to be effective as 'step down' analgesia after 12–24 hours of PCA morphine (Ginsberg et al 2003, **Level IV**).

6.1.2 Non-steroidal anti-inflammatory drugs and COX-2 selective inhibitors

A number of non-steroidal anti-inflammatory drugs (NSAIDs) and COX-2 selective inhibitors have been shown to be effective as sole therapy in a variety of acute pain settings — see Table 6.1. Those for which there is **Level I** evidence of efficacy include: aspirin 600–1200mg (Edwards et al 1999, **Level I**), ibuprofen 200–600mg and diclofenac 50–100mg (Barden et al 2004c, **Level I**; Collins et al 1999b, **Level I**), piroxicam 20–40mg (Edwards et al 2000c, **Level I**), celecoxib 200–400mg (Barden et al 2003a, **Level I**), valdecoxib 20–40mg (Barden et al 2003b, **Level I**), naproxen (Mason et al 2003, **Level I**) and ketorolac (Smith et al 2000, **Level I**).

The NNTs of each of these drugs is listed in Table 6.1.

There is no good evidence that NSAIDs given parenterally or rectally are more effective, or result in fewer side effects, than the same drug given orally for the treatment of postoperative pain (Tramèr et al 1998, **Level I**). Only in the treatment of renal colic do IV NSAIDs result in more rapid analgesia (Tramèr et al 1998, **Level I**).

6.1.3 Paracetamol

Paracetamol is an effective analgesic for acute pain (Barden et al 2004b, **Level I**; Moore et al 1998b, **Level I**).

In the same doses, orally administered paracetamol is less effective and of slower onset than paracetamol given by IV injection (Jarde & Boccard 1997, **Level II**), but more effective and of faster onset than paracetamol administered by the rectal route (see below) (Anderson et al 1996, **Level II**).

6.2 Intravenous route

Analgesic drugs given by the IV route have a more rapid onset of action compared with most other routes of administration.

6.2.1 Opioids and tramadol

Intermittent IV bolus doses

Titration of opioids for severe acute pain is best achieved using intermittent IV bolus doses as it allows more rapid titration of effect and avoids the uncertainty of drug absorption by other routes. The optimal doses and dose intervals for this technique have not yet been established.

In a postoperative care unit, 2mg or 3mg bolus doses of morphine given at 5-minute dose intervals as needed and with no limitation on the number of bolus doses administered, was more effective and resulted in no greater incidence of side effects than the same doses given at 10-minute intervals or when a maximum of 5 doses only was allowed (Aubrun et al 2001, **Level III-3**).

Titration of IV bolus doses of an opioid is frequently accomplished using a treatment algorithm to guide management, which includes age-based bolus doses of opioid given at 3 or 5-minute intervals as needed (Macintyre & Ready 2001).

Large IV bolus doses of tramadol can result in a high incidence of emetic symptoms. This effect can be reduced by slowing delivery of the drug or, in the surgical setting, by giving it before the patient emerges from general anaesthesia (Pang et al 2000, **Level II**).

Continuous infusions

A continuous infusion of opioids results in constant blood levels after approximately 4 half-lives of the opioid used. The aim of an infusion is to avoid the problems associated with the peaks and troughs of intermittent administration techniques. However, the variation in patient response, the changing intensity of acute pain with time and the delay between any alteration of the infusion rate and its subsequent effect, may result in inadequate treatment of incident pain or delayed onset of side effects, such as respiratory depression.

Compared with PCA, continuous IV opioid infusions in a general ward setting resulted in a 5-fold increase in the incidence of respiratory depression (Schug & Torrie 1993, **Level IV**).

6.2.2 Non-steroidal anti-inflammatory drugs and COX-2 selective inhibitors

There are only a limited number of NSAIDs or COX-2 selective inhibitors available for IV injection at present and fewer still where Level I evidence for individual efficacy is available. In single doses as the sole analgesic agent, the COX-2 selective drug parecoxib IV 20–40mg has been shown to be effective (Barden et al 2003b, **Level I**).

IV NSAIDs or COX-2 selective inhibitors are more expensive than oral or rectal NSAIDs although their efficacy and likelihood of side effects is similar (Tramèr et al 1998, **Level I**). Efficacy and times to onset of analgesia are similar with IV and IM parecoxib (Daniels et al 2001, **Level II**).

For renal colic, the onset of action of NSAIDs is faster when given intravenously compared with IM, oral or rectal administration (Tramèr et al 1998, **Level I**).

6.2.3 Paracetamol

IV paracetamol provides effective analgesia after a variety of surgical procedures (Rømsing et al 2002, **Level I**). It is more effective and of faster onset than the same dose given orally (Jarde & Boccard 1997, **Level II**) but, as with IV NSAIDs, is more expensive.

Due to the good bioavailability and tolerability of oral paracetamol, the use of the IV form should be limited to clinical circumstances where use of the enteral route is not appropriate.

CHAPTER 6

6.3 Intramuscular and subcutaneous routes

IM and subcutaneous (SC) injections of analgesic agents (usually opioids) are still commonly employed for the treatment of moderate or severe pain. Absorption may be impaired in conditions of poor perfusion (eg in hypovolaemia, shock, hypothermia or immobility), leading to inadequate early analgesia and late absorption of the drug depot when perfusion is restored.

6.3.1 Opioids and tramadol

IM injection of opioids has been the traditional mainstay of postoperative pain management, despite the fact that surveys have repeatedly shown that pain relief with prn IM opioids is frequently inadequate. Although IM opioids are often perceived to be safer than opioids given by other parenteral routes, the incidence of respiratory depression reported in a recent review ranged from 0.8 (0.2.–2.5)% to 37.0 (22.6–45.9)% using respiratory rate and oxygen saturation, respectively, as indicators (for comparisons with PCA and epidural analgesia see Chapter 7; for comments on respiratory rate as an unreliable indicator of respiratory depression see Section 4.1.3) (Cashman & Dolin 2004, **Level IV**).

Single doses of IM morphine 10mg (McQuay et al 1999, **Level I**) and IM pethidine 100mg (Smith et al 2000, **Level I**) have been shown to be effective in the initial treatment of moderate to severe postoperative pain.

The use of an algorithm allowing administration of IM morphine or pethidine (meperidine) hourly prn and requiring frequent assessments of pain and sedation, led to significant improvements in pain relief compared with longer dose interval prn regimens (Gould et al 1992, **Level III-3**).

The quality of pain relief is less with intermittent IM regimens compared with IV PCA (Walder et al 2001, **Level I**).

The placement of SC plastic cannulae or 'butterfly' needles allows the use of intermittent injections without repeated skin punctures. In elderly adults, the rate of absorption of morphine and the variability in the rate of absorption after a single dose of SC morphine were similar to those reported after IM injection (Semple et al 1997, **Level IV**).

In children, there was no difference in rate of onset, analgesic effect and side effects when SC injections of morphine were compared with IM morphine injections, and there was a significantly higher patient preference for the SC route (Cooper 1996, **Level II**; Lamacraft et al 1997, **Level IV**).

Treatment algorithms for intermittent SC morphine and hydromorphone using age-based dosing with 2-hourly prn dose intervals are available (Macintyre & Ready 2001).

Continuous infusions of opioids via the SC route are as effective as continuous IV infusions (Semple et al 1996, **Level II**).

6.3.2 Non-steroidal anti-inflammatory drugs and COX-2 selective inhibitors

There are only a limited number of NSAIDs or COX-2 selective inhibitors available for IM injection at present and fewer still where Level I evidence for individual efficacy is available. Ketorolac and parecoxib IM are effective analgesic agents (Smith et al 2000, **Level I**; Barden et al 2003b, **Level I**).

6.4 Rectal route

Rectal administration of drugs is useful when other routes are unavailable. It results in uptake into the submucosal venous plexus of the rectum which drains into the inferior, middle and superior rectal veins. Drug absorbed from the lower half of the rectum will pass into the inferior and middle rectal veins and then the inferior vena cava, bypassing the portal system. Any portion of the drug absorbed into the superior rectal vein enters the portal system, subjecting it to hepatic first-pass metabolism.

Potential problems with the rectal route of drug administration relate to the variability of absorption, possible rectal irritation and cultural factors. Some suppositories should not be divided as the drug may not be evenly distributed in the preparation. Contraindications to the use of this route include pre-existing rectal lesions, recent colorectal surgery and immune suppression. Whether the drug is administered to a patient who is awake or under anaesthesia, it is important to obtain prior consent from the patient or guardian.

6.4.1 Opioids

In most instances similar doses of rectal and oral opioids are administered, although there may be differences in bioavailability and the time to peak analgesic effect for the reasons outlined above.

6.4.2 Non-steroidal anti-inflammatory drugs

Rectal administration of NSAIDs provides effective analgesia after a variety of surgical procedures (Rømsing et al 2002, **Level I**). Local effects such as rectal irritation and diarrhoea have been reported following use of the rectal route, but other commonly reported adverse effects such as nausea, vomiting, dizziness and indigestion are independent of the route of administration (Tramèr et al 1998, **Level I**). In a study comparing oral and rectal indomethacin (indometacin) given over a period of 2 weeks, the degree of gastric erosion at endoscopy was the same (Hansen et al 1984, **Level II**). Consequently, there appears to be no advantage in using NSAID suppositories if the oral route is available (Tramèr et al 1998, **Level I**).

6.4.3 Paracetamol

Paracetamol is effective when given by the rectal route (Rømsing et al 2002, **Level I**) although absorption is very variable (Anderson et al 1995, **Level IV**). It is less effective and of slower onset than the same dose administered by the oral route (Anderson et al 1996, **Level II**; Anderson et al 1999, **Level IV**). When available, the oral route is therefore preferable.

6.5 TRANSDERMAL ROUTE

6.5.1 Opioids

The stratum corneum of the epidermis forms a major barrier to the entry of drugs. However, drugs such fentanyl (Jeal & Benfield 1997; Grond et al 2000) and buprenorphine (Sittl et al 2003) are available as transdermal preparations.

Transdermal fentanyl is commonly used in the management of cancer and chronic pain. Due to the formation of a significant intradermal 'reservoir', onset and offset times of this preparation are slow and this makes short-term titration impossible. The time to peak blood concentration is generally between 17 and 48 hours after patch application and the terminal half-life following removal of the patch is 13 to 25 hours (Jeal & Benfield 1997). There is also marked interpatient variation in the maximum blood concentrations reached (Jeal & Benfield 1997; Grond et al 2000).

These factors, in addition to the wide variability of clinical effect (Peng & Sandler 1999) and the high incidence of respiratory depression that can occur in the postoperative setting (Sandler et al 1994, **Level II**; Bulow et al 1995, **Level II**; Grond et al 2000), make transdermal fentanyl preparations unsuitable for acute pain management. Transdermal fentanyl is currently specifically contraindicated for the management of acute or postoperative pain (MIMS 2004).

Iontophoretic transdermal delivery systems for opioids have been investigated (Ashburn et al 1995) but are not in use in clinical practice.

6.5.2 Non-steroidal anti-inflammatory drugs

Topically applied NSAIDs, including ibuprofen, ketoprofen and piroxicam, have been shown to be effective in the treatment of pain caused by soft tissue injuries compared with placebo. Topical indomethacin (indometacin) does not have proven efficacy (Moore at al 1998a, **Level I**).

6.6 TRANSMUCOSAL ROUTES

Drugs administered by transmucosal routes (intranasal, sublingual, buccal, and pulmonary) are rapidly absorbed directly into the systemic circulation, thus bypassing hepatic first-pass metabolism. The drugs most commonly administered by transmucosal routes in acute pain management are the more lipid-soluble opioids.

6.6.1 Intranasal route

A variety of different drugs can be administered by the intranasal (IN) route, including analgesic drugs. The human nasal mucosa contains drug-metabolising enzymes but the extent and clinical significance of human nasal first-pass metabolism is unknown (Dale et al 2002). It is suggested that the volume of a dose of any drug given intranasally should not exceed 150 microlitres in order to avoid run-off into the pharynx (Dale et al 2002).

Opioids

Single-dose pharmacokinetic data in healthy volunteers for a number of opioids administered by the IN route have been summarised by Dale at al (2002). The mean bioavailabilities and times to peak blood concentrations were fentanyl 71% and 5 minutes; sufentanil 78% and 10 minutes; alfentanil 65% and 9 minutes; butorphanol 71% and 49 minutes; oxycodone 46% and 25 minutes; and buprenorphine 48% and 30 minutes. Hydromorphone, when given to volunteers in doses of 1mg or 2mg IN and compared with 2mg IV, had median times to peak blood concentration after the 1mg and 2mg IN doses of 20 minutes and 25 minutes respectively and an overall bioavailability of only 55% (Coda et al 2003).

Clinical data also exist for the effectiveness of several opioids administered via the IN route, including fentanyl (Striebel et al 1996, **Level II**; Toussaint et al 2000, **Level II**; Manjushree et al 2002, **Level II**; Paech et al 2003 **Level II**), butorphanol (Abboud et al 1991, **Level II**), and pethidine (Striebel at al 1993, **Level II**; Striebel at al 1995, **Level II**). Fentanyl has similar analgesic efficacy when given by the IN or IV routes (Striebel et al 1992, **Level II**; Striebel et al 1996, **Level II**; Toussaint et al 2000, **Level II**; Manjushree et al 2002, **Level II**; Paech et al 2003, **Level II**) as does butorphanol (Abboud et al 1991, **Level II**). Intranasal pethidine is more effective than SC injections of pethidine (Striebel et al 1995, **Level II**).

Patient-controlled intranasal analgesia (PCINA) using diamorphine (bolus doses of 0.5mg) was less effective than PCA IV morphine (1mg bolus doses) after joint replacement surgery (Ward et al 2002, **Level II**) but provided better pain relief in doses of

CHAPTER 6

0.1mg/kg compared with 0.2mg/kg IM morphine in children with fractures (Kendall et al 2001, **Level II**).

Adverse effects can be related to the drug itself or to the route of administration. Systemic effects appear to be no higher for IN administration than for other routes with equivalent efficacy; nasal irritation, congestion and bad taste have been reported with the short-term use of butorphanol and pethidine (Dale et al 2002, **Level IV**).

Technical problems with pumps have been reported in up to 10% of cases and dispensing issues for techniques such as PCINA, which could allow ready and unauthorised access to the drugs, have not been addressed (Dale et al 2002).

At the present time, there are insufficient data to support the routine use of IN analgesia for acute pain.

6.6.2 Sublingual and buccal routes

When analgesic drugs are administered by the sublingual (SL) or buccal routes, their efficacy will in part depend on the proportion of drug swallowed.

Opioids

SL buprenorphine, given as a tablet, has an overall bioavailability of 30–35% and a long duration of action (mean half-life 35 hours) (MIMS 2004). SL buprenorphine 0.4mg was found to be as effective as10mg morphine IM (Cuschieri et al 1984, **Level II**) and 75mg pethidine IM after abdominal surgery (Moa & Zetterstrom 1990, **Level II**).

Oral transmucosal fentanyl citrate (OTFC) incorporates fentanyl into a flavoured solid lozenge on a stick and is available in a range of doses from 200 to 1600 micrograms. Overall, the bioavailability of OTFC is about 52% compared with IV fentanyl, with peak blood levels achieved in 22 ± 2.5 minutes (Streisand et al 1991, **Level IV**). The median time to onset of analgesia is about 4 minutes (Lichtor et al 1999, **Level II**).

Only a few studies have investigated the postoperative use of OTFC. It was found to be an effective analgesic after orthopaedic (Ashburn et al 1993, **Level II**) and abdominal surgery (Lichtor et al 1999, **Level II**) and during burns wound care (Sharar et al 1998, **Level II**; Sharar et al 2002, **Level II**).

As a result of the limited data and many alternatives available, the place of OTFC in acute pain settings is not yet established. Because of the risk of achieving high peak plasma levels with unsupervised administration, it is currently specifically contra-indicated for the management of acute pain in opioid naïve patients (MIMS 2004).

6.6.3 Pulmonary

Opioids are rapidly absorbed after nebulised inhalation, reflecting the high blood flow, surface area, and permeability of the lungs.

Clinical data exist for the effectiveness of several opioids administered via the pulmonary route including morphine (Masood & Thomas 1996, **Level II**; Ward et al 1997, **Level II**; Dershwitz et al 2000, **Level IV**; Thipphawong et al 2003, **Level II**) and fentanyl (Worsley et al 1990, **Level II**; Higgins et al 1991, **Level II**).

Peak plasma concentrations following administration of morphine via a standard nebuliser occur within 10 minutes but bioavailability is low with a mean of only 5% (Masood & Thomas 1996, **Level II**). Bioavailability may be improved (up to 59–100%) with peak plasma concentrations occurring at 2 minutes using newer pulmonary drug delivery systems (Ward et al 1997, **Level II**; Dershwitz et al 2000, **Level IV**).

Similarly, using newer pulmonary drug delivery systems, bioavailability of inhaled fentanyl may approach 100% (Mather et al 1998, **Level IV**).

These data are however insufficient to support the routine use of inhaled opioids in acute pain management.

Key messages

1. NSAIDs (including COX-2 selective inhibitors) given parenterally or rectally are not more effective and do not result in fewer side effects than the same drug given orally (**Level I** [Cochrane Review]).
2. Intermittent subcutaneous morphine injections are as effective as intramuscular injections and have better patient acceptance (**Level II**).
3. Continuous intravenous infusion of opioids in the general ward setting are associated with an increased risk of respiratory depression compared with other methods of parenteral opioid administration (**Level IV**).
4. Transdermal fentanyl should not be used in the management of acute pain because of safety concerns and difficulties in short-term dose adjustments needed for titration (**Level IV**).

The following tick boxes ☑ represent conclusions based on clinical experience and expert opinion.

☑ Other than in the treatment of severe acute pain, and providing there are no contraindications to its use, the oral route is the route of choice for the administration of most analgesic drugs.

☑ Titration of opioids for severe acute pain is best achieved using intermittent intravenous bolus doses as it allows more rapid titration of effect and avoids the uncertainty of drug absorption by other routes.

☑ Controlled-release opioid preparations should only be given at set time intervals.

☑ Immediate-release opioids should be used for breakthrough pain and for titration of controlled-release opioids.

☑ The use of controlled-release opioid preparations as the sole agents for the early management of acute pain is discouraged because of difficulties in short-term dose adjustments needed for titration.

☑ Rectal administration of analgesic drugs may be useful when other routes are unavailable but bioavailability is unpredictable and consent should be obtained.

REFERENCES

Abboud TK, Zhu J, Gangolly et al (1991) Transnasal butorphanol: a new method for pain relief of post-cesarean section pain. *Acta Anaesthesiol Scand* 35: 14–18.

Anderson BJ, Woolard GA, Holford NH (1995) Pharmacokinetics of rectal paracetamol after major surgery in children. *Paediatr Anaesth* 5: 237–42.

Anderson B, Kanagasundarum S, Woollard G (1996) Analgesic efficacy of paracetamol in children using tonsillectomy as a pain model. *Anaesth Int Care* 24: 669–73.

Anderson BJ, Holford NH, Woollard GA et al (1999) Perioperative pharmacokinetics of acetaminophen analgesic in children. *Anesthesiology* 90: 411–21.

Ashburn MA, Lind GH, Gillie MH et al (1993) Oral transmucosal fentanyl citrate (OTFC) for the treatment of postoperative pain. *Anesth Analg* 76: 377–81.

Ashburn MA, Streisand J, Zhang J et al (1995) The iontophoresis of fentanyl citrate in humans. *Anesthesiology* 82: 1146–53.

Aubrun F, Monsel S, Langeron O et al (2001) Postoperative titration of intravenous morphine. *Eur J Anaesthesiol* 18: 159–65.

Bandolier (2003) Acute pain. *Bandolier Extra* Feb 2003. (www.ebandolier.com)

Barden J, Edwards JE, McQuay HJ et al (2003a) Single dose oral celecoxib for postoperative pain. *The Cochrane Database of Systematic Reviews*. Issue 1. Art. No.: CD004233. DOI: 10.1002/14651858.CD004233.

Barden J, Edwards JE, McQuay HJ et al (2003b) Oral valdecoxib and injected parecoxib for acute postoperative pain: a quantitative systematic review. *BMC Anesthesiol* 3: 1. (www.biomedcentral.com/1471-2253/3/1).

Barden J, Edwards JE, McQuay HJ et al (2004a) Pain and analgesic response after third molar extraction and other postsurgical pain. *Pain*107: 86–90.

Barden J, Edwards J, Moore A et al (2004b) Single dose oral paracetamol (acetaminophen) for postoperative pain. *The Cochrane Database of Systematic Reviews*. Issue 1. Art. No.: CD004602. DOI: 10.1002/14651858.CD004602.

Barden J, Edwards J, Moore RA et al (2004c) Single dose oral diclofenac for postoperative pain. *The Cochrane Database of Systematic Reviews*. Issue 2. Art. No.: CD004768. DOI: 10.1002/14651858.CD004768.

Bulow HH, Linnemann M, Berg H et al (1995) Respiratory changes during treatment of postoperative pain with high dose of transdermal fentanyl. *Acta Anaesthesiol Scand* 39: 835–39.

Coda BA, Rudy AC, Archer SM et al (2003) Pharmacokinetics and bioavailability of single-dose intranasal hydromorphone hydrochloride in healthy volunteers. *Anesth Analg* 97: 117–23.

Collins SL, Edwards JE, Moore RA et al (1999a) Single dose dextropropoxyphene, alone and with paracetamol (acetaminophen), for postoperative pain. *The Cochrane Database of Systematic Reviews*. Issue 1. Art. No.: CD001440. DOI: 10.1002/14651858.CD001440.

Collins SL, Moore RA, McQuay et al(1999b) Single dose oral ibuprofen and diclofenac for postoperative pain. *The Cochrane Database of Systematic Reviews*, Issue 1. Art. No.: CD001548. DOI: 10.1002/14651858.CD001548.

Cooper IM (1996) Morphine for postoperative analgesia. A comparison of intramuscular and subcutaneous routes of administration. *Anaesth Int Care* 24(5): 574–78.

Cuschieri RJ, Morran CG, McArdle CS (1984) Comparison of morphine and sublingual buprenorphine following abdominal surgery. *Br J Anaesth* 56: 855–59.

Dale O, Hjortkjaer R, Kharasch ED (2002) Nasal administration of opioids for pain management in adults. *Acta Anaesthesiol Scand*46: 759–70.

Daniels SE, Grossman EH, Kuss ME et al (2001) A double-blind, randomized comparison of intramuscularly and intravenously administered parecoxib sodium versus ketorolac and placebo in a post-oral surgery pain model. *Clin Ther* 23: 1018–31.

Dershwitz M, Walsh JL, Morishige RJ et al (2000) Pharmacokinetics and pharmacodynamics of inhaled versus intravenous morphine in healthy volunteers. *Anesthesiology* 93: 619–28.

Edwards JE, Oldman A, Smith L, et al (1999) Single dose oral aspirin for acute pain. *The Cochrane Database of Systematic Reviews* 1999, Issue 4. Art. No.: CD002067. DOI: 10.1002/14651858.CD002067.

Edwards JE, McQuay HJ, Moore RA (2000a) Single dose dihydrocodeine for acute postoperative pain. *The Cochrane Database of Systematic Reviews*. Issue 2. Art. No.: CD002760. DOI: 10.1002/14651858.CD002760.

Edwards JE, Moore RA, McQuay HJ (2000b) Single dose oxycodone and oxycodone plus paracetamol (acetominophen) for acute postoperative pain. *The Cochrane Database of Systematic Reviews*. Issue 2. Art. No.: CD002763. DOI: 10.1002/14651858.CD002763.

Edwards JE, Loke YK, Moore RA et al (2000c) Single dose piroxicam for acute postoperative pain. *The Cochrane Database of Systematic Reviews*. Issue 2. Art. No.: CD002762. DOI: 10.1002/14651858.CD002762.

Ginsberg B, Sinatra RS, Adler LJ et al (2003) Conversion to oral controlled-release oxycodone from intravenous opioid analgesic in the postoperative setting. *Pain Med* 4: 31–38.

Gould TH, Crosby DL, Harmer M et al (1992) Policy for controlling pain after surgery: effect of sequential changes in management. *BMJ* 305: 1187–93.

Grond S, Radbruch L, Lehmann KA (2000) Clinical pharmacokinetics of transdermal opioids: focus on transdermal fentanyl. *Clin Pharmacokinet* 38: 59–89.

Hansen TM, Matzen P, Madsen P (1984) Endoscopic evaluation of the effect of indomethacin capsules and suppositories on the gastric mucosa in rheumatic patients. *J Rheumatol* 11: 484–87.

Higgins MJ, Ashbury AJ, Brodie MJ (1991) Inhaled nebulized fentanyl for post-operative analgesia. *Anaesthesia* 46: 973–76.

Jarde O & Boccard E (1997) Parenteral versus oral route increases paracetamol efficacy. *Clin Drug Invest*14: 474–81.

Jeal W & BenfieldP (1997) Transdermal fentanyl: a review of its pharmacological properties and therapeutic efficacy in pain control. *Drugs* 53: 109–38.

Kampe S, Warm M, Kaufmann J et al (2004) Clinical efficacy of controlled-release oxycodone 20mg administered in a 12-hour dosing schedule on the management of postoperative pain after breast surgery for cancer. *Curr Med Res Opin* 20: 199–202.

Kendall JM, Reeves BC, Latter VS (2001) Multicentre randomised controlled trial of nasal diamorphine for analgesia in children and teenagers with clinical fractures. Nasal Diamorphine Trial Group. *BMJ* 322: 261–65.

Lamacraft G, Cooper MG, Cavalletto BP (1997) Subcutaneous cannulae for morphine boluses in children. *J Pain Sympt Manage* 13: 43–49.

Lichtor JL, Sevarino FB, Joshi GP et al (1999) The relative potency of oral transmucosal fentanyl citrate compared with intravenous morphine in the treatment of moderate to severe postoperative pain. *Anesth Analg* 89: 732–38.

Lim AW & Schug SA (2001) Tramadol versus morphine as oral step down analgesia after postoperative epidural analgesia. *Reg Anesth Pain Med* 26: S133.

Macintyre PE & Ready LB (2001) *Acute Pain Management: A Practical Guide*. 2nd Edition. London: WB Saunders.

Manjushree R, Lahiri A, Ghosh BR et al (2002) Intranasal fentanyl provided adequate postoperative analgesia in paediatric patients. *Can J Anesth* 49: 190–93.

Mason L, Edwards JE, Moore RA et al (2003) Single dose oral naproxen for acute postoperative pain: a quantitative systematic review. *BMC Anesthesiology* 3: 41. (www.biomedcentral.com/1471-2253/3/4).

Masood AR & Thomas SHL (1996) Systemic absorption of nebulized morphine compared with oral morphine in healthy subjects. *Br J Clin Pharmacol* 41: 250–52.

Mather LE, Woodhouse A, Ward ME et al (1998) Pulmonary administration of aerosolised fentanyl: pharmacokinetic analysis of systemic delivery. *Br J Clin Pharmacol* 46: 37–43.

CHAPTER 6

McCormack JP, Warriner CB, Levine M et al (1993) A comparison of regularly dosed oral morphine and on-demand intramuscular morphine in the treatment of postsurgical pain. *Can J Anaesth* 40: 819–24.

McQuay HJ, Carroll D, Moore RA (1999) Injected morphine in postoperative pain: a quantitative systematic review. *J Pain Symptom Manage* 17: 164–74.

McQuay H & Edwards J (2003) Meta-analysis of single dose oral tramadol plus acetaminophen in acute postoperative pain. *Eur J Anaesthesiol* 20 (Suppl 28): 19–22.

Miller RR & Greenblatt DJ (1976) *Drug Effects In Hospitalised Patients*. New York: John Wiley and Sons.

MIMS (2004) *MIMS Annual 2004*. MediMedia Australia Pty Ltd. (www.mims.com.au)

Moa G & Zetterstrom H (1990) Sublingual buprenorphine as postoperative analgesic: a double-blind comparison with pethidine. *Acta Anaesthesiol Scand* 34: 68–71.

Moore RA, McQuay HJ (1997) Single patient data meta-analysis of 3453 postoperative patients: oral tramadol versus placebo, codeine and combination analgesics. *Pain* 69: 287–94.

Moore RA, Tramèr M, Carroll D et al (1998a) Quantitative systematic review of topically-applied nonsteroidal and antiinflammatory drug. *BMJ* 316: 333–38.

Moore A, Collins S, Carroll D (1998b) Single dose paracetamol (acetaminophen), with and without codeine, for postoperative pain. *The Cochrane Database of Systematic Reviews*. Issue 4. Art. No.: CD001547. DOI: 10.1002/14651858.CD001547.

Moore A, Edwards J, Barden J et al (2003) *Bandolier's Little Book of Pain*. New York: Oxford University Press.

Paech MJ, Lim CB, Banks SL et al (2003) A new formulation of nasal spray for postoperative analgesia: a pilot study. *Anaesthesia* 58: 740–44.

Pang WW, Mok MS, Huang S et al (2000) Intraoperative loading attenuates nausea and vomiting of tramadol patient-controlled analgesia. *Can J Anaesth* 47: 968–73.

Peng PW & Sandler AN (1999) A review of the use of fentanyl analgesia in the management of acute pain in adults. *Anesthesiology* 90: 576–79.

Reuben SS, Connelly HR, Maciolek H (1999) Postoperative analgesia with controlled-release oxycodone for outpatient anterior cruciate ligament surgery. *Anesth Analg* 88: 1286–91.

Reuben SS, Steinbery RB, Maciolek H (2002) Preoperative administration of controlled-release oxycodone for the management of pain after ambulatory laparoscopic tubal ligation surgery. *J Clin Anesth* 14: 223–27.

Rømsing J, Møiniche S, Dahl JB (2002) Rectal and parenteral paracetamol, and paracetamol in combination with NSAIDs, for postoperative analgesia. *Br J Anaesth* 88: 215–26.

Sandler AN, Baxter AD, Katz J et al (1994) A double-blind, placebo-controlled trial of transdermal fentanyl after abdominal hysterectomy. Analgesic, respiratory, and pharmacokinetic effects. *Anesthesiology* 81: 1169–80.

Schug SA & Torrie JJ (1993) Safety assessment of postoperative pain management by an acute pain service. *Pain* 55: 387–91.

Semple D, Aldridge LA, Doyle E (1996) Comparison of IV and SC diamorphine infusions for the treatment of acute pain in children. *Br J Anaesth* 6: 310–12.

Semple TJ, Upton RN, Macintyre PE et al (1997) Morphine blood concentrations in elderly postoperative patients following administration via an indwelling subcutaneous cannula. *Anaesthesia* 52: 318–23.

Sharar SR, Bratton SL, Carrougher GJ et al (1998) A comparison of oral transmucosal fentanyl citrate and oral hydromorphone for inpatient pediatric burn wound care analgesia. *J Burn Care Rehabil* 19: 516–21.

Sharar SR, Carrougher GJ, Selzer K et al (2002) A comparison of oral transmucosal fentanyl citrate and oral oxycodone for pediatric outpatient wound care. *J Burn Care Rehabil* 23: 27–31.

Sittl R, Griessinger N, Likar R (2003) Analgesic efficacy and tolerability of transdermal buprenorphine in patients with inadequately controlled chronic pain related to cancer and other disorders: a multicenter, randomized, double-blind, placebo-controlled trial. *Clin Ther* 25: 150–68.

Smith LA, Carroll D, Edwards JE et al (2000) Single-dose ketorolac and pethidine in acute postoperative pain: systematic review with meta-analysis. *Br J Anaesth* 84: 48–58.

Streisand JB, Vavel JR, Stanski DR et al (1991) Absorption and bioavailability of oral transmucosal fentanyl. *Anesthesiology* 75: 223–29.

Striebel HW, Koenigs D, Kramer J (1992) Postoperative pain management by intranasal demand-adapted fentanyl titration. *Anesthesiology* 77: 281–85.

Striebel HW, Malewicz J, Hermanns K et al (1993) Intranasal meperidine titration for postoperative relief. *Anesth Analg* 76: 1047–51.

Striebel HW, Bonillo B, Schwagmeier R et al (1995) Self-administered nasal meperidine for postoperative pain management. *Can J Anesth* 42: 287–91.

Striebel HW, Oelmann T, Spies C et al (1996) Patient-controlled intranasal analgesia: a method for non-invasive postoperative pain management. *Anesth Analg* 83: 548–51.

Sunshine AS, Olson NZ, Colon A et al (1996) Analgesic Efficacy of controlled-release oxycodone in postoperative pain. *J Clin Pharmacol* 36: 595–603.

Thipphawong JB, Babul N, Morishige RJ et al (2003) Analgesic efficacy of inhaled morphine in patients after bunionectomy surgery. *Anesthesiology* 99: 693–700.

Toussaint S, Maidl J, Schwagmeier R et al (2000) Patient-controlled intranasal analgesia: effective alternative to intravenous PCA for postoperative pain relief. *Can J Anaesth* 47: 299–302.

Tramèr SR, Williams JE, Carroll D et al (1998) Comparing analgesic efficacy of non-steroidal anti-inflammatory drugs given by different routes in acute and chronic pain: A qualitative systematic review. *Acta Anaesthesiol Scand* 42: 71–79.

Walder B, Schafer M, Henzi I et al (2001) Efficacy and safety of patient-controlled opioid analgesia for acute postoperative pain. A quantitative systematic review. *Acta Anaesthesiol Scand* 45: 795–804.

Ward ME, Woodhouse A, Mather LE et al (1997) Morphine pharmacokinetics after pulmonary administration from a novel aerosol delivery system, *Clin Pharmacol Ther* 6: 596–609.

Ward M, Minto G, Alexander-Williams JM (2002) A comparison of patient-controlled analgesia administered by the intravenous or intranasal route during the early postoperative period. *Anaesthesia* 57: 48–52.

Worsley MH, Macleod AD, Brodie MJ et al (1990) Inhaled fentanyl as a method of analgesia. *Anaesthesia* 45: 449–51.

7. TECHNIQUES OF DRUG ADMINISTRATION

7.1 PATIENT-CONTROLLED ANALGESIA

Patient-controlled analgesia (PCA) refers to methods of pain relief that allow a patient to self-administer small doses of an analgesic agent as required. Most often, however, the term PCA is associated with programmable infusion pumps that deliver opioid medications intravenously, although a variety of other methods and routes of delivery using opioids as well as other analgesic agents have been described.

7.1.1 Efficacy of intravenous PCA

Analgesia, patient preference and outcomes

Intravenous (IV) opioid PCA provides better analgesia than conventional (intramuscular [IM], subcutaneous [SC]) opioid regimens when all pain outcomes (pain intensity, pain relief and requirement for rescue analgesia) are combined. There is also some evidence of a decreased risk of postoperative pulmonary complications but no differences in opioid consumption, duration of hospital stay or opioid-related adverse effects (Walder et al 2001, **Level I**).

These results may show that there is no great difference between IV PCA and conventional opioid analgesia, or they could indicate that conventional analgesia was managed well under study conditions, with patients given adequate amounts of opioid truly on demand (Walder et al 2001). The enormous variability in PCA parameters (bolus doses, lockout intervals and maximum permitted cumulative doses) used by the various investigators indicates uncertainty as to the ideal PCA program. Adequate analgesia needs to be obtained prior to commencement of PCA and individual PCA prescriptions may need to be adjusted if patients are to receive maximal benefit (Macintyre 2001).

CHAPTER 7

Patient preference for intravenous PCA was significantly higher compared with conventional regimens, although there was no difference in patient satisfaction (Walder et al 2001, **Level I**). Psychological factors that may affect PCA use and efficacy are discussed in Section 1.2.

Cost of PCA

The use of any analgesic technique, even if it is known to provide more effective pain relief, also requires consideration of the cost involved. There are no good consistent data on the cost-effectiveness of PCA compared with conventional opioid analgesic techniques (Walder et al 2001). However, in general PCA comes at a higher cost because of the equipment, consumables and drugs required; nursing time needed is much less (Jacox et al 1997; Choinière et al 1998, **Level II**; Rittenhouse & Choinière 1999).

7.1.2 Drugs used for parenteral PCA

Opioid drugs

In general there is little evidence, on a population basis, to suggest that there are any major differences in efficacy or side effects between morphine and other commonly used opioids such as pethidine (meperidine) (Sinatra et al 1989, **Level II**; Stanley et al 1996, **Level II**; Woodhouse et al 1996, **Level II**), hydromorphone (Rapp et al 1996, **Level II**), fentany (Woodhouse et al 1996, **Level II**) and oxycodone (Silvasti et al 1998, **Level II**), although a greater incidence of pruritus may be seen with morphine (Woodhouse et al 1996, **Level II**). Pain relief on movement may be better with morphine than with pethidine (Sinatra et al 1989, **Level II**; Plummer et al 1997, **Level II**). Remifentanil or pethidine administered via PCA for pain relief during uncomplicated labour resulted in similar pain scores and Apgar scores (Blair et al 2005).

On an individual patient basis, one opioid may be better tolerated than another and a change to an alternative opioid may be beneficial if the patient is experiencing intolerable side effects (Woodhouse et al 1999, **Level II**).

Tramadol may have similar analgesic effect compared with morphine and oxycodone and a similar incidence of nausea and vomiting (Stamer et al 1997, **Level II**; Pang et al 1999, **Level II**; Silvasti et al 1999, **Level II**). It also has a lower risk of respiratory depression and less effect on gastrointestinal motor function compared with other opioids (see Section 4.1.2).

The incidence of opioid-related side effects, including respiratory depression, is the same for both IV PCA and intermittent opioid analgesic regimens (Walder et al 2001, **Level I**). However, in the studies used in this meta-analysis, as with many other studies of opioid analgesia, a variety of definitions of respiratory depression were used (see Section 4.1). In a recent review of published data, the reported incidence of respiratory depression with PCA ranged from 1.2 (0.7–1.9)% to 11.5 (5.6–22.0)% using respiratory rate and oxygen saturation, respectively, as indicators (Cashman & Dolin 2004, **Level IV**). Compared with PCA, continuous IV opioid infusions in a general ward setting resulted in a 5-fold increase in the incidence of respiratory depression (Schug & Torrie 1993, **Level III-2**).

Adjuvant drugs

Antiemetics

Droperidol added to the PCA morphine solution is an effective antiemetic with an NNT of 3; there is no evidence of worthwhile antinauseant effect with the addition of 5-HT_3 receptor antagonists although they may be effective for vomiting, with an NNT of approximately 5 (Tramèr & Walder 1999, **Level I**). Tramèr's group noted no dose-responsiveness with droperidol (Tramèr & Walder 1999, **Level I**). However, in a comparison of the effects of the addition of 0.5mg, 1.5mg and 5mg droperidol to 100mg PCA morphine, the smallest dose had no significant antiemetic effect and the 1.5mg dose was effective against nausea but not vomiting. The 5mg dose significantly reduced both nausea and vomiting, but at the cost of unacceptable sedation, which was not seen at the other doses (Culebras et al 2003, **Level II**).

Droperidol given separately is as effective as adding droperidol to PCA morphine (Gan et al 1995, **Level II**). The cost-benefit and risk-benefit of the routine addition of droperidol to PCA opioids must therefore be considered as all patients receive the drug when not all will need it and some patients might receive inappropriately high doses of droperidol (Macintyre 2001).

Ketamine

The addition of ketamine to PCA morphine does not improve analgesia or reduce the incidence of opioid-related side effects (Subramaniam et al 2004, **Level I**). The addition of s(+) ketamine to PCA morphine was opioid-sparing and reduced pain scores at rest but not with movement; there was no difference in side effects (Snijdelaar et al 2003, **Level II**).

Naloxone

There is no analgesic benefit in adding naloxone to the PCA morphine solution (Sartain et al 2003, **Level II**; Cepeda et al 2002, **Level II**; Cepeda et al 2004, **Level II**); in 'ultra low doses' but not in the higher dose studies, the incidence of nausea and pruritus is decreased (Cepeda 2004, **Level II**).

Other

The addition of clonidine to IV PCA morphine resulted in significantly better pain relief for the first 12 hours only and less nausea and vomiting compared with morphine alone; there was no reduction in morphine requirements (Jeffs et al 2002, **Level II**). The addition of lignocaine (lidocaine) to morphine conferred no benefit in terms of pain relief or side effects (Cepeda at al 1996, **Level II**).

7.1.3 Program parameters for IV PCA

Bolus dose

While the optimal sized bolus dose should provide good pain relief with minimal side effects, there are only limited data available concerning the effects of various dose sizes. In patients prescribed 0.5mg, 1mg and 2mg bolus doses of morphine, most of those who were prescribed 0.5mg were unable to achieve adequate analgesia, while a high incidence of respiratory depression was reported in those who received 2mg (Owen et al 1989, **Level II**). The optimal PCA bolus dose for morphine was therefore 1mg.

Similarly, in patients prescribed 20, 40 or 60 microgram bolus doses of fentanyl, the larger dose was associated with an increased risk of respiratory depression and a conclusion was made that the optimal dose of fentanyl for use in PCA was 40 microgram (Camu et al 1998, **Level II**). However in this study, each dose was infused over 10 minutes, which could alter the effect of that dose.

Rigid adherence to an 'optimal' dose may, however, not lead to the best pain relief for all patients. Initial orders for bolus doses should take into account factors such as a history of prior opioid use (see Section 10.8) and patient age (Macintyre 2001); PCA morphine requirements are known to decrease as patient age increases (Macintyre & Jarvis 1996, **Level IV**). Subsequent bolus doses may require adjustment according to patient pain reports or the onset of any side effects.

The number of demands a patient makes, including the number of 'unsuccessful' demands, is often used as an indication that the patient is in pain and as a guide to adjusting the size of the bolus dose. However, there may be a number of reasons for a high demand rate other than pain, including anxiety, patient confusion, or inappropriate patient use (Macintyre 2001). Even though the length of the lockout interval could allow it, patients may not increase their demand rate enough to compensate for bolus doses that are too small (Owen et al 1989, **Level II**; Owen et al 1990, **Level II**).

Lockout interval

The lockout interval is a safety mechanism which limits the frequency of demands made by the patient. For maximum safety it should be long enough to allow the patient to feel the full effect of one opioid dose before another dose can be delivered. However, if it is too long the effectiveness of PCA could be reduced. There were no differences in pain relief, side effects or anxiety when lockout intervals of 7 or 11 minutes for morphine and 5 or 8 minutes for fentanyl were used (Ginsberg et al 1995, **Level II**).

Concurrent background (continuous) infusions

There is no good evidence to show that the addition of a background infusion to IV PCA improves pain relief or sleep, or reduces the number of demands (Owen et al 1989, **Level II**; Parker et al 1991, **Level II**; Parker et al 1992, **Level II**; Dal et al 2003, **Level II**). Large audits of adult patients have also shown that the risk of respiratory depression is increased when a background infusion is added (Notcutt & Morgan 1990, **Level IV**; Fleming & Coombes 1992, **Level IV**; Schug & Torrie 1993, **Level III-2**; Sidebotham et al 1997, **Level IV**). In adults, the routine use of a background infusion is therefore not recommended, although it may be useful in opioid-tolerant patients (see Section 10.8).

Dose limits

Limits to the maximum amount of opioid that can be delivered over a certain period (commonly 1 or 4 hours) can be programmed into most PCA machines. There is no good evidence of any benefit that can be attributed to these limits.

Loading dose

There is enormous variation in the amount of opioid a patient may need as a 'loading dose' and there is no good evidence of any benefit that can be attributed to the use of the loading dose feature that can be programmed into PCA machines. PCA is essentially a maintenance therapy, therefore a patient's pain should be controlled before PCA is started by administration of individually titrated loading doses (Macintyre 2001). IV opioid loading improved the analgesic efficacy of subsequent oral and PCA opioid therapy in the treatment of acute sickle cell pain (Rees et al 2003, **Level II**).

7.1.4 Efficacy of PCA using other systemic routes of administration

Subcutaneous PCA

Subcutaneous PCA using hydromorphone (Urquhart et al 1988, **Level II**) and morphine (White 1990, **Level II**) is as effective as the same opioids administered by IV PCA; PCA dose requirements via the SC route are higher for hydromorphone compared with IV PCA but there is only a trend to higher SC PCA morphine doses.

Oral PCA

Oral PCA, using a modified IV PCA system, is as effective as IV PCA (Striebel et al 1998, **Level II**).

Intranasal PCA

Intranasal PCA (PCINA) fentanyl can be as effective as IV PCA (Striebel et al 1996, **Level II**; Toussaint et al 2000, **Level II**; Manjushree et al 2002, **Level II**; Paech et al 2003, **Level II**), as is butorphanol (Abboud et al 1991, **Level II**). As would be expected from the data on intranasal (IN) bioavailability of opioids (see Section 6.6.1), higher doses are needed via the IN route (Striebel et al 1996; Manjushree et al 2002). PCINA pethidine is as effective as IV pethidine, although larger doses are needed (Striebel at al 1993, **Level II**), and more effective than SC injections of pethidine (Striebel et al 1995, **Level II**). Diamorphine PCINA (bolus doses of 0.5mg) is less effective than PCA IV morphine (higher bolus doses of 1mg were used) after joint replacement surgery (Ward et al 2002, **Level II**) but provides better pain relief in doses of 0.1mg/kg compared with 0.2mg/kg IM morphine in children with fractures (Kendall et al 2001, **Level II**).

Transdermal PCA

Transdermal PCA fentanyl using iontophoresis is comparable with IV PCA morphine in terms of pain relief and incidence of side effects (Viscusi et al 2004, **Level II**).

Regional PCA

Patient-controlled regional analgesia (PCRA) may also be effective, including after ambulatory surgery. Local anaesthetic agents can be infused into catheters placed subcutaneously into surgical wounds, in nerve plexus sheaths, subacromially and intra-articularly (Rawal et al 1998).

The addition of a background infusion to '3 in 1' PCRA (Singelyn & Gouverneur 2000, **Level II**) or femoral nerve PCRA (Singelyn et al 2001, **Level II**) does not improve pain relief or alter the incidence of side effects but may increase total local anaesthetic consumption. The addition of a background infusion to interscalene brachial plexus PCRA did result in better analgesia (Singelyn et al 1999b, **Level II**).

Patient-controlled analgesic techniques have also been used for the instillation of local anaesthetics into wounds after surgery. After total abdominal hysterectomy, patient-controlled wound instillation of bupivacaine resulted in similar pain scores but less nausea and rescue opioid medications compared with patient-controlled wound instillation of sterile water (Zohar et al 2001, **Level II**). After major abdominal surgery with a midline incision, no such differences were found (Fredman et al 2001, **Level II**).

7.1.5 Epidural PCA

Postoperative patient-controlled epidural analgesia

Comparison with continuous epidural infusions

Patients prescribed patient-controlled epidural analgesia (PCEA) with bupivacaine and fentanyl use lower cumulative doses of the drugs compared with continuous epidural infusions without any differences in pain relief or side effects (Silvasti & Pitkaanen 2001, **Level II**; Standl et al 2003, **Level II**).

Concurrent background (continuous) infusions

The addition of a continuous background infusion to PCEA using bupivacaine and fentanyl following gastrectomy resulted in significantly better dynamic pain scores, higher total doses and a greater incidence of pruritus than PCEA-bolus dose only (Komatsu et al 1998, **Level II**). The use of a night-time-only infusion with PCEA bupivacaine-fentanyl in postgastrectomy patients resulted in better sleep but total cumulative doses were similar and pain scores were only better in the morning of the second postoperative day (Komatsu et al 2001, **Level II**).

However, pain relief is not always improved. After lower abdominal surgery there was no difference in pain scores, but higher total cumulative doses and incidence of side effects when a background infusion was added to PCEA with ropivacaine and fentanyl (Wong et al 2000, **Level II**). The addition of a background infusion to bupivacaine-fentanyl PCEA did not improve pain relief after pelvic reconstruction (Nolan et al 1992, **Level II**).

Drugs used in postoperative patient-controlled epidural analgesia

The drugs used for PCEA are the same as those used for continuous epidural infusions (see Chapter 5 and Section 7.2). Generalisations about the efficacy of different drugs and drug combinations administered via PCEA are difficult because of the wide variety of analgesic agents and concentrations used in the various studies.

Obstetric PCEA

Comparison with continuous epidural infusions

Patients who receive PCEA using the same local anaesthetic drug or local anaesthetic/opioid combination require lower doses of local anaesthetic, have less motor block and are less likely to need anaesthetic interventions (eg clinician 'top up') than those prescribed continuous epidural infusions for labour analgesia (van der Vyver et al 2002, **Level I**).

Concurrent continuous (background) infusions

Evidence of benefit for the addition of a continuous infusion in the obstetric setting is limited. PCEA with a background infusion resulted in greater analgesic consumption without improved pain relief (Ferrante et al 1994, **Level II**; Boselli et al 2004, **Level II**).

Drugs used in obstetric patient-controlled epidural analgesia

Results for the effectiveness of PCEA with different local anaesthetics or local anaesthetic-opioid solutions are mixed (see Section 10.2.2).

7.1.6 Equipment

Information regarding complications due to equipment problems is case-based; examples from a range of the cases reported are given.

Uncontrolled syphoning of syringe contents when the PCA machine was above patient level has been reported following cracked glass PCA syringes (Thomas & Owen 1988; ECRI 1996), failure of a damaged drive mechanism to retain the syringe plunger (Kwan 1995), and improperly secured PCA cassettes (ECRI 1995). To minimise the risk of syphoning, the use of antisyphon valves is recommended (Kluger & Owen 1990; Harmer 1994; ECRI 1996; Macintyre 2001).

Anti-reflux valves are essential if the PCA infusion is not connected to a dedicated IV line. The non-PCA infusion tubing should have an anti-reflux (one-way) valve upstream from the connection with the PCA line to prevent back-flow up the non-PCA line should distal obstruction occur; otherwise, inappropriate dosing could occur (Rutherford & Patri 2004).

7.1.7 Patients and staff factors

Patient factors

Much of the information regarding complications due to patient factors is case-based — examples from a range of the cases reported are given.

Education

Few controlled studies have evaluated the influence of information on PCA use. Of 200 patients surveyed who used PCA, approximately 20% were worried that they may become addicted, and 20% and 30% respectively felt that the machine could give them too much drug or that they could self-administer too much opioid (Chumbley et al 1998, **Level IV**). In a follow-up study, the same group conducted focus groups with previous PCA users, developed a new information leaflet and then undertook a randomised study comparing the old and new leaflet. They found that patients wanted more information on the medication in the PCA, the possible side effects and assurance that they would not become addicted (Chumbley et al 2002, **Level II**).

Inappropriate use of PCA

The safety of PCA depends on an adequate understanding of the technique by the patient and the fact that unauthorised persons do not press the demand button.

Oversedation with PCA has followed mistaking the PCA handset for the nurse-call button and family or unauthorised nurse-activated demands (Wakerlin & Larson 1990; Fleming & Coombes 1992; Chisukata 1993; Schug & Torrie 1993; Ashburn et al 1994; Sidebotham et al 1997; Tsui et al 1997).

There have been case reports expressing concerns that patients can use PCA to treat increasing pain and therefore mask problems such as compartment syndrome (Harrington et al 2000; Richards et al 2004), urinary retention (Hodsman et al 1988), pulmonary embolism (Meyer & Eagle 1992) and myocardial infarction (Finger & McLeod 1995).

However, appropriate routine patient monitoring should detect changes in pain scores and analgesic consumption enabling identification of such complications.

Nursing and medical staff

Much of the information regarding complications due to nursing and medical staff factors is case-based — examples from a range of the cases reported are given.

Operator error is a common safety problem related to PCA use. Mortality from programming errors has been estimated to range from 1 in 33,000 to 1 in 338,800 patients prescribed PCA (Vincente et al 2003). There are now several case reports in the literature outlining serious programming errors with PCA, including fatalities (Notcutt et al 1992; Ashburn et al 1994; Heath 1995; ECRI 1997; Vincente et al 2003).

A number of reports involve the programming of drug concentrations that were lower than the concentration ordered, with the resultant delivery of an excessive amount of opioid leading to respiratory depression and sometimes death (ECRI 1997; ECRI 2002). The use of an incorrect prefilled 'standard syringe' for PCA (morphine 5mg/mL instead of the prescribed 1mg/mL) also had a fatal outcome (Vincente et al 2003). It has been suggested that drug concentrations should be standardised within institutions to reduce the chance of administration and programming errors (ECRI 2002).

Inappropriate prescriptions of supplementary opioids (by other routes) and sedative drugs can lead to oversedation and respiratory depression (Ashburn et al 1994; Etches 1994; Tsui et al 1997).

7.1.8 PCA in specific patient groups

For PCA in the paediatric patient, the elderly patient, the patient with obstructive sleep apnoea and the opioid-tolerant patient, see Sections 10.1, 10.3, 10.6 and 10.8 respectively.

Key messages

1. Intravenous opioid PCA provides better analgesia than conventional parenteral opioid regimens (**Level I**).
2. Patient preference for intravenous PCA is higher when compared with conventional regimens (**Level I**).
3. Opioid administration by IV PCA does not lead to lower opioid consumption, reduced hospital stay or a lower incidence of opioid-related adverse effects compared with traditional methods of intermittent parenteral opioid administration (**Level I**).
4. The addition of ketamine to PCA morphine does not improve analgesia or reduce the incidence of opioid-related side effects (**Level I**).
5. Patient-controlled epidural analgesia for pain in labour results in the use of lower doses of local anaesthetic, less motor block and fewer anaesthetic interventions compared with continuous epidural infusions (**Level I**).

6. There is little evidence that one opioid via PCA is superior to another with regards to analgesic or adverse effects in general; on an individual patient basis one opioid may be better tolerated than another (**Level II**).
7. There is no analgesic benefit in adding naloxone to the PCA morphine solution, however the incidence of nausea and pruritus may be decreased (**Level II**).
8. The addition of a background infusion to IV PCA does not improve pain relief or sleep, or reduce the number of PCA demands (**Level II**).
9. Subcutaneous PCA opioids can be as effective as IV PCA (**Level II**).
10. Intranasal PCA opioids can be as effective as IV PCA (**Level II**).
11. Patient-controlled epidural analgesia results in lower cumulative doses of the drugs compared with continuous epidural infusions without any differences in pain relief or side effects (**Level II**).
12. The risk of respiratory depression with PCA is increased when a background infusion is used (**Level IV**).

The following tick boxes ☑ represent conclusions based on clinical experience and expert opinion.

☑ Adequate analgesia needs to be obtained prior to commencement of PCA. Initial orders for bolus doses should take into account individual patient factors such as a history of prior opioid use and patient age. Individual PCA prescriptions may need to be adjusted.

☑ The routine addition of anti-emetics to PCA opioids is not encouraged, as it is of no benefit compared with selective administration.

☑ PCA infusion systems must incorporate antisyphon valves and in non-dedicated lines, antireflux valves.

☑ Drug concentrations should be standardised within institutions to reduce the chance of programming errors.

CHAPTER 7

7.2 EPIDURAL ANALGESIA

Epidural analgesia (ie the provision of pain relief by continuous administration of pharmacological agents into the epidural space via an indwelling catheter) has become a widely used technique for the management of acute pain in adults and children, particularly after surgery and sometimes trauma, and in parturients.

7.2.1 Efficacy

The difficulty with interpretation of available data is that epidural analgesia is not a single entity but can be provided by a number of pharmacological agents administered into different levels of the epidural space for a wide variety of operations.

However, the universal efficacy of epidural analgesia has been well demonstrated. Regardless of analgesic agent used, location of catheter, type of surgery and type or time of pain assessment, it provides better pain relief than parenteral opioid administration (Block et al 2003, **Level I**; Werawatganon & Charuluxanum 2004, **Level I**). Improved pain relief with epidural local anaesthetic drugs leads to increased PaO_2 levels and a decreased incidence of pulmonary infections and pulmonary complications overall when compared with systemic opioids (Ballantyne et al 1998, **Level I**).

Thoracic epidural analgesia in combination with non-steroidal anti-inflammatory drugs (NSAIDs) and IV nutritional support after major abdominal surgery has been shown to prevent protein loss compared with epidural analgesia alone, or PCA with or without nutritional support (Barratt 2000, **Level II**).

7.2.2 Drug used for epidural analgesia

With regard to choice of pharmacological agents, relevant differences in effects and adverse effects can be found with use of local anaesthetics and opioids.

Opioids

Opioids alone via the epidural route seem to be of limited benefit. In particular, when administered via a thoracic approach, opioids failed to demonstrate any advantage over parenteral opioids except for a slight reduction in the rate of atelectasis (Ballantyne et al 1998, **Level I**) and there is no benefit with regard to bowel recovery (Steinbrook 1998; Jørgensen et al 2001, **Level I**). On the basis of the available studies, the benefits of administering lipophilic opioids alone by the epidural route would appear to be marginal, or unproven in the case of upper abdominal surgery, and in many situations will not outweigh the risks of the more invasive route of administration (for detailed discussion see Wheatley et al 2001 and Section 5.2.1).

Epidural pethidine has been used predominantly in the obstetric setting. After caesarean section epidural pethidine resulted in better pain relief and less sedation than IV pethidine(Paech 1994, **Level II**) but inferior analgesia compared with intrathecal morphine, albeit with less pruritus, nausea and drowsiness (Paech 2000, **Level II**).

Local anaesthetic-opioid combinations

Combinations of low concentrations of local anaesthetic agents and opioids have been shown to provide consistently superior pain relief compared with either of the drugs alone (Curatolo 1998, **Level I**).

Adjuvant drugs

The addition of small amounts of adrenaline (epinephrine) to such mixtures has resulted in improved analgesia and reduced systemic opioid concentrations (Niemi & Breivik 1998; Niemi & Breivik 2002, **Level II**) (see also Section 5.3).

7.2.3 Level of administration

Thoracic

Thoracic epidural analgesia is widely used for the treatment of pain after major abdominal and thoracic surgery. Administration of local anaesthetics into the thoracic epidural space results in improved bowel recovery after abdominal surgery, while these benefits are not consistent with lumbar administration (Steinbrook 1998; Jørgensen et al 2004, **Level I**). If epidural analgesia is extended for more than 24 hours, a further benefit is a significant reduction in the incidence of postoperative myocardial infarction (Beattie & Badner 2001, **Level I**). In patients with multiple rib fractures, provision of epidural analgesia has been shown to reduce the risk of nosocomial pneumonia and the number of ventilator days (Bulger et al 2004, **Level II**).

High thoracic epidural analgesia, used for coronary artery bypass graft surgery, can result in reduced postoperative pain (both at rest and with activity), risk of dysrhythmias, pulmonary complications and time to extubation when compared with IV opioid analgesia. Mortality and the rate of myocardial infarction was not reduced (Liu et al 2004, **Level I**).

Lumbar

Lumbar epidural analgesia is widely used to provide analgesia after orthopaedic and vascular operations to the lower limbs and urological and other pelvic surgery.

After hip or knee replacement, epidural analgesia provides better pain relief than parenteral opioids, in particular with movement (Choi et al 2003, **Level I**). Although epidural infusions of local anaesthetics alone or combined with opioids are better than opioids alone, there is insufficient evidence to make conclusions about other outcomes. Used in vascular surgery, lumbar epidural analgesia improves outcome by reducing incidence of graft occlusion (Tuman et al 1991, **Level II**; Christopherson et al 1993; **Level II**).

CHAPTER 7

7.2.4 Patient controlled epidural analgesia

The use of PCEA has become increasingly popular; it is based on similar concepts as other patient-controlled techniques. It has been shown to be safe and effective in standard ward settings (Liu et al 1998, **Level IV**) and results in reduced epidural analgesic requirements (Silvasti & Pikkanen 2001; Standl et al 2003, **Level II**) (see Section 7.1).

7.2.5 Adverse effects

Neurological injury

Permanent neurological damage is the most feared complication of epidural analgesia. Reported incidences in large case series are in the range of 0.005–0.05% (Kane 1981, **Level IV**; Dahlgren & Tornebrandt 1995, **Level IV**; Aromaa et al 1997, **Level IV**; Giebler et al 1997, **Level IV**). A recent retrospective survey from Sweden puts the risk of a severe neurological complication after obstetric epidural analgesia at 1:25,000 and for all other patients at 1:3600; 67% resulted in permanent neurologic deficit (Moen et al 2004, **Level IV**). It also identified osteoporosis as a previously neglected risk factor.

The incidence of transient neuropathy after epidural analgesia in large case series was in the range of 0.013–0.023% (Xie & Liu 1991, **Level IV**; Tanaka et al 1993, **Level IV**; Auroy et al 1997, **Level IV**).

Epidural haematoma

A major concern is the development of an epidural haematoma with subsequent, potentially permanent, spinal cord injury. A review including case series involving over

1,335,000 patients with epidural analgesia reported 7 cases of haematoma (0.0005%) (Wulf 1996, **Level IV**). On the basis of this case series the possible incidence is in the order of 1 in 100,000 at the upper limit of the 95% confidence interval. The Swedish case series quoted above puts the overall risk of epidural haematoma after epidural blockade at 1 in 10,300 (Moen et al 2004, **Level IV**). A higher incidence of epidural haematoma (1:3,100) has been estimated for epidural analgesia in association with inappropriate low molecular weight heparin dose regimens (Horlocker & Wedel 2000) (see Section 7.4).

Early diagnosis and, if indicated, immediate decompression (less than 8 hours after the onset of neurological signs) increases the likelihood of partial or good neurological recovery (Horlocker et al 2003, **Level IV**).

Epidural abscess

Serious neuraxial infections following epidural anaesthesia have previously been reported as rare. However, prospective studies have found rates in the range of 0.015–0.05% (Kindler et al 1996, **Level IV**; Rygnestad et al 1997, **Level IV**; Wang et al 1999, **Level IV**). It is of note that in the studies with these high incidences, patients had long durations of epidural catheterisation; the mean duration in patients with an epidural space infection was 11 days (no infection occurred in any patient whose catheter was in situ for less than 2 days and the majority of patients were immunocompromised) (Wang et al 1999, **Level IV**).

Only 5.5% of 915 cases of epidural abscess published between 1954 and 1997 developed following epidural anaesthesia and analgesia; 71% of all patients had back pain as the initial presenting symptom and only 66% were febrile (Reihsaus et al 2000, **Level IV**). The classic triad of symptoms (back pain, fever and neurological changes) was present in only 13% of patients with an epidural abscess (in a study unrelated to epidural catheterisation); diagnostic delays occurred in 75% of these patients and such delays led to a significantly higher incidence of residual motor weakness (Davies et al 2004, **Level IV**).

The presence of severe or increasing back pain, even in the absence of a fever, may indicate epidural space infection and should be investigated promptly.

Respiratory depression

The incidence of respiratory depression with epidural analgesia depends on the criteria used to define respiratory depression. In a recent review of published case series and audit data, the reported incidence of respiratory depression ranged from 1.1 (0.6–1.9)% to 15.1 (5.6–34.8)% using respiratory rate and oxygen saturation, respectively, as indicators (see Section 4.1.3 for comments on respiratory rate as an unreliable indicator of respiratory depression); this was very similar to the incidence reported for PCA (Cashman & Dolin 2004, **Level IV**).

Hypotension

The incidence of hypotension depends on the dose of local anaesthetic and criteria used to define hypotension. In the same review as above, the reported incidence of hypotension was 5.6(3.0–10.2%) (Cashman & Dolin 2004, **Level IV**). It is often the result of hypovolaemia (Wheatley et al 2001).

Post dural puncture headache

Headache following dural puncture may occur with an incidence of 0.4–24%. Post dural puncture headache (PDPH) is classically postural in nature and is more common in patients under 50 years of age and in the parturient. Up to 90% of cases improve spontaneously within 10 days (Candido & Stevens 2003).

For discussion of possible prevention and treatment see Section 9.6.5.

Treatment failure

Epidural analgesia may not always be successful due to a number of factors including catheter malposition or displacement, or technical and patient factors resulting in an inability to achieve effective analgesia. Intolerable side effects may also be an indication for premature discontinuation. In a large prospective audit, 22% of patients had premature termination of postoperative epidural infusions: the most common causes were dislodgement (10%) and inadequate analgesia (3.5%), sensory or motor deficit (2.2%). Most of these failures occurred on or after postoperative day 2 (Ballantyne et al 2003, **Level IV**).

Other

There has been concern among surgeons about increased risk of anastomotic leakage after bowel surgery due to the stimulating effects of epidural administration of local anaesthetics; so far there is no evidence to support these claims (Holte & Kehlet 2001, **Level I**).

CHAPTER 7

Key messages

1. All techniques of epidural analgesia for all types of surgery provide better postoperative pain relief compared with parenteral opioid administration (**Level I** [Cochrane Review]).
2. Epidural local anaesthetics improve oxygenation and reduce pulmonary infections and other pulmonary complications compared with parenteral opioids (**Level I**).
3. Thoracic epidural analgesia utilising local anaesthetics improves bowel recovery after abdominal surgery (**Level I**).
4. Thoracic epidural analgesia extended for more than 24 hours reduces the incidence of postoperative myocardial infarction (**Level I**).
5. Epidural analgesia is not associated with increased risk of anastomotic leakage after bowel surgery (**Level I**).
6. Thoracic epidural analgesia reduces incidence of pneumonia and need for ventilation in patients with multiple rib fractures (**Level II**).
7. The combination of thoracic epidural analgesia with local anaesthetics and nutritional support leads to preservation of total body protein after upper abdominal surgery (**Level II**).
8. Lumbar epidural analgesia reduces graft occlusion rates after peripheral vascular surgery (**Level II**).

9. Combinations of low concentrations of local anaesthetics and opioids provide better analgesia than either component alone (**Level II**).

10. The risk of permanent neurologic damage in association with epidural analgesia is very low; the incidence is higher where there have been delays in diagnosing an epidural haematoma or abscess (**Level IV**).

11. Immediate decompression (within 8 hours of the onset of neurological signs) increases the likelihood of partial or good neurological recovery (**Level IV**).

The following tick box ☑ represents conclusions based on clinical experience and expert opinion.

☑ The provision of epidural analgesia by continuous infusion or patient-controlled administration of local anaesthetic-opioid mixtures is safe on general hospital wards, as long as supervised by an anaesthesia-based pain service with 24-hour medical staff cover and monitored by well-trained nursing staff.

7.3 INTRATHECAL ANALGESIA

7.3.1 Drugs used for intrathecal analgesia

Local anaesthetics

Local anaesthetics given intrathecally provide only short-term postoperative analgesia. The use of spinal microcatheters (<24 gauge) for postoperative infusions of local anaesthetics became controversial when multiple cases of cauda equina syndrome were reported (Bevacqua 2003).

Opioids

Intrathecal opioids have been used for surgical procedures ranging from lower limb orthopaedic surgery to coronary artery bypass grafting because of their ability to provide prolonged postoperative analgesia following a single dose. Clinical experience with morphine, fentanyl and sufentanil has shown no neurotoxicity or behavioural changes at normal intrathecal doses (Hodgson et al 1999, **Level IV**).

Efficacy

A prospective study of 5,969 patients given intrathecal morphine (200–800 micrograms) for pain relief following a range of surgical procedures reported a high degree of patient satisfaction and effective analgesia in the first 24 hours. The incidence of pruritus was 37%, nausea and vomiting 25% and respiratory depression 3% ($PaCO_2$ > 50mmHg and/or respiratory rate <8) (Gwirtz et al 1999, **Level IV**). Intrathecal morphine after abdominal surgery (200–400 micrograms) (Kong et al 2002, **Level II**; Devys et al 2003, **Level II**; Fleron et al 2003, **Level II**) and prostatic surgery (50-200 micrograms ± clonidine) (Brown et al 2004, **Level II**) resulted in better analgesia and lower opioid requirements than morphine PCA during the first 24 hours postoperatively.

After coronary artery bypass surgery, intrathecal morphine reduced systemic morphine use and global pain scores, but increased pruritus; there were no significant effects on

CHAPTER 7

mortality, myocardial infarction, dysrhythmias, nausea and vomiting, or time to tracheal extubation (Liu et al 2004, **Level I**). Following hip and knee arthroplasty, intrathecal morphine (100–300 micrograms) provided excellent analgesia for 24 hours after surgery with no difference in side effects; after hip arthroplasty only there was a significant reduction postoperative morphine requirements (Rathmell et al 2003, **Level II**). Also after hip arthroplasty, 100 microgram and 200 microgram doses of intrathecal morphine produced good and comparable pain relief and reductions in postoperative morphine requirements; 50 micrograms was ineffective (Murphy et al 2003, **Level II**).

After caesarean section a single dose of morphine (100 microgram) added to a spinal anaesthetic prolonged the time to first postoperative analgesic administration resulting in at least 11 hours of effective analgesia. Adverse effects included pruritus (43%), nausea (10%) and vomiting (12%). The rate of respiratory depression with intrathecal opioids (all opioids and all doses) was low and not significantly different from controls, with a NNH of 476 for respiratory depression. In these patients, sufentanil and fentanyl showed no analgesic benefits (Dahl et al 1999, **Level I**).

Side effects

Typical side effects of intrathecal opioids include nausea and vomiting, pruritus and delayed respiratory depression. The definition of 'respiratory depression' in different investigations often lacks uniformity with a quarter of the studies cited in a review using respiratory rate as a marker (Ko et al 2003). Patients may be hypoxic or hypercapnic with a normal respiratory rate (Bailey et al 1993, **Level IV**), while others may be able to maintain normocarbia with a lower respiratory rate (Boezaart et al 1999, **Level II**). See Section 4.1 for the use of sedation as a better clinical early indicator of respiratory depression.

Intrathecal morphine produces dose dependent analgesia and respiratory depression. In opioid naïve volunteers, maximum respiratory depression occurred at 3.5–7.5 hours following intrathecal morphine at 200–600 microgram doses (Bailey et al 1993, **Level IV**). Volunteers given 600 micrograms had significant depression of the ventilatory response to carbon dioxide up to 19.5 hours later. Clinical signs or symptoms including respiratory rate, sedation and pupil size, did not reliably indicate hypoventilation or hypoxaemia, unlike peripheral pulse oximetry.

Postoperative nausea and vomiting is common after intrathecal morphine. The combination of ondansetron with either dexamethasone or droperidol had a better antiemetic effect after gynaecological surgery when compared with droperidol plus dexamethasone (Sanchez-Ledesma et al 2002, **Level II**).

Pruritus can be difficult to treat, and a variety of agents have been used including naloxone, nalbuphine, ondansetron, propofol and antihistamines. The itch is thought to be caused by stimulation of spinal and supraspinal mu opioid receptors. Nalbuphine and ondansetron (Charuluxananan et al 2003, **Level II**; Tzeng et al 2003, **Level II**) are effective in reducing spinal opioid-induced pruritus.

Adjuvant drugs

A variety of adjuvant drugs have been used with intrathecal analgesia. Many drugs are not licensed for use as spinal analgesic agents; however adequate evidence from the literature may make their use acceptable (for more detail see Section 5.3).

7.3.2 Combined spinal-epidural versus epidural analgesia in labour

Combined spinal epidural (CSE) analgesia provided faster onset of analgesia and increased maternal satisfaction compared with epidural analgesia (Hughes et al 2003, **Level I**). There was an increased incidence of pruritus in the CSE group but no difference was found with forceps delivery, maternal mobility, post dural puncture headache, caesarean section rates or admission of babies to a neonatal unit. Both standard CSE or epidural techniques provided high maternal satisfaction (see also Section 10.2).

Key messages

1. Combination of spinal opioids with local anaesthetics reduces dose requirements for either drug alone (**Level I**).
2. Intrathecal morphine at doses of 100–200 microgram offers effective analgesia with a low risk of adverse effects (**Level II**).

The following tick box ☑ represents conclusions based on clinical experience and expert opinion.

☑ Clinical experience with morphine, fentanyl and sufentanil has shown no neurotoxicity or behavioural changes at normal clinical intrathecal doses.

7.4 Regional analgesia and concurrent anticoagulant medications

7.4.1 Neuraxial blockade

The low event rate of epidural haematoma makes randomised controlled trials and subsequent evidence-based statements impossible. Information comes only from case reports and case series.

Such information suggests that the incidence is possibly smaller than that of spontaneous epidural haematoma. Between 1962 and 1992, 326 case reports of spontaneous epidural haematoma were published (Schmidt & Nolte 1992), while between 1906 and 1996 only 51 cases of epidural haematoma following epidural anaesthesia or analgesia were reported (Wulf 1996).

Anticoagulation (48% of cases) was the most important risk factor for epidural haematoma following insertion of an epidural needle/catheter, followed by coagulopathy (38% of cases) (Wulf 1996, **Level IV**). This is confirmed by the series of epidural haematomas that followed epidural anaesthesia/analgesia in combination with inappropriate low molecular weight heparin regimens in the USA, where the incidence was reported to be 1 in 3,000 (Horlocker et al 2003).

In view of the increased risk of epidural haematoma associated with the concurrent use of epidural analgesia and anticoagulants, the American Society of Regional Anesthesia and Pain Medicine (ASRA) published a number of consensus statements (Horlocker et al 2003). These statements have to be seen as 'a panel of experts' best faith efforts to offer reasonable pathways for patient management' (Bergqvist et al 2003) and not as a standard of care. They will not substitute for an individual risk/benefit assessment of every patient by the individual anaesthetist. The most relevant statements are summarised as follows (Horlocker et al 2003).

- *Antiplatelet medications* — NSAIDs alone do not significantly increase the risk of spinal haematoma, but should be regarded as a risk factor if combined with other classes of anticoagulants. In such situations COX-2 inhibitors should be considered. Recommended time intervals between discontinuation of other antiplatelet medications and neuraxial blockade are 4–8 hours for eptifibatide and tirofiban, 24–48 hours for abciximab, 7 days for clopidogrel and 14 days for ticlopidine.
- *Unfractionated IV and SC heparin* — Thromboprophylaxis with SC heparin is not a contraindication to neuraxial blockade. To identify heparin-induced thrombocytopenia, a platelet count should be done prior to removal of an epidural catheter in patients who have had more than 4 days of heparin therapy. Intraoperative anticoagulation with IV heparin should start no sooner that 1 hour after placement of the epidural or spinal needle. Epidural catheters should be removed 2–4 hours after the last heparin dose and following an evaluation of the patient's coagulation status. A bloody tap may increase the risk, but there are insufficient data to support cancellation of a case.
- *Low molecular weight heparin* (LMWH) — Epidural catheter placement should occur at least 12 hours after standard prophylactic LMWH doses. The first postoperative dose of LMWH dose should be given 6–8 hours after surgery and subsequent doses every 24 hours after that. The epidural catheter should be removed at least 12 hours after the last dose of LMWH and the next dose should not be given until at least 2 hours after removal.
- *Oral anticoagulants* (warfarin) — Established warfarin therapy should be discontinued at least 4–5 days prior to neuraxial blockade and the International Normalised Ratio (INR) measured. Preoperative initiation of warfarin therapy requires an INR check prior to neuraxial blockade if a single dose of warfarin 5mg was given more than 24 hours preoperatively or a second dose was given. INR should also be checked prior to removal of indwelling epidural catheters if warfarin was administered more than 36 hours preoperatively. An INR < 1.5 is a value estimated to be safe, while INR > 3 requires withholding or reducing warfarin therapy before the catheter is removed.

- *Fibrinolysis and thrombolysis* — Patients receiving fibrinolytic or thrombolytic drugs should not undergo neuraxial blockade except in highly unusual circumstances; no data are available on a safe time interval after use of such drugs. No definite recommendations are given for the removal of neuraxial catheters after initiation of such therapy, although determination of fibrinogen level might be useful in such situations.
- *Herbal therapy* — Although garlic, ginkgo and ginseng have effects on haemostasis, there are currently no specific concerns about their use with neuraxial blockade.
- *New anticoagulants* — The situation with regard to the newer anticoagulants is unclear and for most, recommendations cannot be made at present. Caution is advised with all forms of major regional analgesia until further information is available.

7.4.2 Plexus and other peripheral regional blockade

Significant blood loss rather than neurological deficit seems to be the main risk when plexus or other regional blocks are performed in patients taking anticoagulant medications (Horlocker et al 2003). The previously quoted consensus statements may also be applied to plexus and other peripheral regional techniques, but such application may be more restrictive than necessary (Horlocker et al 2003).

Key messages

1. **Anticoagulation is the most important risk factor for the development of epidural haematoma after neuraxial blockade (Level IV).**

The following tick box ☑ represents conclusions based on clinical experience and expert opinion.

☑ **Consensus statements of experts guide the timing and choice of regional anaesthesia and analgesia in the context of anticoagulation, but do not represent a standard of care and will not substitute the risk/benefit assessment of the individual patient by the individual anaesthetist.**

7.5 Other regional and local analgesic techniques

7.5.1 Continuous peripheral nerve blockade

Continuous peripheral nerve blockade (CPNB) extends the duration of postoperative analgesia beyond the finite period that single injection techniques provide. Important technical issues include the technique used for nerve location, the type of continuous catheter equipment, and local anaesthetic infusion choice and management. Grant et al (2001) describe a CPNB catheter delivery system using an insulated Tuohy needle that allows peripheral nerve stimulation, aspiration for blood, injection of local anaesthesia and catheter passage without having to change needle position or disconnect tubing. Several similar kits are available commercially.

Upper limb

Interscalene

Continuous interscalene analgesia improved analgesia and patient satisfaction and reduced opioid-related side effects compared with IV PCA (Borgeat et al 1997, **Level II**; Borgeat et l 1998, **Level II**; Borgeat et al 2000, **Level II**). Continuous interscalene analgesia provided better analgesia and reduced opioid requirements following shoulder surgery compared with single injection interscalene blockade (Ilfield et al 2000, **Level II;** Klein et al 2000a, **Level II**).

Permanent neurological injury has been reported following injection of local anaesthetic into the cervical spinal cord when an interscalene block was performed under general anaesthesia (Benumof 2000).

Axillary

There is no consistent evidence that continuous axillary analgesia is better than a single axillary brachial plexus injection of a long-acting local anaesthetic. After elective hand surgery continuous axillary infusions of 0.1%, 0.2% ropivacaine or saline were not sufficient to adequately treat pain without the addition of adjunct agents (Salonen et al 2000, **Level II**).

Lower limb

Femoral nerve

Continuous femoral nerve blockade (often called a '3 in 1' block as a catheter placed in the femoral nerve sheath may allow local anaesthetic to reach both the lateral femoral cutaneous and obturator nerves as well as the femoral nerve) provided postoperative analgesia and functional recovery that was better than IV PCA morphine and comparable with epidural analgesia following total knee arthroplasty (Capdevila et al 1999, **Level II**; Singelyn et al 1998, **Level II**). It decreased nausea and vomiting compared with IV morphine and decreased hypotension and urinary retention compared with epidural analgesia (Capdevila et al 1999, **Level II**; Singelyn et al 1998, **Level II**).

Generalisations about the efficacy of different drugs and drug combinations administered via continuous '3 in 1' blocks are difficult because of the wide variety of analgesic agents and concentrations used in various studies. However 0.2% bupivacaine at 10 mL/h reduced morphine consumption and improved functional recovery when compared with 0.1% bupivacaine at 10 mL/hr following total knee arthroplasty (Ganapathy et al 1999, **Level II**) and venous bupivacaine and metabolite concentrations were below toxic levels for 3 days postoperatively.

Femoral nerve block (either single shot or continuous) was more effective than intra-articular local anaesthesia following arthroscopic anterior cruciate ligament reconstruction (Dauri et al 2003; Iskendar et al 2003, **Level II**).

Audit data of patients following total hip replacement indicated that continuous '3 in 1' blocks provided pain relief that was comparable to IV morphine and epidural analgesia; the incidence of nausea, vomiting, pruritis and sedation was reduced compared with IV morphine and there was a reduced incidence of urinary retention and hypotension compared with epidural analgesia (Singelyn & Gouverneur 1999a, **Level III-2**).

Fascia iliaca block

Continuous fascia iliaca block provides similar analgesia to a '3-in-1' block following anterior cruciate ligament repair and the catheter was considered technically easier to insert (Morau et al 2003, **Level II**). It is likely that many catheters placed as a classic '3-in-1' block were in fact relying on local anaesthetic spread along the plane of the fascia iliaca (Capdevila et al 1998; **Level II**). Fascia iliaca block is also of benefit in some paediatric procedures (see Section 10.1.7).

Sciatic nerve

Following total knee arthroplasty, combined sciatic and femoral nerve blockade did not improve analgesia compared with femoral block alone (Allen et al 1998, **Level II**). However, after lower extremity surgery (Ilfeld et al 2002, **Level II**) and foot surgery (White et al 2003a, **Level II**), continuous popliteal sciatic nerve analgesia resulted in better pain relief , lower opioid requirements and fewer side effects compared with opioids alone.

Lumbar plexus

Both continuous posterior lumbar plexus and femoral analgesia significantly reduced 48-hour opioid requirements and pain scores following total knee joint replacement surgery compared with IV PCA morphine (Kaloul et al 2004, **Level II**). There were no differences in pain scores or morphine consumption between the two regional analgesia groups.

Continuous psoas compartment blockade can be used for postoperative analgesia following total hip replacement (Capdevilla et al 2002, **Level IV**) and surgical repair of hip fractures (Chudinov et al 1999, **Level II**).

Thoracic paravertebral blocks

Following cosmetic breast surgery thoracic paravertebral blockade resulted in modest benefits only; reduced nausea (at 24 hours) and opioid requirements compared with general anaesthesia (Klein 2000, **Level II**).

Thoracic paravertebral blockade is more effective than thoracic epidural analgesia for the management of post-thoracotomy pain and leads to better pulmonary function as assessed by peak expiratory flow rate, neuroendocrine stress response, and a lower incidence of side effects (urinary retention, nausea, vomiting) and pulmonary morbidity (Richardson et al 1999, **Level II**).

Intercostal and interpleural blocks

There is no evidence that interpleural analgesia provides superior analgesia compared with thoracic epidural analgesia following thoracotomy for minimally invasive direct coronary artery bypass surgery (Mehta et al 1998, **Level II**). Continuous epidural analgesia is superior to continuous intercostal analgesia following thoracotomy (Debreceni et al 2003, **Level II**).

Patient-controlled regional analgesia

Continuous regional analgesia techniques can be provided with continuous infusion alone, a combination of continuous infusion and patient-controlled bolus doses or patient-controlled bolus doses alone. In a comparison with continuous infusions for '3 in 1' nerve blockade, patient-controlled regional analgesia (PCRA) was associated with similar pain scores and patient satisfaction but reduced consumption of local anaesthetic (Singelyn & Governeur 2000, **Level II**). A study in patients having open shoulder surgery concluded that a baseline infusion, with PCRA added to reinforce the block before physiotherapy, was the best choice (Singelyn & Governeur 2000, **Level II**).

The addition of a background infusion to '3 in 1' PCRA (Singelyn & Gouverneur 2000, **Level II**) or femoral nerve PCRA (Singelyn et al 2001, **Level II**) does not improve pain relief or alter the incidence of side effects but may increase total local anaesthetic consumption. The addition of a background infusion to interscalene brachial plexus PCRA did result in better analgesia (Singelyn et al 1999b, **Level II**).

7.5.2 Intra-articular analgesia

A preliminary small study compared continuous interscalene analgesia with continuous intra-articular analgesia following rotator cuff surgery in an outpatient setting. Both study groups had logistical problems and relatively high pain scores following resolution of the surgical block (Klein et al 2003, **Level II**).

There is evidence of a small benefit only of intra-articular local anaesthesia for postoperative pain after anterior cruciate ligament repair (Møiniche et al 1999, **Level I**). Femoral nerve block (either single shot or continuous) is more effective than intra-articular local anaesthesia following arthroscopic repair (Dauri et al 2003, **Level II**; Iskendar et al 2003, **Level II**).

Intra-articular opioids following knee joint arthroscopy are moderately effective for up to 24 hours if at least 5mg morphine is injected into the joint (Kalso et al 2002, **Level I**). Intra-articular analgesia with opioids is not effective following total knee joint replacement surgery (Badner1997, **Level II**; Maurerhan et al 1997; Klassen et al 1999).

7.5.3 Wound infiltration including wound catheters

Wound infiltration with long-acting local anaesthetics has been shown to lengthen the time until first analgesic request in a number of investigations. A systematic review found that this was most effective following surgery for inguinal hernia repair, where up to 7 hours relief was obtained in comparison with saline. Procedures involving deeper or intracavity structures such as hysterectomy or cholecystectomy showed no benefit (Møiniche et al 1998, **Level I**).

The effectiveness of continuous wound infusion with local anaesthetics administered using an infusion pump or elastomeric device has not been reviewed, but many small randomised trials exist. Although not effective after abdominal surgery (Leong et al 2002, **Level II**), continuous wound infiltration with local anaesthetic for 24–48 hours has been shown to improve pain relief and decrease opioid requirements following anterior cruciate ligament reconstruction, shoulder surgery, spinal surgery and median sternotomy following cardiac surgery (Hoenecke et al 2002, **Level II**; Dowling et al 2003, **Level II**; Gottschalk et al 2003, **Level II**; White et al 2003b, **Level II**; Bianconi et al 2004, **Level II**).

Infusion of ropivacaine into the site of iliac crest bone graft harvest resulted in better pain relief in the postoperative period compared with IV PCA alone and significantly less pain in the iliac crest during movement at 3 months (Blumenthal et al 2005, **Level II**).

7.5.4 Topical application of local anaesthetics

Topical EMLA® cream (eutectic mixture of lignocaine [lidocaine] and prilocaine) is effective in reducing the pain associated with venous ulcer debridement (Briggs 2003, **Level I**). See Section 10.1.4 for use in children and Section 9.9.2 for use in the emergency department.

7.5.5 Safety

Anticoagulation

Caution should be applied in the use of some peripheral nerve or plexus blocks in patients with impaired coagulation (see Section 7.4). This is particularly important for blocks where direct pressure in the event of a traumatised blood vessel is not possible (eg lumbar plexus, psoas compartment, infraclavicular). This risk is highlighted in a recent case report of plexopathy following lumbar plexus blockade in a patient receiving low molecular weight heparin (Capdevila et al 2002).

Nerve injury

Most nerve injury after these techniques presents as residual paraesthesia and rarely as permanent paralysis. In a prospective study, the incidence of neurologic injury following peripheral nerve blocks was 1.9 per 10,000 (Auory et al 1997, **Level IV**). The overall incidence of long-term injury following brachial plexus block ranges between 0.02% and 0.4% depending on the definition of injury and length of follow-up (Borgeat et al 2001, **Level IV**; Klein et al 2002, **Level IV**; Neal et al 2002, **Level IV**).

Permanent neurological injury has been reported following injection of local anaesthetic into the cervical spinal cord when an interscalene block was performed under general anaesthesia (Benumof 2000).

Toxicity

Local anaesthetic toxicity due to accidental intravascular injection or rapid absorption is a known complication of all peripheral nerve blocks, and was associated with cardiac arrest (1.4 per 10,000) or seizures (7.5 per 10,000) in a prospective survey of over 21,000 cases (Auroy et al 1997, **Level IV**). Surveys specifically investigating brachial plexus blocks have reported a higher rate of seizures (0.2%) (Brown et al 1995, **Level IV**; Borgeat et al 2001, **Level IV**).

Key messages

1. Intra-articular local anaesthetics reduce postoperative pain only minimally (**Level I**).

2. Intra-articular opioids following knee arthroscopy provide analgesia for up to 24 hours (**Level I**).

3. Wound infiltration with long-acting local anaesthetics provides effective analgesia following inguinal hernia repair but not open cholecystectomy or hysterectomy (**Level I**).

4. Topical EMLA® cream (eutectic mixture of lignocaine [lidocaine] and prilocaine) is effective in reducing the pain associated with venous ulcer debridement (**Level I** [Cochrane Review]).

5. Continuous interscalene analgesia provides better analgesia, reduced opioid-related side effects and improved patient satisfaction compared with IV PCA after open shoulder surgery (**Level II**).

6. Continuous femoral nerve blockade provides postoperative analgesia and functional recovery superior to IV morphine, with fewer side effects, and comparable to epidural analgesia following total knee joint replacement surgery (**Level II**).

7. Continuous posterior lumbar plexus analgesia is as effective as continuous femoral analgesia following total knee joint replacement surgery (**Level II**).

8. Wound infiltration with continuous infusions of local anaesthetics improves analgesia and reduces opioid requirements following a range of non-abdominal surgical procedures (**Level II**).

REFERENCES

Abboud TK, Zhu J, Gangolly et al (1991) Transnasal butorphanol: a new method for pain relief of post-cesarean section pain. *Acta Anaesthesiol Scand* 35: 14–18.

Allen HW, Liu SS, Ware PD et al (1998) Peripheral nerve blocks improve analgesia after total knee replacement surgery. *Anesth Analg* 87: 93–97.

Aromaa U, Lahdensuu M, Cozanitis DA (1997) Severe complications associated with epidural and spinal anaesthesias in Finland 1987–1993. A study based on patient insurance claims. *Acta Anaesthesiol Scand* 41: 445–52.

Ashburn MA, Love G, Pace NL (1994) Respiratory-related critical events with intravenous patient-controlled analgesia. *Clin J Pain* 10: 52–56.

Auroy Y, Narchi P, Messiah A et al (1997) Serious complications related to regional anesthesia: results of a prospective survey in France. *Anesthesiology* 87: 479–86.

Badner NH, Bourne RB, Rorabeck CH et al (1997) Addition of morphine to intra-articular bupivacaine does not improve analgesia following knee joint replacement. *Reg Anesth* 22: 347–50.

Bailey PL, Rhondeau S, Schafer PG et al (1993) Dose-response pharmacology of intrathecal morphine in human volunteers. *Anesthesiology* 79: 49–59.

Ballantyne JC, Carr DB, deFerranti S et al (1998) The comparative effects of postoperative analgesic therapies on pulmonary outcome: cumulative meta-analyses of randomized, controlled trials. *Anesth Analg* 86: 598–612.

Ballantyne JC, McKenna JM, Ryder E (2003) Epidural analgesia – experience of 5628 patients in a large teaching hospital derived audit. *Acute Pain* 4: 89–97.

Barratt SMS, Smith RC, Kee AJ et al (2000) Multimodal analgesia and intravenous nutrition preserves total body protein following major abdominal surgery *Reg Anesth Pain Med* 27: 15–22.

Beattie WS, Badner NH, Choi P (2001) Epidural analgesia reduces postoperative myocardial infarction: a meta-analysis. *Anesth Analg* 93: 853–58.

Benumof JL (2000) Permanent loss of cervical spinal cord function associated with interscalene block performed under general anesthesia. *Anesthesiology* 93:1541–44.

Bergqvist D, Wu CL, Neal JM (2003) Anticoagulation and neuraxial regional anesthesia: perspectives. *Reg Anesth Pain Med* 28: 163–66.

Bevacqua BK (2003) Continuous spinal anaesthesia: what's new and what's not. *Best Practice & Research. Clinical Anaesthesiology* 17: 393–406.

Bianconi M, Ferraro L, Ricci R et al (2004) The pharmacokinetics and efficacy of ropivacaine continuous wound instillation after spine fusion surgery. *Anesth Analg* 98: 166–72.

Blair JM, Dobson GT, Hill DA et al (2005) Patient controlled analgesia for labour: a comparison of remifentanil with pethidine. *Anaesthesia* 60: 22–27.

Block BM, Liu SS, Rowlingson AJ et al (2003) Efficacy of postoperative epidural analgesia: A meta-analysis. *JAMA* 290: 2455–63.

Blumenthal S, Dullenkopf A, Rentsch K et al (2005). Continuous infusion of ropivacaine for pain relief after iliac crest bone grafting for shoulder surgery. *Anesthesiology* 102: 392–97.

Boezaart AP, Eksteen JA, Spuy GVD et al (1999) Intrathecal morphine double-blind evaluation of optimal dosage for analgesia after major lumbar spinal surgery. *Spine* 24: 1131–37.

Borgeat A, Schappi B, Biasca N et al (1997) Patient-controlled analgesia after major shoulder surgery: patient-controlled interscalene analgesia versus patient-controlled analgesia. *Anesthesiology* 87: 1343–47.

Borgeat A, Tewes E, Biasca N et al (1998) Patient-controlled interscalene analgesia with ropivacaine after major shoulder surgery: PCIA vs PCA. *Br J Anaesth* 81: 603–05.

Borgeat A, Perschak H, Bird P et al (2000) Patient-controlled interscalene analgesia with ropivacaine 0.2% versus patient-controlled intravenous analgesia after major shoulder surgery: effects on diaphragmatic and respiratory function. *Anesthesiology* 92: 102–08.

Borgeat A, Ekatodramis G, Kalberer F et al (2001) Acute and nonacute complications associated with interscalene block and shoulder surgery: a prospective study. *Anesthesiology* 95: 875–80.

Boselli E, Debon R, Cimino Y et al (2004) Background infusion is not beneficial during labor patient-controlled analgesia with ropivacaine 0.1% plus 0.5 μg/ml sufentanil. *Anesthesiology* 100: 968–72.

Briggs M, Nelson EA. Topical agents or dressings for pain in venous leg ulcers. *The Cochrane Database of Systematic Reviews* 2003, Issue 1. Art. No.: CD001177. DOI: 10.1002/14651858.CD001177.

Brown DL, Ransom DM, Hall JA et al (1995) Regional anesthesia and local anesthetic-induced systemic toxicity: seizure frequency and accompanying cardiovascular changes. *Anesth Analg* 81: 321–28.

Brown DR, Hofer RE, Patterson DE et al (2004) Intrathecal anesthesia and recovery from radical prostatectomy. *Anesthesiology* 100: 926–34.

Bulger EM, Edwards T, Klotz P et al (2004) Epidural analgesia improves outcome after multiple rib fractures. *Surgery* 136: 426–30.

Camu F, Van Aken H, Bovill JG (1998) Postoperative analgesic effects of three demand-dose sizes of fentanyl administered by patient-controlled analgesia. *Anesth Analg* 87: 890–95.

Candido K & Stevens R (2003) Post-dural puncture headache: pathophysiology, prevention and treatment. *Best Pract Res Clin Anaesthesiol* 17: 451–69.

Capdevila, XP. Biboulet P, Morau D et al (1998) Comparison of the three-in-one and fascia iliaca compartment blocks in adults: clinical and radiographic analysis. *Anesth Analg* 86: 1039–44.

CHAPTER 7

Capdevila X, Barthelet Y, Biboulet P et al (1999) Effects of perioperative analgesic technique on the surgical outcome and duration of rehabilitation after major knee surgery. *Anesthesiology* 91: 8–15.

Capdevila X, Macaire P, Dadure C et al (2002) Continuous psoas compartment block for postoperative analgesia after total hip arthroplasty: new landmarks, technical guidelines, and clinical evaluation. *Anesth Analg* 94: 1606–13.

Cashman JN, Dolin SJ (2004) Respiratory and haemodynamic effects of acute postoperative pain management: evidence from published data. *Br J Anaesth* 93: 212–23.

Cepeda MS, Delgado M, Ponce M et al (1996) Equivalent outcomes during postoperative patient-controlled intravenous analgesia with lidocaine plus morphine versus morphine alone. *Anesth Analg* 83: 102–06.

Cepeda MS, Africano JM, Manrique AM et al (2002) The combination of low dose of naloxone and morphine in PCA does not decrease opioid requirements in the postoperative period. *Pain* 96: 73–79.

Cepeda MS, Alvarez H, Morales O et al (2004) Addition of ultralow dose naloxone to postoperative morphine PCA: unchanged analgesia and opioid requirements but decreased incidence of opioid side effects. *Pain* 107: 41–46.

Charuluxananan S, Kyokong O, Somboonviboon W et al (2003) Nalbuphine versus ondansetron for prevention of intrathecal morphine-induced pruritus after cesarean delivery. *Anesth Analg* 96: 1789–93.

Chisukata AM (1993) Nurse-call button on a patient-controlled analgesia pump? *Anaesthesia* 48: 90.

Choi PT, Bhandari M, Scott J, Douketis J (2003) Epidural analgesia for pain relief following hip or knee replacement. *The Cochrane Database of Systematic Reviews*, Issue 3. Art. No.: CD003071. DOI: 10.1002/14651858.CD003071.

Choinière M, Rittenhouse BE, Perreault S et al (1998) Efficacy and costs of patient-controlled analgesia versus regularly administered intramuscular opioid therapy. *Anesthesiology* 89: 1377–88.

Christopherson R, Beattie C, Frank SM et al (1993) Perioperative morbidity in patients randomized to epidural or general anesthesia for lower extremity vascular surgery. Perioperative Ischemia Randomized Anesthesia Trial Study Group. *Anesthesiology* 79: 422–34.

Chudinov A, Berkenstadt H, Salai M et al (1999) Continuous psoas compartment block for anesthesia and perioperative analgesia in patients with hip fractures. *Reg Anesth Pain Med* 24: 563–68.

Chumbley GM, Hall GM, Salmon P (1998) Patient-controlled analgesia: an assessment by 200 patients. *Anaesthesia* 53: 216–21.

Chumbley GM, Hall GM, Salmon P (2002) Patient-controlled analgesia: what information does the patient want? *Nursing* 39: 459–71.

Culebras X, Corpataux JB, Gaggero G et al (2003) The antiemetic effect of droperidol added to morphine patient-controlled analgesia: a randomized, controlled, multicenter dose-finding study. *Anesth Analg* 97:816–21.

Curatolo M, Petersen-Felix S, Scaramozzino P et al (1998) Epidural fentanyl, adrenaline and clonidine as adjuvants to local anaesthetics for surgical analgesia:meta-analysis of analgesia and side-effects. *Acta Anaesth Scand* 42: 910–20.

Dahl JB, Jeppesen IS, Jorgensen H et al (1999) Intraoperative and postoperative analgesic efficacy and adverse effects of intrathecal opioids in patients undergoing cesarean section with spinal anesthesia. A qualitative and quantitative systematic review of randomised controlled trials. *Anesthesiology* 91: 1919–27.

Dahlgren N & Tornebrandt K (1995) Neurological complications after anaesthesia. A follow-up of 18,000 spinal and epidural anaesthetics performed over three years. *Acta Anaesthesiol Scand* 39: 872–80.

Dal D, Kanbak M, Caglar M et al (2003) A background infusion of morphine does not enhance postoperative analgesia after cardiac surgery. *Can J Anaesth* 50: 476–79.

Dauri M, Polzoni M, Fabbi E et al (2003) Comparison of epidural, continuous femoral block and intraarticular analgesia after anterior cruciate ligament reconstruction. *Acta Anaesthesiol Scand* 47: 20–25.

Davies DP, Wold RM, Patel RJ et al (2004) The clinical presentation and impact of diagnostic delays on emergency department patients with spinal epidural abscess. *J Emerg Med* 26: 285–91.

Debreceni G, Molnar Z, Szelig L et al (2003) Continuous epidural or intercostal analgesia following thoracotomy: a prospective randomized double-blind clinical trial. *Acta Anaesthesiol Scand* 47: 1091–95.

Devys JM, Mora A, Plaud B et al (2003) Intrathecal + PCA morphine improves analgesia during the first 24 h after major abdominal surgery compared to PCA alone. *Can J Anesth* 50: 355–61.

Dowling R, Thielmeier K, Ghaly A et al (2003) Improved pain control after cardiac surgery: results of a randomized, double-blind, clinical trial. *J Thorac Cardiovasc Surg* 126: 1271–78.

ECRI (1995) Improper cassette attachment allows gravity free-flow from SIMS-Deltec CADD-series pumps. *Health Devices* 24: 84–86.

ECRI (1996) Overinfusion caused by gravity free-flow from a damaged prefilled glass syringe. *Health Devices* 25: 476–77.

ECRI (1997) Abbott PCA Plus II patient-controlled analgesic pumps prone to misprogramming resulting in narcotic overinfusions. *Health Devices* 26: 389–91.

ECRI (2002) Medication safety: PCA pump programming errors continue to cause fatal infusion. *Health Devices* 31: 342–46.

Etches RC (1994) Respiratory depression associated patient-controlled analgesia: a review of eight cases. *Can J Anesth* 41: 125–32.

Etches RC, Gammer T-L, Cornish R (1996) Patient-controlled epidural analgesia after thoracotomy: A comparison of meperidine with and without bupivacaine. *Anesth Analg* 93: 81–86.

Ferrante M, Rosinia FA, Gordon C et al (1994) The role of continuous background infusions in patient-controlled epidural analgesia for labor and delivery. *Anesth Analg* 79: 80–84.

Finger MJ & McLeod DG (1995) Postoperative myocardial infarction after radical cystoprostatectomy masked by patient-controlled analgesia. *Urology* 45: 155–57.

Fleming BM & Coombs DW (1992) A survey of complications documented in a quality-control analysis of patient-controlled analgesia in the postoperative patient. *J Pain Symptom Manage* 7: 463–69.

Fleron M, Weiskopf R, Bertrand M et al (2003) A comparison of intrathecal opioid and intravenous analgesia for the incidence of cardiovascular, respiratory, and renal complications after abdominal aortic surgery. *Anesth Analg* 97: 2–12.

Fredman B, Zohar E, Tarabykin A et al (2001) Bupivacaine wound instillation via an electronic patient-controlled analgesia device and a double-catheter system does not decrease postoperative pain or opioid requirements after major abdominal surgery. *Anesth Analg* 92: 189–93.

Gan TJ, Alexander R, Fennelly M et al (1995) Comparison of different methods of administering droperidol in patient-controlled analgesia in the prevention of postoperative nausea and vomiting. *Anesth Analg* 80: 81–85.

Ganapathy S, Wasserman RA, Watson JT et al (1999) Modified continuous femoral three-in-one block for postoperative pain after total knee arthroplasty. *Anesth Analg* 89: 1197–202.

Giebler RM, Scherer RU, Peters J (1997) Incidence of neurologic complications related to thoracic epidural catheterization. *Anesthesiology* 86: 55–63.

Ginsberg B, Gil KM, Muir M et al (1995) The influence of lockout intervals and drug selection on patient-controlled analgesia following gynaecological surgery. *Pain* 62: 95–100.

Gottschalk A, Burmeister MA, Radtke P et al (2003) Continuous wound infiltration with ropivacaine reduces pain and analgesic requirement after shoulder surgery. *Anesth Analg* 97: 1086–91.

Grant SA, Nielsen KC, Greengrass RA et al (2001) Continuous peripheral nerve block for ambulatory surgery. *Reg Anesth Pain Med* 26: 209–14.

Gwirtz K, Young J, Byers R et al (1999) The safety and efficacy of intrathecal opioid analgesia for acute postoperative pain: Seven years experience with 5969 surgical patients at Indiana University Hospital. *Anesth Analg* 88: 599–604.

Harmer M (1994) Overdosage during patient controlled analgesia. Follow manufacturers' instructions. *BMJ* 309: 1583.

Harrington P, Bunola J, Jennings AJ et al (2000) Acute compartment syndrome masked by intravenous morphine from a patient-controlled analgesia pump. *Injury* 31: 387–89.

Heath ML (1995) Safety of patient-controlled analgesia. *Anaesthesia* 50: 573.

Hodgson PS, Neal JM, Pollock JE et al (1999) The neurotoxicity of drugs given intrathecally (spinal). *Anesth Analg* 88: 797–809.

Hodsman NB, Kenny GN, McArdle CS (1988) Patient controlled analgesia and urinary retention. *Br J Surg* 75: 212.

Hoenecke HR Jr, Pulido PA, Morris BA et al (2002) The efficacy of continuous bupivacaine infiltration following anterior cruciate ligament reconstruction. *Arthroscopy* 18: 854–58.

Holte K & Kehlet H (2001) Epidural analgesia and risk of anastomotic leakage. *Reg Anesth Pain Med* 26: 111–17.

Horlocker TT & Wedel DJ (2000) Neurologic complications of spinal and epidural anesthesia. *Reg Anesth Pain Med* 25: 83–98.

Horlocker TT, Wedel DJ, Benzon H et al (2003) Regional anesthesia in the anticoagulated patient: defining the risks (the second ASRA Consensus Conference on Neuraxial Anesthesia and Anticoagulation). *Reg Anesth Pain Med* 28: 172–97.

Hughes D, Simmons SW, Brown J et al (2003) Combined spinal-epidural versus epidural analgesia in labour. *The Cochrane Database of Systematic Reviews.* Issue 4. Art. No.: CD003401. DOI: 10.1002/14651858.CD003401.

Ilfeld BM, Morey TE, Wand RD et al (2002) Continuous popliteal sciatic nerve block for postoperative pain control at home. *Anesthesiology* 97: 959–65.

Ilfeld BM, Morey TE, Wright TW et al (2003) Continuous interscalene brachial plexus block for postoperative pain control at home: a randomized, double-blinded, placebo-controlled study. *Anesth Analg* 96:1089–95.

Iskandar H, Benard A, Ruel-Raymond J et al (2003) Femoral block provides superior analgesia compared with intra-articular ropivacaine after anterior cruciate ligament reconstruction. *Reg Anesth Pain Med* 28: 29–32.

Jacox A, Carr DB, Mahrenholz DM et al (1997) Cost considerations in patient-controlled analgesia. *Pharmacoeconomics* 12: 109–20.

Jeffs SA, Hall JE, Morris S (2002) Comparison of morphine alone with morphine plus clonidine for postoperative patient-controlled analgesia. *Br J Anaesth* 89: 424–27.

Jørgensen H, Wetterslev J, Møiniche S, Dahl JB (2001) Epidural local anaesthetics versus opioid-based analgesic regimens for postoperative gastrointestinal paralysis, PONV and pain after abdominal surgery. *The Cochrane Database of Systematic Reviews*, Issue 1. Art. No.: CD001893. DOI: 10.1002/14651858.CD001893.

Kaloul I, Guay J, Cote C et al (2004) The posterior lumbar plexus (psoas compartment) block and the three-in-one femoral nerve block provide similar postoperative analgesia after total knee replacement. *Can J Anaesth* 51: 45–51.

Kalso E, Smith L, McQuay HJ et al (2002) No pain, no gain: clinical excellence from scientific rigour – lessons learned from IA morphine. *Pain* 98: 269–75.

Kampe S, Weigand C, Kaufmann J et al (1999) Postoperative analgesia with no motor block by continuous epidural infusion of ropivacaine 0.1% and sufentanil after total hip replacement. *Anesth Analg* 89: 395–98.

Kane RE (1981) Neurologic deficits following epidural or spinal anesthesia. *Anesth Analg* 60: 150–61.

Kendall JM, Reeves BC, Latter VS (2001) Multicentre randomised controlled trial of nasal diamorphine for analgesia in children and teenagers with clinical fractures. Nasal Diamorphine Trial Group. *BMJ* 322: 261–65.

Kindler C, Seeberger M, Siegemund M et al (1996) Extradural abscess complicating lumbar extradural anaesthesia and analgesia in an obstetric patient. *Acta Anaesthesiol Scand* 40: 858–61.

Klasen JA, Opitz SA, Melzer C et al (1999) Intraarticular, epidural, and intravenous analgesia after total knee arthroplasty. *Acta Anaesthesiol Scand* 43: 1021–26.

Klein SM, Grant SA, Greengrass RA et al (2000a) Interscalene brachial plexus block with a continuous catheter insertion system and a disposable infusion pump. *Anesth Analg* 91: 1473–78.

Klein SM, Bergh A, Steele SM et al (2000b) Thoracic paravertebral block for breast surgery. *Anesth Analg* 90: 1402–05.

Klein SM, Nielsen KC, Greengrass RA et al (2002) Ambulatory discharge after long-acting peripheral nerve blockade: 2382 blocks with ropivacaine. *Anesth Analg* 94: 65–70.

Klein SM, Steele SM, Nielsen KC et al (2003) The difficulties of ambulatory interscalene and intra-articular infusions for rotator cuff surgery: a preliminary report. *Can J Anaesth* 50: 265–69.

Kluger MT & Owen H (1990) Antireflux valves in patient-controlled analgesia. *Anaesthesia* 45: 1057–61.

Ko S, Goldstein DH, VanDenKerkhof EG (2003) Definitions of 'respiratory depression' with intrathecal morphine postoperative analgesia: a review of the literature. *Can J Anaesth* 50: 679–88.

Komatsu H, Matsumoto S, Mitsuhata H et al (1998) Comparison of patient-controlled epidural analgesia with and without background infusion after gastrectomy. *Anesth Analg* 87: 907–10.

Komatsu H, Matsumoto S, Mitsuhata H (2001) Comparison of patient-controlled epidural analgesia with and without night-time infusion after gastrectomy. *Br J Anaesth* 87: 633–35.

Kong SK, Onsiong SMK, Chui WK et al (2002) Use of intrathecal morphine for postoperative pain relief after elective laparoscopic colorectal surgery. *Anaesthesia* 57: 1168–73.

Kwan A (1995) Overdose of morphine during PCA. *Anaesthesia* 50: 919.

Leeson-Payne CG, Towell T (1996) Magnetic mayhem. *Anaesthesia* 51: 1081–82.

Leong WM, Lo WK, Chiu JW (2002) Analgesic efficacy of continuous delivery of bupivacaine by an elastomeric balloon infusor after abdominal hysterectomy: a prospective randomised controlled trial. *Aust N Z J Obstet Gynaecol* 42: 515–18.

Liu S, Angel JM, Owens BD et al (1995) Effects of epidural bupivacaine after thoracotomy. *Reg Anesth* 20: 303–10.

Liu SS, Allen HW, Olsson GL (1998) Patient-controlled epidural analgesia with bupivacaine and fentanyl on hospital wards: prospective experience with 1,030 surgical patients. *Anesthesiology* 88: 688–95.

Liu SS, Block BM, Wu CL (2004) Effects of perioperative central neuraxial analgesia on outcome after coronary artery bypass surgery: a meta-analysis. *Anesthesiology* 101: 153–61.

Lowson SM, Alexander JI, Black AMS et al (1994) Epidural diamorphine infusions with and without 0.167% bupivacaine for post-operative analgesia. *Eur J Anaesthesiol* 11: 345–52.

Macintyre PE &Jarvis DA (1996) Age is the best predictor of postoperative morphine requirements. *Pain* 64: 357–64.

Macintyre PE (2001) Safety and efficacy of patient-controlled analgesia. *Br J Anaesth* 87: 36–46.

Manjushree R, Lahiri A, Ghosh BR et al (2002) Intranasal fentanyl provided adequate postoperative analgesia in paediatric patients. *Can J Anesth* 49: 190–93.

Mauerhan DR, Campbell M, Miller JS et al (1997) Intra-articular morphine and/or bupivacaine in the management of pain after total knee arthroplasty. *J Arthroplasty* 12: 546–52.

Mehta Y, Swaminathan M, Mishra Y et al (1998)A comparative evaluation of intrapleural and thoracic epidural analgesia for postoperative pain relief after minimally invasive direct coronary artery bypass surgery. *J Cardiothorac Vasc Anesth* 12: 162–65.

Meyer GS & Eagle KA (1992) Patient-controlled analgesia masking pulmonary embolus in a postoperative patient. *Crit Care Med* 20: 1619–21.

Moen V, Dahlgren N, Irestedt L (2004) Severe neurological complications after central neuraxial blockades in Sweden 1990-1999. *Anesthesiology* 101: 950–59.

Møiniche S, Mikkelsen S, Wetterslev J et al (1998) A systematic review of incisional local anesthesia for postoperative pain relief after abdominal operations. *Br J Anaesth* 81: 377–83.

Møiniche S, Mikkelsen S, Wetterslev J et al (1999) A systematic review of intra-articular local anesthesia for postoperative pain relief after arthroscopic knee surgery. *Reg Anesth Pain Med* 24: 430–37.

Morau D, Lopez S, Biboulet P et al (2003) Comparison of continuous 3-in-1 and fascia Iliaca compartment blocks for postoperative analgesia: feasibility, catheter migration, distribution of sensory block, and analgesic efficacy. *Reg Anesth Pain Med* 28: 309–14.

Murphy PM, Stack D, Kinirons B et al (2003) Optimising the dose of intrathecal morphine in older patients undergoing hip arthroplasty. *Anesth Analg* 97: 1709–15.

Neal JM, Hebl JR, Gerancher JC et al (2002) Brachial plexus anesthesia: essentials of our current understanding. *Reg Anesth Pain Med* 27: 402–28.

Niemi G & Breivik H (1998) Adrenaline markedly improves thoracic epidural analgesia produced by a low-dose infusion of bupivacaine, fentanyl and adrenaline after major surgery. A randomised, double-blind, cross-over study with and without adrenaline. *Acta Anaesthesiol Scand* 42: 897–909.

Niemi G & Breivik H (2002) Adrenaline markedly improves thoracic epidural analgesia produced by a low-dose infusion of ropivacaine, fentanyl and adrenaline after major surgery. A randomised, double-blind, cross-over study with and without epinephrine. *Anesth Analg* 94: 1598–1605.

Nolan JP, Dow AAC, Parr MJA et al (1992) Patient-controlled analgesia following post-traumatic pelvic reconstruction. *Anaesthesia* 47: 1037–41.

Notcutt WG & Morgan RJ (1990) Introducing patient-controlled analgesia for postoperative pain control into a district general hospital. *Anaesthesia* 45: 401–06.

Notcutt WG, Knowles P, Kaldas R (1992) Overdose of opioid from patient-controlled analgesia pumps. *Br J Anaesth* 69: 95–97.

Owen H, Plummer JL, Armstrong I et al (1989) Variables of patient-controlled analgesia 1. bolus size. *Anaesthesia* 44: 7–10.

Owen H, Kluger MT, Plummer JL (1990) Variables of patient-controlled analgesia 4: the relevance of bolus dose size to supplement a background infusion. *Anaesthesia* 45: 619–22.

Paech MJ, Moore JS, Evans SF (1994 Meperidine for patient-controlled analgesia after cesarean section. Intravenous versus epidural administration. *Anesthesiology*. 80: 1268–76.

Paech MJ, Pavy TJ, Orlikowski CE et al (2000) Postoperative intraspinal opioid analgesia after caesarean section; a randomised comparison of subarachnoid morphine and epidural pethidine. *Int J Obstet Anesth* 9: 238–45.

Paech MJ, Lim CB, Banks SL et al (2003) A new formulation of nasal spray for postoperative analgesia: a pilot study. *Anaesthesia* 58: 740–44.

Pang WW, Mok MS, Lin CH et al (1999) Comparison of patient-controlled analgesia (PCA) with tramadol or morphine. *Can J Anaesth* 46: 1030–35.

Parker RK, Holtmann B, White PF (1991) Patient-controlled analgesia. Does a concurrent opioid infusion improve pain management after surgery? *JAMA* 266: 1947–52.

Parker RK, Holtmann B, White PF (1992) Effects of a nighttime opioid infusion with PCA therapy on patient comfort and analgesic requirements after abdominal hysterectomy. *Anesthesiology* 76: 362–67.

Plummer JL, Owen H, Ilsley AH et al (1997) Morphine patient-controlled analgesia is superior to meperidine patient-controlled analgesia for postoperative pain. *Anesth Analg* 84: 794–99.

Rapp SE, Egan KJ, Ross BK et al (1996) A multidimensional comparison of morphine and hydromorphone patient-controlled analgesia. *Anesth Analg* 82: 1043–48.

Rathmell JP, Pino CA, Taylor R et al (2003) Intrathecal morphine for postoperative analgesia: a randomized, controlled, dose-ranging study after hip and knee arthroplasty. *Anesth Analg* 97: 1452–57.

Rawal N, Axelsson K, Hylander et al (1998) Postoperative patient-controlled local anesthetic administration at home. *Anesth Analg* 86: 86–89.

Rees DC, Olujohungbe AD, Parker NE et al (2003) Guidelines for the management of the acute painful crisis in sickle cell disease. *Br J Haematol* 120: 744–52.

Reeves M, Lindholm DE, Myles PS et al (2001) Adding ketamine to morphine for patient-controlled analgesia after major abdominal surgery: A double-blinded, randomized controlled trial. *Anesth Analg* 93: 116–20.

Reihsaus E, Waldbaur H, Seeling W (2000) Spinal epidural abscess; a meta-analysis of 915 patients. *Neurosurg Rev* 23: 175–204.

Richards H, Langston A, Kulkarni R et al (2004) Does patient controlled analgesia delay the diagnosis of compartment syndrome following intramedullary nailing of the tibia. *Injury* 35: 296–98.

Richardson J, Sabanathan S, Jones J et al (1999) A prospective, randomized comparison of preoperative and continuous balanced epidural or paravertebral bupivacaine on post-thoracotomy pain, pulmonary function and stress responses. *Br J Anaesth* 83: 387–92.

Rittenhouse BE & Choinière M (1999) An economic evaluation of pain therapy after hysterectomy: patient-controlled analgesia versus regular intramuscular opioid therapy. *Int J Tech Assess Health Care* 15: 548–62.

Rutherford J & Patri M (2004) Failure of antireflux valve in a Vygon PCA set. *Anaesthesia* 59: 511.

Rygnestad T, Borchgrevink PC, Eide E (1997) Postoperative epidural infusion of morphine and bupivacaine is safe on surgical wards. Organisation of the treatment, effects and side-effects in 2000 consecutive patients. *Acta Anaesthesiol Scand* 41: 868–76.

Salonen MH, Haasio J, Bachmann M et al (2000) Evaluation of efficacy and plasma concentrations of ropivacaine in continuous axillary brachial plexus block: high dose for surgical anesthesia and low dose for postoperative analgesia. *Reg Anesth Pain Med* 25: 47–51.

Sanchez-Ledesma MJ, López-Olaondo L, Pueyo FJ et al (2002) A comparison of three antiemetic combinations for the prevention of postoperative nausea and vomiting. *Anesth Analg* 95: 1590–95.

Sartain JB, Barry JJ, Richardson CA et al (2003) Effect of combining naloxone and morphine for intravenous patient-controlled analgesia, *Anesthesiology* 99: 148–51.

Schmidt A & Nolte H (1992) [Subdural and epidural hematomas following epidural anesthesia. A literature review]. *Anaesthesist* 41: 276–84.

Schug SA & Torrie JJ (1993) Safety assessment of postoperative pain management by an acute pain service. *Pain* 55: 387–91.

Scott DA, Blake D, Buckland M et al (1999) A comparison of epidural ropivacaine infusion alone and in combination with 1, 2, and 4 microg/mL fentanyl for seventy-two hours of postoperative analgesia after major abdominal surgery. *Anesth Analg* 88: 857–64.

Scott NB, Mogensen T, Bigler D et al (1989) Continuous thoracic extradural 0.5% bupivacaine with or without morphine: effect on quality of blockade, lung function and the surgical stress response. *Br J Anaesth* 62: 253–57.

Sidebotham D, Dijkhuizen MR, Schug SA (1997) The safety and utilization of patient-controlled analgesia. *J Pain* Symptom Manage 14: 202–09.

Silvasti M, Rosenberg P, Seppala T et al (1998) Comparison of analgesic efficacy of oxycodone and morphine in postoperative intravenous patient-controlled analgesia. *Acta Anaesthesiol Scand* 42: 576–80.

Silvasti M, Tarkkila P, Tuominen M et al (1999) Efficacy and side effects of tramadol versus oxycodone for patient-controlled analgesia after maxillofacial surgery. *Eur J Anaesthesiol* 16: 834–39.

Silvasti M & Pitkanen M (2001) Patient-controlled epidural analgesia versus continuous epidural analgesia after total knee arthroplasty. *Acta Anaesthesiol Scand* 45: 471–76.

Sinatra RS, Lodge K, Sibert K et al (1989) A comparison of morphine, meperidine and oxymorphone as utilized in patient-controlled analgesia following Cesarean delivery. *Anesthesiology* 70: 585–90.

Singelyn FJ, Aye F, Gouverneur JM (1997) Continuous popliteal sciatic nerve block: an original technique to provide postoperative analgesia after foot surgery. *Anesth Analg* 84: 383–86.

Singelyn FJ, Deyaert M, Joris D et al (1998) Effects of intravenous patient-controlled analgesia with morphine, continuous epidural analgesia, and continuous three-in-one block on postoperative pain and knee rehabilitation after unilateral total knee arthroplasty. *Anesth Analg* 87: 88–92.

Singelyn FJ & Gouverneur JM (1999a) Postoperative analgesia after total hip arthroplasty: i.v. PCA with morphine, patient-controlled epidural analgesia, or continuous '3-in-1' block?: a prospective evaluation by our acute pain service in more than 1,300 patients. *J Clin Anesth* 11: 550–54.

Singelyn FJ, Seguy S, Gouverneur JM (1999b) Interscalene brachial plexus analgesia after open shoulder surgery: continuous versus patient-controlled infusion. *Anesth Analg* 89: 1216–20.

Singelyn FJ & Gouverneur JM (2000) Extended 'three-in-one' block after total knee arthroplasty: continuous versus patient-controlled techniques. *Anesth Analg* 91: 176–80.

Singelyn FJ, Venderelst PE, Gouverneur JM (2001) Extended 'femoral nerve sheath block after total hip arthroplasty: continuous versus patient-controlled techniques. *Anesth Analg* 92: 455–59.

Snijdelaar DG, Cornelisse HB, Schmid RL et al (2004) A randomised, controlled study of peri-operative low dose s(+) ketamine in combination with postoperative patient-controlled s(+) ketamine and morphine after radical prostatectomy *Anaesthesia* 59: 222–28.

Stamer UM, Maier C, Grond S et al (1997) Tramadol in the management of postoperative pain: A double blind placebo and active drug controlled study. *Eur J Anaesthesiol* 14: 646–54.

Standl T, Burmeister MA, Ohnesorge H et al (2003) Patient-controlled epidural analgesia reduces analgesic requirements compared to continuous epidural infusion after major abdominal surgery. *Can J Anaesth* 50: 258–64.

Stanley G, Appadu B, Mead M et al (1996) Dose requirements, efficacy and side effects of morphine and pethidine delivered by patient-controlled analgesia after gynaecological surgery. *Br J Anaesth* 76: 484–86.

Steinbrook RA (1998) Epidural anesthesia and gastrointestinal motility. *Anesth Analg* 86: 830–36.

Striebel SW, Malewicz J, Hermanns K et al (1993) Intranasal meperidine titration for postoperative pain relief. *Anesth Analg* 76: 1042–51.

Striebel SW, Bonillo B, Schwagmeier R et al (1995) Self-administered nasal meperidine for postoperative pain management. *Can J Anesth* 42: 287–91.

Striebel SW, Oelmann T, Spies C et al (1996) Patient-controlled intranasal analgesia: a method for non-invasive postoperative pain management. *Anesth Analg* 83: 548–51.

Striebel HW, Scheitza W, Philippi W et al (1998) Quantifying oral analgesic consumption using a novel method and comparison with patient-controlled intravenous analgesic consumption. *Anesth Analg* 86: 1051–53.

Subramaniam K, Subramaniam B, Steinbrook RA (2004) Ketamine as adjuvant analgesic to opioids: a quantitative and qualitative systematic review. *Anesth Analg* 99: 482–95.

Tanaka K, Watanabe R, Harada T et al (1993) Extensive application of epidural anesthesia and analgesia in a university hospital: incidence of complications related to technique. *Reg Anesth* 18: 34–38.

Thomas DW &Owen H (1988) Patient-controlled analgesia--the need for caution. A case report and review of adverse incidents. *Anaesthesia* 43: 770–72.

Toussaint S, Maidl J, Schwagmeier R et al (2000) Patient-controlled intranasal analgesia: effective alternative to intravenous PCA for postoperative pain relief. *Can J Anaesth* 47: 299–302.

Tramèr MR & Walder B (1999) Efficacy and adverse effects of prophylactic antiemetics during patient-controlled analgesia therapy: A quantitative systematic review. *Anesth Analg* 88: 1354–61.

Tsui SL, Irwinmg, Wong CM et al (1997) An audit of the safety of an acute pain service. *Anaesthesia* 52: 1042–47.

Tuman KJ, McCarthy RJ, March RJ et al (1991) Effects of epidural anesthesia and analgesia on coagulation and outcome after major vascular surgery. *Anesth Analg* 73: 696–704.

Tzeng JI, Chu KS, Ho ST et al (2003) Prophylactic iv ondansetron reduces nausea, vomiting and pruritus following epidural morphine for postoperative pain control. *Can J Anaesth* 50: 1023–26.

Urquhart ML, Klapp K, White PF (1988) Patient-controlled analgesia: a comparison of intravenous versus subcutaneous hydromorphone. *Anesthesiology* 69: 428–32.

Van der Vyver M, Halpern S, Joseph G (2002) Patient-controlled epidural analgesia versus continuous infusion for labour analgesia: a meta-analysis. *Br J Anaesth* 89: 459–65.

Vincente KJ, Kada-Bekhaled K, Hillel G et al (2003) Programming errors contribute to death from patient-controlled analgesia: case report and estimate of probability. *Can J Anesth* 50: 328–32.

Viscusi ER, Reynolds L, Chung F et al (2004) Patient-controlled transdermal fentanyl hydrochloride vs intravenous morphine pump for postoperative pain. *JAMA* 291: 1333–41.

Wakerlin G & Larson CP (1990) Spouse-controlled analgesia. *Anesth Analg* 70: 119.

Walder B, Schafer M, Henzi H et al (2001) Efficacy and safety of patient-controlled opioid analgesia for acute postoperative pain. *Acta Anaesthesiol Scand* 45: 795–804.

Wang LP, Hauerberg J, Schmidt JF (1999) Incidence of spinal epidural abscess after epidural analgesia: a national 1-year survey. *Anesthesiology* 91: 1928–36.

Ward M, Minto G, Alexander-Williams JM (2002) A comparison of patient-controlled analgesia administered by the intravenous or intranasal route during the early postoperative period. *Anaesthesia* 57: 48–52.

Werawatganon T, Charuluxanun S (2004). Patient controlled intravenous opioid analgesia versus continuous epidural analgesia for pain after intra-abdominal surgery. *The Cochrane Database of Systematic Reviews*. Issue 3. Art. No.: CD004088. DOI: 10.1002/14651858.CD004088.pub2.

Wheatley RG, Schug SA, Watson D (2001) Safety and efficacy of postoperative epidural analgesia. *Br J Anaesth* 87: 47–61.

White PF (1990) Subcutaneous-PCA: an alternative to IV-PCA for postoperative pain management. *Clin J Pain* 6: 297–300

White PF, Issioui T, Skrivanek GD et al (2003a) The use of a continuous popliteal sciatic nerve block after surgery involving the foot and ankle: does it improve the quality of recovery? *Anesth Analg* 97:1303–09.

White PF, Shivani S, Latham P et al (2003b) Use of a continuous local anesthetic infusion for pain management after median sternotomy. *Anesthesiology* 99: 918–23.

Wong K, Chong JL, Lo WK et al (2000) A comparison of patient-controlled epidural analgesia following gynaecological surgery with and without a background infusion. *Anesthesia* 55: 212–16.

Woodhouse A, Hobbes AFT, Mather LE et al (1996) A comparison of morphine, pethidine and fentanyl in the postsurgical patient-controlled analgesia (PCA) environment. *Pain* 64: 115–21.

Woodhouse A, Ward ME, Mather LE (1999) Intra subject variability in postoperative patient-controlled analgesia (PCA): Is the patient equally satisfied with morphine, pethidine and fentanyl? *Pain* 80: 545–53.

Wulf H (1996) Epidural anaesthesia and spinal haematoma. *Can J Anaesth* 43: 1260–71.

Xie R & Liu YP (1991) Survey of the use of epidural analgesia in China. *Chin Med J* 104: 510–15.

Zohar E, Fredman B, Phillipov A et al (2001) The analgesic efficacy if patient-controlled bupivacaine wound instillation after total abdominal hysterectomy with bilateral salpingo-oopherectomy. *Anesth Analg* 93: 482–87.

8. NON-PHARMACOLOGICAL TECHNIQUES

8.1 Psychological interventions

Psychological interventions used in the management of acute pain are generally seen as adjuncts to pharmacological and physical therapeutic modalities, but there is growing evidence for the value of their contribution.

Psychological interventions may be grouped into the following categories: information provision (procedural or sensory); relaxation and attentional strategies; and hypnosis and cognitive-behavioural interventions.

8.1.1 Provision of information

Procedural information is information given to a patient before any treatment that summarises what will happen during that treatment. *Sensory information* is information that describes the sensory experiences the patient may expect during the treatment. The benefits or otherwise of providing procedural and/or sensory information may vary according to patient group.

Combined sensory-procedural information is effective in reducing negative affect and reports of procedure-related pain and distress in patients undergoing various diagnostic, dental, experimental pain and other procedures (Suls & Wan 1989, **Level I**). Only a small number of studies included in this analysis investigated the effects in patients having surgery where the combination led to improved pain relief and postoperative activity (Miro & Raich 1999, **Level II**).

However, results regarding the efficacy of the individual techniques are conflicting. In patients undergoing surgery, procedural information was reported to be effective in reducing negative affect, pain report, pain medication use and behavioural and clinical recovery (Johnston & Vogele 1993, **Level I**) while it is of no significant benefit after a variety of mainly non-surgical procedures (Suls & Wan 1989, **Level I**).

In patients undergoing surgery the provision of sensory information has no significant benefit (Campbell et al 1999, **Level II**) but it may have some, albeit inconsistent, value in other procedures (Suls & Wan 1989, **Level I**).

In some patients, especially those with an avoidant coping style, providing too much information or the need to make too many decisions may exacerbate anxiety and pain (Wilson 1981, **Level II**) although this may not be a strong effect (Miro & Raich 1999, **Level II**). Nevertheless, it may be useful to assess a patient's normal approach to managing stress (coping style) in order to identify the best options for that patient (Wilson 1981, **Level II**; Miro & Raich 1999, **Level II**).

8.1.2 Relaxation and attentional strategies

Relaxation

Relaxation training usually involves teaching a patient ways to calm him/herself, either by listening to a recorded audiotape or following written or spoken instructions, which may then be memorised by the patient. Some methods focus on altering muscle tension, often sequentially, while others concentrate on altering breathing patterns. Regardless of the approach used, repeated practice of the technique by the patient is regarded as critical. Relaxation techniques are closely related to, and often indistinguishable from, forms of meditation and self-hypnosis.

The use of relaxation techniques in cancer patients undergoing acute medical treatment was effective in reducing treatment-related pain as well as pulse rate, blood pressure and emotional adjustment variables (depression, anxiety and hostility) (Luebbert et al 2001, **Level I**). However, a systematic review of the use of relaxation techniques in the perioperative setting, in which a lack of appropriate data meant that a meta-analysis was not undertaken, showed that there is currently little convincing evidence of benefit (Seers & Carroll 1998).

Attentional techniques

Attentional techniques aim to alter a patient's attention in relation to their pain. A range of such strategies have been reported from those involving distraction using imaginary scenes or sensations, to those that focus on external stimuli such as music, scenes or smells. Some techniques also involve modification or re-interpretation of the experience of pain (Logan et al 1995). Attempting to alter the patient's emotional state, from stress or fear to comfort or peace, is also a common feature of many of these practices, which are often used in conjunction with relaxation methods (Williams 1996).

In acute postoperative pain there is some evidence to support the use of some attentional techniques, often in combination with relaxation, to reduce reported pain and analgesic use (Daake & Gueldner 1989, **Level II**; Good et al 1999, **Level II**; Miro & Raich 1999, **Level II**; Voss et al 2004, **Level II**). Music does not reduce anxiety levels or pain in patients undergoing surgery or invasive procedures (Evans 2002, **Level I**).

There is also some evidence to suggest that rather than shifting a patient's attention away from the pain, instructions to focus on the sensory rather than emotional stimuli during a painful procedure can alter pain perception and reduce pain in patients classified as having a high desire for control but low perceived control (Baron et al 1993, **Level II**; Logan et al 1995, **Level II**). Instructing patients to focus their attention on the pain site was more effective than listening to music in reducing pain associated with burns dressing (Haythornthwaite et al 2001, **Level II**).

8.1.3 Hypnosis

The essential components of hypnosis are considered to be a"narrowed focus of attention, reduced awareness of external stimuli, with absorption in and increased responsiveness to hypnotic suggestions" (Gamsa 2003). The variable or unstandardised nature of hypnotic procedures makes it difficult to compare studies or draw general conclusions about the effectiveness of the technique (Ellis & Spanos 1994).

Hypnosis has been shown to provide effective relief of pain in both laboratory and clinical settings (Montgomery et al 2000, **Level I**). Most of the studies using hypnosis for the management of clinical acute pain have focused on acute procedural pain. A review of the use of hypnosis in the management of clinical pain concluded that it was effective in reducing acute pain associated with medical procedures, such as that during burn wound care and bone marrow aspiration, and childbirth (Patterson & Jensen 2003; Cyna et al 2004, **Level I**). In patients with cancer, hypnosis also reduces the pain associated with procedures such as breast biopsy, lumbar puncture and bone marrow aspiration (Wall & Womack 1989, **Level II**; Liossi & Hatira 1999, **Level II**; Montgomery et al 2002, **Level II**; Liossi & Hatira 2003, **Level II**). Hypnosis may be as effective as cognitive behavioural interventions in these settings (Liossi & Hatira 1999, **Level II**).

Hypnosis used in labour leads to a decreased requirement for pharmacological analgesia, increased incidence of spontaneous vaginal delivery and decreased use of labour augmentation (Cyna et al 2004, **Level I**).

8.1.4 Cognitive-behavioural interventions

Cognitive-behavioural interventions involve the application of principles derived from the study of learning (or behaviour change) and experimentally derived methods to change the ways in which pain sufferers perceive and react to their pain (and other stressors) (Bradley 1996).

Cognitive-behavioural interventions focus on overt behaviours and cognitions (thought processes) in patients as well as on environmental contexts. Interactions between the patient and others, especially health care providers and family members, may need to be changed to support the desired response in the patient. These interventions may be helpful in promoting an increased sense of control and reducing the sense of hopelessness and helplessness common among patients with acute pain.

Critically, cognitive-behavioural principles require the patient to be an active participant in the process, rather than a passive recipient. In addition to a technique like relaxation, methods taught involve active problem-solving and addressing unhelpful beliefs and responses.

Specific pain coping strategies

Coping strategies include all ways in which a person attempts to respond (cognitively or behaviourally) to pain. Patients who respond with overly alarmist or catastrophic thoughts tend to experience more pain and distress (Jensen et al 1991; Haythornthwaite et al 2001, **Level II**; Sullivan et al 2001). A given coping strategy may not be useful in all circumstances (Turk & Monarch 2002). For example, ignoring or denying the presence of pain may be helpful when first injured (to reduce distress), but could later delay appropriate diagnosis and treatment.

Training in coping methods or behavioural instruction prior to surgery results in improved measures of pain, negative affect and reduced analgesic use (Johnston & Vogele 1993, **Level I**).

Broader cognitive-behavioural interventions

Cognitive-behavioural interventions commonly used to reduce procedure-related pain in children and adolescents include breathing exercises, relaxation, distraction, imagery, filmed modelling, reinforcement/incentive, behavioural rehearsal and active coaching by a parent or health care provider (Powers 1999). In children, adolescents or adults undergoing cancer-related diagnostic and treatment procedures, similar interventions may result in a clinically significant reduction in pain (Ellis & Spanos 1994; DuHamel et al 1999; Liossi & Hatira 1999, **Level II**; Redd et al 2001).

Reports of benefit after surgery are much less common. However, a recent study of adolescent patients after spinal fusion surgery showed that information plus training in coping strategies achieved the greatest pain reduction, compared with information only, coping strategies only, and a control. The effect was most evident in subjects aged 11–13 years, compared with the 14–18 year age group, where no differences between interventions were found (La Montagne et al 2003, **Level II**).

Key messages

1. Combined sensory-procedural information is effective in reducing pain and distress (**Level I**).
2. Training in coping methods or behavioural instruction prior to surgery reduces pain, negative affect and analgesic use (**Level I**).
3. Hypnosis and attentional techniques reduce procedure-related pain (**Level II**).

8.2 TRANSCUTANEOUS ELECTRICAL NERVE STIMULATION

A systematic review published in 1996 concluded that transcutaneous electrical nerve stimulation (TENS) was not effective for the relief of postoperative pain (Carroll et al 1996). The authors noted that non-randomised studies overestimated the beneficial effects of TENS.

Another group later argued that some of the studies reporting no benefit from TENS may have used ineffective treatment doses — low and possibly ineffective current intensities or sensory threshold intensity. They performed a systematic review of publications using TENS after surgery where 'assumed optimal TENS parameters' were used; that is, if TENS was administered at an intensity described by the patients as 'strong and/or definite subnoxious, and/or maximal non-painful, and/or maximal tolerable', or at a current amplitude of greater than 15 mA. They concluded that strong, subnoxious intensity TENS significantly reduced postoperative analgesic requirements (Bjordal et al 2003, **Level I**).

It has also been suggested that the frequencies used in TENS might affect outcome. When used as an adjunct to patient-controlled analgesia (PCA) morphine, TENS reduced PCA morphine requirements, duration of PCA therapy and the incidence of nausea, dizziness and itching after lower abdominal surgery (Hamza et al 1999, **Level II**). A combination of mixed frequencies (2Hz and 100Hz) was more effective than either frequency alone. Similarly, mixed-frequency TENS of 50Hz and 100Hz as a supplement to pharmacological analgesia improved dynamic pain relief (Rakel & Frantz 2003, **Level II**).

High-frequency TENS is of value in the treatment of primary dysmenorrhoea (Proctor et al 2002, **Level I**).

There appears to be no good evidence for any analgesic effect of TENS during labour (Carroll et al 1997, **Level I**).

Key message

1. Certain stimulation patterns of TENS may be effective in some acute pain settings (**Level I**).

8.3 ACUPUNCTURE

Reviews of the effectiveness of acupuncture in an acute pain setting suggest that it may be useful for managing pain during childbirth (Smith et al 2003, **Level I**), idiopathic headache (Melchart et al 2001, **Level I**) and dental pain (Ernst & Pittler 1998, **Level I**).

It may also be effective in treating postoperative pain. Both preoperative low and high-frequency electro-acupuncture reduced postoperative analgesic requirements and the incidence of nausea and dizziness after lower abdominal surgery (Lin et al 2002, **Level II**).

Acupuncture needles inserted preoperatively were also found to reduce postoperative pain, opioid consumption and nausea as well as plasma cortisol and adrenaline (epinephrine) levels (Kotani et al 2001, **Level II**).

Key message

1. Acupuncture may be effective in some acute pain settings (**Level I**).

8.4 PHYSICAL THERAPIES

8.4.1 Manual and massage therapies

Most publications relating to manual (eg physiotherapy and chiropractic) and massage therapies involve the use of these treatments in low back pain and other musculoskeletal pain. The evidence for these therapies is covered in detail in *Evidence-based Management of Musculoskeletal Pain*, published by the Australian Acute Musculoskeletal Pain Guidelines Group (2003) and endorsed by the NHMRC. For a summary of some of the key messages from this document see Sections 9.4 and 9.5.

There is little consistent evidence of any benefit for the use of massage in the treatment of postoperative pain. Foot massage and guided relaxation did not lower pain scores after cardiac surgery (Hatten et al 2002, **Level II**). Similarly, massage after abdominal or thoracic (via a sternotomy) surgery did not reduce pain scores or analgesic use, although a significant reduction in the unpleasantness of pain (the affective component of pain) was reported (Piotrowski et al 2003, **Level II**). In patients after abdominal surgery, the use of a mechanical massage device which leads to intermittent negative pressure on the abdominal wall resulted in significantly lower pain scores and analgesic use on the second and third days after surgery as well as reduced time to first flatus (Le Blanc-Louvry et al 2002, **Level II**).

8.4.2 Heat and cold

Evidence for any benefits from postoperative local cooling is mixed. Significant reductions in opioid consumption and pain scores after a variety of orthopaedic operations have been reported (Brandner et al 1996; **Level II**; Barber et al 1998, **Level II**; Saito et al 2004, **Level II**); other studies have shown no such reductions (Leutz & Harris 1995, **Level II**; Edwards et al 1996, **Level II**; Konrath et al 1996, **Level II**).

Similarly, no benefit in terms of pain relief or opioid requirements was seen after total abdominal hysterectomy (Finan et al 1992, **Level II**) or caesarean section (Hanjani et al 1992, **Level II**).

REFERENCES

Australian Acute Musculoskeletal Pain Guidelines Group (2003) Evidence-based Management of Musculoskeletal Pain. National Health and Medical Research Council. (www.health.gov.au/nhmrc/publications/synopses/cp94syn.htm)

Barber FA, McGuire DA, Click S (1998) Continuous-flow therapy for outpatient anterior cruciate ligament reconstruction *Arthroscopy* 14: 130–35.

Baron RS, Logan H, Hoppe S (1993) Emotional and sensory focus as mediators of dental pain among patients differing in desired and felt dental control. *Health Psych* 12: 381–89.

Bjordal JM, Johnson MI, Ljunggreen AE (2003) Transcutaneous electrical nerve stimulation (TENS) can reduce postoperative analgesic consumption. A meta-analysis with assessment of optimal treatment parameters for postoperative pain. *Eur J Pain* 7: 181–88.

Bradley LA (1996) Cognitive-behavioural therapy for chronic pain. In: Gatchel RJ, Turk DC, (Eds) *Psychological Approaches to Pain Management*. New York: Guilford Press, pp 131–47.

Brandner B, Munro B, Bromley L et al (1996) Evaluation of the contribution to postoperative analgesia by local cooling of the wound. *Anaesthesia* 51: 1021–25.

Campbell C, Guy A, Banim M (1999) Assessing surgical patients' expectations and subsequent perceptions of pain in the context of exploring the effects of preparatory information: raising issues of gender and status. *Eur J Pain* 3: 211–19.

Carroll D, Tramèr M, McQuay H et al (1996) Randomization is important in studies with pain outcomes: systematic review of transcutaneous electrical nerve stimulation in acute postoperative pain. *Br J Anaesth* 77: 798–803.

Carroll D, Tramèr M, McQuay H et al (1997) Transcutaneous electrical nerve stimulation in labour pain: a systematic review. *Br J Obstet Gynaecol* 104(2): 169–75.

Cyna AM, McAuliffe GL, Andrew M (2004) Hypnosis for pain relief in labour and childbirth: a systematic review. *Brit J Anaesth* 93: 505–11.

Daake DR & Gueldner SH (1989) Imagery instruction and the control of post surgical pain. *Appl Nurse Res* 2: 114–20.

DuHamel KN, Redd WH, Johnson Vickberg SM (1999) Behavioural interventions in the diagnosis, treatment and rehabilitation of children with cancer. *Acta Oncol* 38: 719–34.

Edwards DJ, Rimmer M, Keene GC (1996) The use of cold therapy in the postoperative management of patients undergoing arthroscopic anterior cruciate ligament reconstruction. *Am J Sports Med* 24: 193–95.

Ellis JA & Spanos NP (1994) Cognitive-behavioural interventions for children's distress during bone marrow aspirations and lumbar punctures: a critical review. *J Pain Symptom Manage* 9: 96–108.

Ernst E & Pittler MH (1998) The effectiveness of acupuncture in treating acute dental pain. *Br Dent J* 184: 443–47.

Evans D (2002) The effectiveness of music as an intervention for hospital patients: a systematic review. *J Adv Nursing* 37: 8–18.

Finan MA, Roberts WS, Florica MS et al (1993) The effects of cold therapy on postoperative pain in gynaecologic patients: a prospective randomized study. *Am J Obstet Gynecol* 168: 542–44.

Gamsa A (2003) Hypnotic Analgesia. In: Melzack R, Wall PD (Eds) *Handbook of Pain Management*. Sydney:Churchill Livingstone.

Good M, Stanton-Hicks M, Grass JA et al (1999) Relief of post operative pain with jaw relaxation, music and their combination. *Pain* 81: 163–72.

Hamza MA, White PF, Hesham EA et al (1999) Effect of the frequency of transcutaneous electrical nerve stimulation on the postoperative opioid analgesic requirements and recovery profile. *Anesthesiology* 91: 1232–38.

Hanjani A, Corcoran S, Chatwani A (1992) Cold therapy in the management of postoperative cesarean section pain. *Am J Obstet Gynecol* 167: 108–09.

Hattan J, King L, Griffiths P (2002) The impact of foot massage and guided relaxation following cardiac surgery: a randomized controlled trial. *J Adv Nursing* 37(2): 199–207.

Haythronthwaite JA, Lawrence JW, Fauerbach JA (2001) Brief cognitive intervention for burn pain. *Ann Behav Med* 23: 42–49.

Jensen MP, Turner JA, Romano JM et al (1991) Coping with chronic pain: A critical review of the literature. *Pain* 47: 249–83.

Johnston M & Vogele C (1993) Benefits of psychological preparation for surgery: a meta analysis. *Ann Behav Med* 15: 245–56.

Konrath GA, Lock T, Goitz HT et al (1996) The use of cold therapy after anterior cruciate ligament reconstruction: a prospective, randomized study and literature review. *Am J Sports Med* 24: 629–33.

Kotani N, Hashimoto H, Sato Y et al (2001) Preoperative intradermal acupuncture reduces postoperative pain, nausea and vomiting, analgesic requirement and sympathoadrenal responses. *Anesthesiology* 95: 349–56.

LaMontagne LL, Hepworth JT, Cohen F et al (2003) Cognitive-behavioural intervention effects on adolescents' anxiety and pain following spinal fusion surgery. *Nursing Res* 52: 183–90.

Le Blanc-Louvry I, Costaglioli B, Boulon C et al (2002) Does mechanical massage of the abdominal wall after colectomy reduce postoperative pain and shorten the duration of ileus. Results of a randomised study. *J Gastrointest Surg* 6: 43–49.

Leutz DW, Harris H (1995) Continuous cold therapy in total knee arthroplasty. *Am J Knee Surg* 8: 121–23.

Lin JG, Lo MW, Wen YR et al (2002) The effect of high and low frequency electroacupuncture in pain after lower abdominal surgery. *Pain* 99: 509–14.

Liossi C & Hatira P (1999) Clinical hypnosis versus cognitive-behavioural training for pain management with pediatric cancer patients undergoing bone marrow aspiration. *Int J Clin Exp Hypn* 47: 104–116.

Liossi C & Hatira P (2003) Clinical hypnosis in the alleviation of procedure-related pain in pediatric oncology patients. *Int J Clin Exp Hypn* 51: 4–28.

Logan H, Baron R, Kohout F (1995) Sensory focus as therapeutic treatment for acute pain. *Psychosom Med* 57: 475–84.

Luebbert K, Dahme B, Hasenbring M (2001) The effectiveness of relaxation training in reducing treatment-related symptoms and improving emotional adjustment in acute non-surgical cancer treatment: a meta-analytical review. *Psychooncology* 10: 490–502.

Melchart D, Linde K, Fischer P et al (2001)Acupuncture for idiopathic headache. *The Cochrane Database of Systematic Reviews*. Issue 1. Art. No.: CD001218. DOI: 10.1002/14651858.CD001218.

Miro J & Raich RM (1999) Preoperative preparation for surgery: an analysis of the effects of relaxation and information provision. *Clin Psych Psychother* 6: 202–09.

Montgomery GH, DuHamel KN, Redd WH (2000) A meta analysis of hypnotically induced analgesia: how effective is hypnosis? *Int J Clin Exp Hypn*48: 138–53.

Montgomery GH, Weltz CR, Seltz M et al (2002) Brief presurgery hypnosis reduces distress and pain in excisional breast biopsy patients. *Int J Clin Exp Hypn* 50: 17–32.

Patterson DR & Jensen MP (2003) Hypnosis and clinical pain. *Psych Bull* 129: 495–521.

Piotrowski MM, Paterson C, Mitchinson A et al (2003) Massage as adjuvant therapy in the management of acute postoperative pain. *Am J Coll Surg* 197: 1037–46.

Powers SW (1999) Empirically supported treatment in pediatric psychology: procedure-related pain. *J Ped Psych* 24: 131–45.

Proctor ML, Smith CA, Farquhar CM et al (2002) Transcutaneous electrical nerve stimulation and acupuncture for primary dysmenorrhoea. *The Cochrane Database of Systematic Reviews*. Issue 1. Art. No.: CD002123. DOI: 10.1002/14651858.CD002123.

Rakel B & Frantz R (2003) Effectiveness of transcutaneous electrical nerve stimulation on postoperative pain with movement. *J Pain* 4: 455–64.

Redd WH, Montgomery GH, DuHamel KN (2001) Behavioural intervention for cancer treatment side effects. *JNCI* 92: 810–23.

Saito N, Horiuchi H, Kobayashi S et al (2004) Continuous local cooling for pain relief following total hip arthroplasty. *J Arthroplasty* 19: 334–37.

Seers K & Carroll D (1998) Relaxation techniques for acute pain management: a systematic review. *J Adv Nursing* 27: 466–75.

Smith CA, Collins CT, Cyna AM et al (2003) Crowther CA. Complementary and alternative therapies for pain management in labour. *The Cochrane Database of Systematic Reviews*. Issue 2. Art. No.: CD003521. DOI: 10.1002/14651858.CD003521.

Smith LA & Oldman AD (1999) Acupuncture and dental pain. *Br Dent J* 186: 158–59.

Sullivan MJL, Thorn B, Haythornthwaite JA et al (2001) Theoretical perspective on the relation between catastrophising and pain. *Clin J Pain* 17: 52–64.

Suls J & Wan CK (1989) Effects of sensory and procedural information on coping with stressful medical procedures and pain. A meta analysis. *J Consult Clin Psychol* 57: 372–79.

Turk DC & Monarch ES (2002) Biopsychosocial perspective on chronic pain. In: Turk DC & Gatchel RJ (Eds) *Psychological Approaches to Pain Management*. 2nd edition, New York: Guilford.

Voss JA, Good M, Yates B et al (2004) Sedative music reduces anxiety and pain during chair rest after open-heart surgery. *Pain* 112: 197–203.

Wall VJ & Womack W (1989) Hypnotic versus active cognitive strategies for alleviation of procedural distress in pediatric oncology patients. *Am J Clin Hypn* 31: 181–91.

Williams DA (1996) Acute pain management. In: Gatchel RJ, Turk DC (Eds) *Psychological Approaches to Pain Management*. New York: Guilford Press. pp 55–77.

Wilson JF (1981) Behavioural preparation for surgery: benefit or harm? *J Behav Med* 4: 79–102.

9. SPECIFIC CLINICAL SITUATIONS

9.1 POSTOPERATIVE PAIN

One of the most common sources of pain is postoperative pain and a large amount of the evidence presented so far in this document is based on studies of pain relief in the postoperative setting. However, many of the management principles derived from these studies can be applied to the management of acute pain in general, as outlined in the sections that follow.

In addition to this approach, there is also a need for information on postoperative pain management that relates to the site of surgery and specific surgical procedures (Rowlingson & Rawal 2003). The development of such procedure-specific guidelines has just begun: they require considerable effort and resources and have not been addressed in this document. An ambitious project to develop such evidence-based guidelines for the management of postoperative pain has been initiated by the PROSPECT group. The first of these guidelines can be found at their website: www.postoppain.org.

Similarly, operative site-specific acute pain management has been addressed in the Clinical Practice Guideline for the Management of Postoperative Pain' published by the Veterans Health Administration and Department of Defense in the USA (Rosenquist et al 2003). A copy of these guidelines can be found at www.oqp.med.va.gov/cpg/PAIN/PAIN_base.htm (VHA/DoD 2002).

9.1.1 Risks of postoperative neuropathic pain

CHAPTER 9

Neuropathic pain has been defined as 'pain initiated or caused by a primary lesion or dysfunction in the nervous system' (Merskey & Bogduk 1994). Acute causes of neuropathic pain can be iatrogenic, traumatic, inflammatory or infective. Nerve injury is a risk in many surgical procedures and may present as acute neuropathic pain in the postoperative period. The incidence of acute neuropathic pain has been reported as 1–3%, based on patients referred to an acute pain service, primarily after surgery or trauma (Hayes et al 2002, **Level IV**). The majority of these patients had persistent pain at 12 months, suggesting that acute neuropathic pain is a risk factor for chronic pain. There is some evidence that specific early analgesic interventions may reduce the incidence of chronic pain (often neuropathic pain) after some operations (eg thoracotomy, amputation). For more details see Sections 1.3 and 9.1.2.

The prompt diagnosis (Rasmussen & Sindrup 2004) of acute neuropathic pain is therefore important. Management is based on extrapolation of data from the chronic pain setting (see Sections 4.3.2 to 4.3.6).

Key messages

1. Acute neuropathic pain occurs after trauma and surgery (**Level IV**).

The following tick box ☑ represents conclusions based on clinical experience and expert opinion.

☑ Diagnosis and subsequent appropriate treatment of acute neuropathic pain might prevent development of chronic pain.

9.1.2 Acute postamputation pain syndromes

Following amputation of a limb, and also breast, tongue, teeth, genitalia and even inner organs such as the rectum, or a deafferentiation injury such as brachial plexus avulsion (Bates & Stewart 1991; Boas et al 1993; Kroner et al 1994), a number of phenomena can develop. These require differentiation.

- Stump pain is pain localised to the site of amputation. It can be acute (usually nociceptive) or chronic (usually neuropathic) and is most common in the immediate postoperative period (Jensen et al 1985; Nikolajsen & Jensen 2001). The overall incidence of stump pain is uncertain; early stump pain is increased by the presence of severe preamputation pain (Nikolajsen et al 1997).
- Phantom sensation is defined as any sensory perception of the missing body part with the exclusion of pain. Almost all patients who have undergone amputation experience phantom sensations (Jensen et al 1983). These sensations range from a vague awareness of the presence of the organ via associated paraesthesia to complete sensation including size, shape, position, temperature and movement.
- Phantom limb pain is defined as any noxious sensory phenomenon in the missing limb or organ. The incidence of phantom limb pain is estimated to be 30–85% after limb amputation and occurs usually in the distal portion of the missing limb (Jensen et al 1985; Perkins & Kehlet 2000; Nikolajsen & Jensen 2001). Pain can be immediate — 75% of patients will report phantom pain within the first few days after amputation (Nikolajsen et al 1997) — or delayed in onset. The pain is typically intermittent and diminishes with time after amputation. Factors that may be predictive of postamputation phantom pain are the severity of preamputation pain, the degree of postoperative stump pain and chemotherapy (see Section 1.3). If preamputation pain was present, phantom pain may resemble that pain in character and localisation (Katz & Melzack 1990).

There is a strong correlation between phantom limb and stump or site pain and they may be inter-related (Jensen et al 1983; Kooijman et al 2000). All three of the above phenomena can coexist (Nikolajsen et al 1997).

Prevention

Evidence for the benefit of epidural analgesia in the prevention of all phantom limb pain is inconclusive (Halbert et al 2002, **Level I**). However, a recent analysis of studies on phantom limb pain prophylaxis, showed that perioperative (pre-, intra- and postoperative) epidural analgesia reduced the incidence of *severe* phantom limb pain (NNT 5.8) (Gehling & Tryba 2003, **Level III-2**).

A small observational study found that while the overall incidence of long-term phantom limb pain was similar in patients given ketamine (bolus dose followed by an infusion, started prior to skin incision and continued for 72 hours postoperatively) compared with no ketamine, the incidence of *severe* phantom limb pain was reduced in the ketamine group (Dertwinkel et al 2002, **Level III-3**). A more recent study also looking at the effects of ketamine reported that the incidence of phantom limb pain at 6 months after amputation was 47% in the ketamine group and 71% in the control group, but this difference did not reach statistical significance (Hayes et al 2004, **Level II**).

Infusions of local anaesthetics via peripheral nerve sheath catheters, usually inserted by the surgeon at the time of amputation, are a safe method of providing excellent analgesia in the immediate post-operative period (Pinzur et al 1996, **Level II**; Lambert et al 2001, **Level II**). However, they are of no proven benefit in preventing phantom pain or stump pain (Halbert et al 2002, **Level I**).

Therapy

A survey in 1980 identified over 50 different therapies currently in use for the treatment of phantom limb pain (Sherman et al 1980), suggesting limited evidence for effective treatments. This was confirmed by a systematic review (Halbert et al 2002).

- Calcitonin by intravenous (IV) infusion is effective in the treatment of phantom limb pain (Jaeger & Maier 1992, **Level II**). Calcitonin may also be given subcutaneously or intranasally (Wall & Heyneman 1999).
- Ketamine, an N-methyl D-aspartate (NMDA) receptor antagonist (see Section 4.3.2), provided short-term relief of stump and phantom limb pain (Nikolajsen et al 1996, **Level II**).
- Oral slow-release morphine (Huse et al 2001, **Level II**) and IV infusions of morphine reduced phantom limb pain (Wu et al 2002, **Level II**).
- Gabapentin reduced phantom limb pain (Bone et al 2002, **Level II**).
- IV lignocaine (lidocaine) significantly reduced stump pain but had no effect on phantom pain (Wu et al 2002, **Level II**).

Non-pharmacological treatment options for phantom limb pain are also effective (eg sensory discrimination training) (Flor et al 2001, **Level II**).

Key messages

1. There is little evidence from randomised controlled trials to guide specific treatment of postamputation pain syndromes (**Level I**)
2. Continuous regional blockade via nerve sheath catheters provides effective postoperative analgesia after amputation, but has no preventive effect on phantom limb pain (**Level II**).
3. Calcitonin, morphine, ketamine, gabapentin and sensory discrimination training reduce phantom limb pain (**Level II**).

4. Ketamine and lignocaine (lidocaine) reduce stump pain (**Level II**).

5. Perioperative epidural analgesia reduces the incidence of severe phantom limb pain (**Level III-2**).

The following tick box ☑ represents conclusions based on clinical experience and expert opinion.

☑ Perioperative ketamine may prevent severe phantom limb pain.

9.1.3 Day surgery

Over 60% of surgery is now performed on a day-stay basis. Adequate postoperative pain management is often the limiting factor when determining whether a patient can have surgery performed as a day procedure.

Predictors of pain

The incidence of severe pain after day surgery has been reported to be 5.3% in the first postoperative 24 hours; orthopaedic patients had the highest incidence of severe pain and increased body mass index and duration of anaesthesia were significant predictors of severe pain (Chung et al 1997, **Level IV**). Another important predictor of severe pain is type of surgery, particularly open inguinal hernia repair, laparoscopy and plastic surgery (Pavlin et al 2002, **Level IV**). The best predictor of severe pain at home is inadequate pain control in the first few hours following surgery (Beauregard et al 1998, **Level IV**).

Adverse effects of pain

Inadequate analgesia may delay patient discharge; pain was the most common cause of Phase 1 recovery delays affecting 24% of patients overall (Pavlin et al 2002, **Level IV**). Uncontrolled pain is also a major cause of nausea and vomiting, further extending the patient's stay in the recovery room (Eriksson et al 1996: Michaloliakou et al 1996), and of unplanned admissions and readmissions (Gold et al 1989, **Level IV**).

Inadequate pain management may cause sleep disturbance (Strassels et al 2002, **Level IV**) and limit early mobilisation, which may be crucial for early return to normal function and work (Beauregard et al 1998, **Level IV**).

Local anaesthesia techniques

Local infiltration

Infiltration of local anaesthetic reduces requirements for opioid analgesics after day surgery and leads to a lower incidence of nausea and vomiting (Eriksson et al 1996, **Level II**; Michaloliakou et al 1996, **Level II**).

IV regional anaesthesia

A systematic review of adjuncts added to the solutions for IV regional anaesthesia for surgical procedures has shown the following (Choyce & Peng 2002, **Level I**):

- non-steroidal anti-inflammatory drugs (NSAIDs), particularly ketorolac, improve postoperative analgesia;

- clonidine improves postoperative analgesia and prolongs tourniquet tolerance; and
- opioids show no clinically relevant benefit.

Dexmedetomidine added to solutions for IV regional anaesthesia improves the quality of anaesthesia and perioperative analgesia without adverse effects (Memis et al 2004, **Level II**).

Intra-articular

Intra-articular injection of local anaesthetic into the knee has limited analgesic efficacy and the effect is small to moderate and short-lived, however it may be of clinical significance in day-case surgery (Møiniche et al 1999, **Level I**). An analgesic effect of intra-articular morphine was evident up to 24 hours postoperatively (Gupta et al 2001, **Level I**; Kalso et al 2002, **Level I**). This effect was probably not dose dependent and a systemic effect of intra-articular morphine could not be excluded (see Section 5.2).

Intra-articular NSAIDs such as tenoxicam and ketorolac have consistently shown a reduction in postoperative pain (Reuben & Connelly 1995, **Level II**; Elhakim et al 1996, **Level II**; Reuben & Connelly1996, **Level II**; Cook et al 1997, **Level II**, Convery et al 1998, **Level II**; Colbert et al 1999, **Level II**; Gupta et al 1999, **Level II**). However there is some concern that their use may hinder bone healing. Uncertainty remains as no long-term follow-up study in humans has been undertaken.

Intra-articular clonidine reduced pain in the majority of studies; however, the reduction in pain intensity is mild, while dose-related hypotension is of concern (Gentili et al 1996, **Level II**; Reuben & Connelly1999, **Level II**; Buerkle et al 2000, **Level II**; Iqbal et al 2000, **Level II**; Joshi et al 2000, **Level II**; Gentili et al 2001, **Level II**) (see Section 5.3).

Single dose peripheral nerve blockade

Peripheral nerve blocks are useful in ambulatory surgery as they provide site-specific anaesthesia with prolonged analgesia and minimal haemodynamic changes. The decision to discharge ambulatory patients following peripheral nerve blockade with long-acting local anaesthesia is controversial as there is always the potential risk of harm to an anaesthetised limb.

A prospective study including 1,119 upper and 1,263 lower extremity blocks demonstrated that long-acting peripheral nerve blocks are safe and that patients can be discharged with an insensate limb (Klein et al 2002a, **Level IV**). Provided patients are given verbal and written information regarding the risks as well as appropriate follow-up, it would seem reasonable to discharge these patients with the benefit of prolonged analgesia.

Ilioinguinal and iliohypogastric nerve block

Herniorrhaphy performed under ilioinguinal and iliohypogastric nerve block leads to superior pain relief, less morbidity, less urinary retention and cost advantages (Ding & White1995, **Level II**).

Paravertebral block

Paravertebral blocks also provide good analgesia after inguinal herniorrhaphy with earlier discharge, high patient satisfaction and few side effects (Klein et al 2002b, **Level II**). The key feature of this block after breast surgery is that analgesia is prolonged beyond 24 hours (Klein et al 2000b, **Level II**).

Upper and lower limb plexus blocks

A single dose femoral nerve block with bupivacaine for anterior cruciate ligament reconstruction provides 20–24 hours of postoperative analgesia (Mulroy et al 2001, **Level II**). There is an associated decreased requirement for recovery room stay and unplanned hospital admission, thereby having the potential to create significant hospital cost savings (Williams et al 2004, **Level III-3**).

Continuous peripheral nerve blockade

Patients may suffer intense pain following resolution of a peripheral nerve block although it maximises pain relief in the first 12–24 hours (Chung et al 1997, **Level IV**). Perineural catheters are commonly placed for interscalene, infraclavicular, femoral and popliteal blocks. Significant patient advantages are sustained postoperative analgesia, opioid sparing and less sleep disturbance (Ilfeld et al 2002a, **Level II**) and improved rehabilitation (Capdevila et al 1999, **Level II**).

Local anaesthetic perfusion of the wound for 48 hours following subacromial decompression led to improved pain scores for 5 days postoperatively, compared with patients who received saline infusions (Savoie et al 2000, **Level II**).

Inadvertent intravascular catheter placement should be excluded prior to patient discharge using a test dose of local anaesthetic and adrenaline (epinephrine) (Rawal et al 2002). A medical officer should be available (24 hours a day) to answer questions as necessary, as 30% of patients make unscheduled phone calls regarding catheter infusions despite been given adequate written and verbal instructions (Ilfeld et al 2002b, **Level II**). Patients may also have significant anxiety about catheter removal at home (Ilfeld et al 2004, **Level IV**).

Non-pharmacological techniques

Non-pharmacological techniques such as transcutaneous electric nerve stimulation (TENS), acupuncture, hypnosis, ultrasound, laser and cryoanalgesia have also been used in the treatment of acute pain management after ambulatory surgery. Pressure on acupoints decreased pain following knee arthroscopy (Felhendler & Lisander 1996, **Level II**). Continuous-flow cold therapy has been shown to be effective following outpatient anterior cruciate ligament reconstruction, also reducing analgesic requirements (Barber et al 1998, **Level II**).

Key messages

1. The use of NSAIDs or clonidine as adjuncts to local anaesthetic agents in intravenous regional anaesthesia improves postoperative analgesia (**Level I**).
2. Infiltration of the wound with local anaesthetic agents provides good and long-lasting analgesia after ambulatory surgery (**Level II**).
3. Peripheral nerve blocks with long-acting local anaesthetic agents provide long-lasting postoperative analgesia after ambulatory surgery (**Level II**).
4. Continuous peripheral nerve blocks provide extended analgesia after ambulatory surgery and have been shown to be safe if adequate resources and patient education are provided (**Level II**).
5. Optimal analgesia is essential for the success of ambulatory surgery (**Level IV**).

9.2 ACUTE SPINAL CORD INJURY

Acute pain following spinal cord injury is common, with over 90% of patients experiencing pain in the first 2 weeks following injury (Siddall et al 1999, **Level IV**). Acute pain may also develop during the rehabilitation phase due to intercurrent disease (eg renal calculus) or exacerbation of a chronic pain syndrome.

Pain associated with spinal cord injury usually falls into two main categories: *neuropathic pain* either at or below the level of the spinal cord injury, and *nociceptive pain*, from somatic and visceral structures (Siddall et al 2002). Neuropathic pain associated with a lesion of the central nervous system is termed *central pain* (Merskey & Bogduk 1994). Phantom pain and complex regional pain syndromes may also develop in patients with spinal cord injury.

The taxonomy of spinal cord injury pain in Table 9.1 is based on Siddall (2002).

Table 9.1 Taxonomy of spinal cord injury pain

Pain type	Location relative to level of injury	Description, structures and pathology
Neuropathic pain	*Above level*	*pain located in area of sensory preservation* peripheral nerve or plexus injury
	At level	*'segmental pain' at level of the injury* spinal cord lesion (central pain) nerve root lesion (cauda equina) combined cord and root lesions syringomyelia

CHAPTER 9

Pain type	Location relative to level of injury	Description, structures and pathology
	Below level	*pain below the level of injury* spinal cord lesion (eg central dysaesthesia syndrome) phantom pain
	Other	complex regional pain syndrome
Nociceptive pain	*Somatic*	musculoskeletal pain (eg vertebral fracture, muscle spasms, overuse syndromes) procedure-related pain (eg pressure sore dressings) dysreflexic headache
	Visceral	urinary tract (eg calculi) gastrointestinal tract

Treatment of acute neuropathic pain after spinal cord injury

There are limited studies examining the treatment of acute neuropathic pain after spinal cord injury. Treatment must therefore largely be based on evidence from studies of chronic central pain and other neuropathic pain syndromes.

Opioids

IV alfentanil decreased central pain following spinal cord injury compared with placebo and ketamine (Eide et al 1995, **Level II**). IV morphine decreased tactile allodynia but had no effect on other neuropathic pain components in spinal cord injury and post-stroke patients (Attal et al 2002, **Level II**).

Ketamine

Ketamine infusion decreased neuropathic pain in spinal cord injury patients (Eide et al 1995, **Level II**).

Membrane stabilisers

IV lignocaine (lidocaine) was superior to placebo in reducing spontaneous pain and brush allodynia in patients with central pain, including spinal cord injury (Attal et al 2000, **Level II**). IV lignocaine was also effective in the treatment of neuropathic pain of peripheral nerve lesions (Kalso et al 1998, **Level I**). Mexiletine was not effective in reducing neuropathic spinal cord injury pain (Chiou Tan et al 1996, **Level II**).

Antidepressants

While antidepressants are useful in other neuropathic pain states, there was no significant difference in pain or disability with amitriptyline compared with placebo in spinal cord injury patients with chronic pain (Cardenas et al 2002, **Level II**). There are no studies of SSRIs in the treatment of central pain (Sindrup & Jensen 1999, **Level I**).

Anticonvulsants

Lamotrigine reduced spontaneous and evoked pain in patients with *incomplete* spinal cord injury (Finnerup et al 2002, **Level II**).

Valproate was ineffective in the treatment of spinal cord injury pain (Drewes et al 1994, **Level II**) whereas gabapentin decreased pain intensity and frequency, and improved quality of life (Levendoglu et al 2004, **Level II**).

Treatment of nociceptive and visceral pain after spinal cord injury

There is no specific evidence for the treatment of acute nociceptive and visceral pain in spinal cord injury patients. Treatment must therefore be based on evidence from other studies of nociceptive and visceral pain.

Key messages

1. IV opioids, ketamine and lignocaine (lidocaine) decrease acute spinal cord injury pain (**Level II**).
2. Gabapentin is effective in the treatment of acute spinal cord injury pain (**Level II**).

The following tick box ☑ represents conclusions based on clinical experience and expert opinion.

☑ Treatment of acute spinal cord pain is largely based on evidence from studies of other neuropathic and nociceptive pain syndromes.

9.3 Acute burns injury pain

CHAPTER 9

Acute pain following burns injury can be nociceptive and/or neuropathic in nature and may be constant (background pain), intermittent or procedure-related. There is limited evidence for the management of pain in burns injury and treatment is largely based on evidence from case reports and case series or data extrapolated from other relevant areas of pain medicine.

Burns pain is often undertreated, particularly in the elderly (Choinière 2001). However, effective pain management after acute burns injury is essential, not only for humanitarian and psychological reasons, but also to facilitate procedures such as dressing changes and physiotherapy and possibly to minimise the development of chronic pain, which is reported in 35–58% of burns patients (Choinière et al 1989; Dauber et al 2002).

Immediately after the injury, simple measures such as cooling (Davies 1982), covering and immobilising the burn may provide analgesia (Kinsella & Booth 1991; Gallagher et al 2000a). With severe burns pain, analgesia is best achieved by titration of IV opioids.

Opioid doses do not require adjustment as the pharmacokinetics of morphine are unchanged in burns patients (Perreault et al 2001). Absorption of intramuscular (IM) and subcutaneous (SC) opioids may be unreliable in the presence of hypovolaemia and vasoconstriction associated with burns (Kinsella & Rae 2003). Patient-controlled morphine is effective for burns pain in adults (Choinière et al 1992, **Level II**) and children (Gaukroger et al 1991, **Level IV**). Conversion to oral opioids is possible once normal gut function has returned.

Opioids may be supplemented with non-opioid drugs. There is experimental evidence for beneficial effects of ketamine (Ilkjaer et al 1996) and dextromethorphan (Ilkjaer et al 1997) on hyperalgesia and clinical evidence of an opioid-sparing effect with clonidine (Viggiano et al 1998, **Level II**).

Management of procedural pain

Procedural pain may be difficult to manage in burns patients. Dressing changes may be associated with frequent and prolonged periods of pain; up to 84% of burns patients reporting extreme, intense pain during therapeutic procedures (Ashburn 1995).

Opioid therapy is the mainstay of analgesia for burns procedures. However, very high doses may be required (Linneman et al 2000, **Level IV**) and opioid-related sedation and respiratory depression may develop when the pain stimulus decreases following the procedure.

Short-acting opioids such as fentanyl (Prakash 2004, **Level II**) and alfentanil (Sim et al 1996, **Level IV**) administered via patient-controlled analgesia (PCA) and target-controlled infusions (Gallagher et al 2000b, **Level IV**) have been used successfully to provide analgesia during burns dressing changes. Sedation, as an adjunct to analgesia, can improve pain relief. This has been shown for lorazepam combined with morphine (Patterson et al 1997, **Level II**); patient-controlled sedation with propofol may also be effective (Coimbra et al 2003, **Level IV**).

Nitrous oxide, ketamine and IV lignocaine (lidocaine) infusions (Jonsson et al 1991, **Level IV**) have also been used to provide analgesia for burns procedures (see Sections 4.3.1 and 4.3.2).

Topical analgesic techniques, such as lignocaine (lidocaine) (Brofelt et al 1989, **Level IV**) and morphine-infused silver sulfadiazine cream (Long et al 2001, **Level IV**) may be effective.

Non-pharmacological management

Hypnosis, distraction, auricular electrical stimulation, therapeutic touch techniques and massage therapy have been used for the treatment of burns pain, including procedural pain; a lack of prospective randomised trials makes comparisons with conventional therapies difficult (Kinsella & Rae 2003) (see Section 8.1.3). A study comparing two psychological support interventions, hypnosis and stress-reducing strategies, found that VAS anxiety scores were significantly better after hypnosis although there was no significant difference in pain reports (Frenay et al 2001, **Level II**).

Key messages

1. Opioids, particularly via PCA, are effective in burns pain, including procedural pain (**Level IV**).

The following tick boxes ☑ represent conclusions based on clinical experience and expert opinion.

☑ Acute pain following burns injury can be nociceptive and/or neuropathic in nature and may be constant (background pain), intermittent or procedure-related.

☑ Acute pain following burns injury requires aggressive multimodal and multidisciplinary treatment.

9.4 ACUTE BACK PAIN

Acute back pain in the cervical, thoracic, or, in particular, lumbar and sacral regions, is a common problem affecting most adults at some stage of their lives. The causes are rarely serious, most often non-specific and the pain is usually self-limiting.

Appropriate investigations are indicated in patients who have signs or symptoms that might indicate the presence of a more serious condition ('red flags'). Such 'red flags' include symptoms and signs of infection (eg fever), risk factors for infection (eg underlying disease process, immunosuppression, penetrating wound), history of trauma or minor trauma (if > 50 years, history of osteoporosis and taking corticosteroids), past history of malignancy, age > 50 years, failure to improve with treatment, unexplained weight loss, pain at multiple sites or at rest and absence of aggravating features (Australian Acute Musculoskeletal Pain Guidelines Group 2003). A full neurological examination is warranted in the presence of lower limb pain and other neurological symptoms.

Psychosocial and occupational factors ('yellow flags') appear to be associated with an increased risk of progression from acute to chronic pain; such factors should be assessed early in order to facilitate appropriate interventions (Australian Acute Musculoskeletal Pain Guidelines Group 2003).

NHMRC guidelines for the *Evidence-based Management of Acute Musculoskeletal Pain* include chapters on acute neck, thoracic spinal and low back pain (Australian Acute Musculoskeletal Pain Guidelines Group 2003). In view of the high quality and extensiveness of these guidelines, no further assessment of these topics has been undertaken for this document. The following is an abbreviated summary of key messages from these guidelines; the practice points recommended for musculoskeletal pain in general are listed in Section 9.5 and represent the consensus of the Steering Committee of these guidelines.

The guidelines can be found at www.health.gov.au/nhmrc/publications/pdf/cp94.pdf.

Key messages

1. Acute low back pain is non-specific in about 95% of cases and serious causes are rare; common examination and investigation findings also occur in asymptomatic controls and may not be the cause of pain (**Level I**).
2. Advice to stay active, heat wrap therapy, 'activity-focused' printed and verbal information and behavioural therapy interventions are beneficial in acute low back pain (**Level I**).
3. Advice to stay active, exercises, multimodal therapy and pulsed electromagnetic therapy are effective in acute neck pain (**Level I**).
4. Soft collars are not effective for acute neck pain (**Level I**).
5. Appropriate investigations are indicated in cases of acute low back pain when alerting features ('red flags') of serious conditions are present (**Level III-2**).
6. Psychosocial and occupational factors ('yellow flags') appear to be associated with progression from acute to chronic back pain; such factors should be assessed early to facilitate intervention (**Level III-2**).

9.5 ACUTE MUSCULOSKELETAL PAIN

Other than acute back pain, acute shoulder and anterior knee pain are two common painful musculoskeletal conditions.

A summary of findings relating to acute musculoskeletal pain can be found in *Evidence-based Management of Acute Musculoskeletal Pain*, published by the Australian Acute Musculoskeletal Pain Guidelines Group (Australian Acute Musculoskeletal Pain Guidelines Group 2003) and endorsed by the NHMRC (Australian Acute Musculoskeletal Pain Guidelines Group 2003). In view of the high quality and extensiveness of these guidelines, no further assessment of these topics has been undertaken for this document.

The following is an abbreviated summary of key messages from these guidelines and represent the consensus of the Steering Committee of these guidelines.

The guidelines can be found at www.health.gov.au/nhmrc/publications/pdf/cp94.pdf.

Key messages

1. Topical and oral NSAIDs improve acute shoulder pain (**Level I**).
2. Subacromial corticosteroid injection relieves acute shoulder pain in the early stages (**Level I**).
3. Exercises improve acute shoulder pain in patients with rotator cuff disease (**Level I**).
4. Therapeutic ultrasound may improve acute shoulder pain in calcific tendonitis (**Level I**).

5. Advice to stay active, exercises, injection therapy and foot orthoses are effective in acute patellofemoral pain (**Level I**).
6. Low-level laser therapy is ineffective in the management of patellofemoral pain (**Level I**).

The following tick boxes ☑ represent conclusions based on clinical experience and expert opinion.

☑ A management plan for acute musculoskeletal pain should comprise the elements of assessment (history and physical examination, but ancillary investigations are not generally indicated), management (information, assurance, advice to resume normal activity, pain management) and review to reassess pain and revise management plan.

☑ Information should be provided to patients in correct but neutral terms with the avoidance of alarming diagnostic labels to overcome inappropriate expectations, fears or mistaken beliefs.

☑ Regular paracetamol, then if ineffective, NSAIDs, may be used for acute musculoskeletal pain.

☑ Oral opioids, preferably short-acting agents at regular intervals, may be necessary to relieve severe acute musculoskeletal pain; ongoing need for such treatment requires reassessment.

☑ Adjuvant agents such as anticonvulsants, antidepressants and muscle relaxants are not recommended for the routine treatment of acute musculoskeletal pain.

9.6 Acute medical pain

CHAPTER 9

9.6.1 Abdominal pain

Acute abdominal pain may originate from visceral or somatic structures or may be referred; neuropathic pain states should also be considered. Recurrent acute abdominal pain may be a manifestation of a chronic visceral pain disorder such chronic pancreatitis or irritable bowel syndrome and may require a multidisciplinary pain management approach.

A common misconception is that analgesia masks the signs and symptoms of abdominal pathology and should be withheld until a diagnosis is established. Pain relief does not interfere with the diagnostic process in acute abdominal pain in adults (McHale & LoVecchio 2001, **Level I**; Thomas et al 2003, **Level II**) or in children (Kim et al 2002, **Level II**).

Renal colic

Pethidine has commonly been used in the treatment of renal colic in the belief that it causes less smooth muscle spasm. However, there was no difference in analgesia when IV morphine and pethidine were compared in the treatment of renal colic (O'Connor et al 2000; **Level II**).

NSAIDs are effective analgesics in renal colic (Labrecque et al 1994, **Level I**), providing superior pain relief, less vomiting and decreased requirements for rescue analgesia compared with parenteral opioids (Holdgate & Pollock 2004, **Level I**). The onset of analgesia was more rapid when NSAIDs were given intravenously (Tramèr et al 1998, **Level I**). NSAIDs reduced the incidence of recurrent renal colic in emergency department patients (Kapoor et al 1989, **Level II**; Laerum et al 1995, **Level II**).

Anticholinergic, antispasmodic drugs such as hyoscine-N-butylbromide were less effective analgesics than NSAIDs (al-Waili & Saloom 1998, **Level II**) and failed to provide additional pain relief when combined with NSAIDs in the treatment of renal colic (Jones et al 2001, **Level II**).

Biliary colic and acute pancreatitis

All opioids increase sphincter of Oddi tone and bile duct pressures in animal and human experimental models (Thompson 2001). Morphine increased sphincter of Oddi contractions more than pethidine during cholecystectomy (Thune et al 1990, **Level IV**). There are no clinical studies comparing opioids in the treatment of pain associated with biliary spasm or acute pancreatitis (Thompson 2001).

Parenteral NSAIDs such as ketorolac, tenoxicam and diclofenac were at least as effective as parenteral opioids and more effective than hyoscine-N-butylbromide in providing analgesia for biliary colic (Goldman et al 1989, **Level II**; Al-Waili & Saloom 1998, **Level II**; Dula et al 2001, **Level II**; Henderson et al 2002, **Level II**; Kumar et al 2004, **Level II**) and may also prevent progression to cholecystitis (Goldman et al 1989, **Level II**; Akriviadis et al 1997, **Level II**; Al-Waili & Saloom 1998, **Level II**; Kumar et al 2004, **Level II**).

Irritable bowel syndrome

Smooth muscle relaxants (Poynard et al 2001, **Level I**) and peppermint oil (NNT=3.1) (Pittler & Ernst 1998, **Level I**) provide good pain relief in patients with irritable bowel disease.

Primary dysmenorrhea

NSAIDS are of benefit in the treatment of dysmenorrhoea (Marjoribanks et al 2003, **Level I**) including naproxen (NNT= 2.4), ibuprofen (NNT=2.6) and mefenamic acid (NNT=3.0); ibuprofen had the least adverse effects. Aspirin and paracetamol were less effective than NSAIDs (Zhang & Li Wan Po 1998, **Level I**).

Vitamin B_1 (Proctor & Murphy 2002, **Level I**) and fennel (Namavar Jahromi et al 2003, **Level III-2**) have been shown to be of benefit in the treatment of pain associated with dysmenorrhoea.

Key messages

1. Provision of analgesia does not interfere with the diagnostic process in acute abdominal pain (**Level I**).
2. NSAIDs are superior to parenteral opioids in the treatment of renal colic (**Level I** [Cochrane Review]).
3. The onset of analgesia is faster when NSAIDs are given IV for the treatment of renal colic (**Level I**).

4. Antispasmodics and peppermint oil are effective in the treatment of acute pain in irritable bowel syndrome (**Level I**).
5. NSAIDS and vitamin B_1 are effective in the treatment of primary dysmenorrhoea (**Level I** [Cochrane Review]).
6. There is no difference between pethidine and morphine in the treatment of renal colic (**Level II**).
7. Parenteral NSAIDs are as effective as parenteral opioids in the treatment of biliary colic (**Level II**).

9.6.2 Acute herpes zoster infection

Acute herpes zoster infection (shingles) is common, occurring in 50% of those over 50 years of age. It causes severe acute pain in dermatomes supplied by spinal or cranial dorsal root ganglia, which have been infected by the varicella zoster virus. Early management of acute zoster infection may reduce the incidence of post-herpetic neuralgia (PHN). PHN is defined as pain that persists from more than 3 months after the onset of acute herpes zoster; it is more common in the immunocompromised patient and the elderly, following acute herpes zoster in 75% of those aged over 70 years (Johnson & Whitton 2004).

Treatment of acute herpes zoster associated pain

Antiviral agents

Acyclovir given within 72 hours of onset of the rash accelerates the resolution of pain and reduces the risk of PHN (Wood et al 1996, **Level I**; Jackson et al 1997, **Level I**). Similar data are available for famciclovir (Dworkin et al 1998, **Level I**) and valaciclovir (Tyring et al 2000, **Level II**).

Antidepressants

Amitriptyline for 90 days, started at the onset of acute zoster, reduced pain prevalence at 6 months post-zoster infection (Bowsher 1997, **Level II**).

Corticosteroids

Corticosteroids may reduce the acute pain of herpes zoster and accelerate the healing of skin lesions, but they neither prevent nor reduce the duration of PHN (Ernst et al 1998). They are not routinely used due to the potential for dissemination of the zoster virus if given without a concurrent antiviral agent and the multitude of potential medical complications associated with their administration.

Anticonvulsants

There is no evidence that anticonvulsants are beneficial in the pain of acute herpes zoster but they are effective in the treatment of PHN (see Section 4.3.4).

Aspirin

Topical aspirin, in either moisturiser or diethyl ether, is an effective analgesic in acute zoster, whereas oral aspirin and topical NSAIDS are not as effective (De Bennedittis & Lorenzetti 1996, **Level II**; Balakrishnan et al 2001, **Level II**).

Neuraxial and sympathetic blockade

A recent review of the use of neuraxial and sympathetic blockade concluded that epidural local anaesthetic plus steroids was effective for the treatment of pain from acute zoster and, if given within 2 months of the onset of the zoster, may reduce the incidence of postherpetic neuralgia at 1 year; evidence for benefit of sympathetic blocks was conflicting (Kumar et al 2004).

Key messages

1. **Antiviral agents started within 72 hours of onset of rash accelerate acute pain resolution and may reduce severity and duration of postherpetic neuralgia (Level I).**
2. **Amitriptyline use in low doses from onset of rash for 90 days reduces incidence of postherpetic neuralgia (Level II).**
3. **Topical aspirin is an effective analgesic in acute zoster (Level II).**

The following tick box ☑ represents conclusions based on clinical experience and expert opinion.

☑ Provision of early and appropriate analgesia is an important component of the management of acute zoster and may have benefits in reducing postherpetic neuralgia.

9.6.3 Acute cardiac pain

Acute coronary syndrome refers to a range of acute myocardial ischaemic states including unstable angina and myocardial infarction. Typically, myocardial ischaemia causes central chest pain, which may radiate into the arm, neck and/ or jaw; non-typical presentations can occur, particularly in the elderly patient (see Section 10.3). Reducing the ischaemia by optimising myocardial oxygen delivery, reducing myocardial oxygen consumption and restoring coronary blood flow will reduce ischaemic pain and limit myocardial tissue damage. The mainstay of analgesia in acute coronary syndrome is the restoration of adequate myocardial oxygenation as outlined above, including the use of supplemental oxygen (Braunwald 2002; Rapaport 2002; Ornato 2003; Pollack 2003).

Nitroglycerine was found to be effective in relieving acute ischaemic chest pain; however, the analgesic response did not predict a diagnosis of active coronary artery disease (Henrikson et al 2003, **Level IV**).

In patients with suspected acute coronary syndrome, IV morphine significantly reduced pain within 20 minutes of administration; morphine doses were low (average of 7mg over 3 days) and 52% of patients required no morphine at all. Independent predictors of increased morphine requirements included suspicion or confirmation of infarction, ST changes on the admission electrocardiogram, male sex and a history of angina or cardiac failure (Everts et al 1998, **Level IV**).

Morphine provided better analgesia than IV metoprolol (Everts et al 1999, **Level II**) and was associated with better cardiovascular outcomes during acute hospital admission and later follow-up when compared with a fentanyl-droperidol mixture administered early in the treatment of patients with acute ischaemic chest pain (Burduk et al 2000, **Level II**).

IV bolus doses of morphine and alfentanil were equally effective in relieving acute ischaemic chest pain but the onset of analgesia was faster with alfentanil (Silvast & Saarnivaara 2001, **Level II**). Morphine was similar to buprenorphine (Weiss & Ritz 1988, **Level II**) and pethidine (Neilsen et al 1984, **Level II**) in terms of analgesia and adverse effects.

IV tramadol provided adequate analgesia with minimal changes in clinical cardiorespiratory parameters in acute myocardial infarction (Rettig & Kropp, **Level III-2**), although it was associated with a significant decrease in left ventricular stroke work index, but stable respiratory parameters when compared with morphine in these patients (Stankov 1995, **Level III-2**).

In patients with chest pain due to cocaine-induced acute coronary syndrome, the addition of IV diazepam or lorazepam to treatment with sublingual nitroglycerine provided superior analgesia (Baumann et al 2000 **Level II**; Honderick et al 2003, **Level II**).

Nitrous oxide in oxygen was effective in relieving acute ischaemic chest pain, with a significant reduction in beta-endorphin levels (O'Leary et al 1987, **Level II**).

NSAIDs may be useful in the treatment of the acute pain of pericarditis (Schifferdecker & Spodick 2003).

Key messages

1 Morphine is an effective and appropriate analgesic for acute cardiac pain (**Level II**).

2 Nitroglycerine is an effective and appropriate agent in the treatment of acute ischaemic chest pain (**Level IV**).

The following tick box ☑ represents conclusions based on clinical experience and expert opinion.

☑ The mainstay of analgesia in acute coronary syndrome is the restoration of adequate myocardial oxygenation, including the use of supplemental oxygen, nitroglycerine, beta blockers and strategies to improve coronary vascular perfusion.

9.6.4 Acute pain and haematological disorders

Sickle cell disease

Sickle cell disease is a common inherited disorder of abnormal haemoglobin production. Haemoglobin S polymerises when deoxygenated, causing rigidity of the erythrocytes, blood hyperviscosity and occlusion of the microcirculation with resultant tissue ischaemia and infarction.

Sickle cell disease most commonly presents with painful vaso-occlusive crises, occurring either spontaneously or due to dehydration, infection, temperature change or low oxygen tension. There is great interindividual variability in the frequency and severity of crises. Pain during an acute crisis is typically severe and most frequently reported in the back, legs, knees, arms, chest and abdomen and may last from hours to weeks

(Ballas & Delengowski 1993, **Level IV**). Sickle cell crises involving abdominal organs can mimic an acute surgical abdomen. Acute chest syndrome secondary to sickle cell disease may present with chest pain, cough, dyspnoea and fever.

Treatment of pain

Biopsychosocial assessment and multidisciplinary pain management may be required when treating patients with frequent, painful sickle cell crises. A pain management plan in the form of a letter, card or portfolio carried by the patient is also recommended (Rees et al 2003).

Detailed clinical guidelines for managing acute painful crises in sickle cell disease are listed in Rees et al (2003).

Oxygen

Although oxygen supplementation is often prescribed during acute sickle cell crises, there was no difference in pain duration, number of pain sites or opioid consumption in patients treated with either air or oxygen (Robieux et al 1992, **Level II**; Zipursky et al 1992, **Level II**). However, nocturnal oxygen desaturation was associated with a significantly higher rate of painful sickle cell crises in children (Hargrave et al 2003, **Level IV**).

NSAIDs

Single dose parenteral ketorolac does not reduce opioid requirements in painful vaso-occlusive crisis (Wright et al 1992, **Level II**; Hardwick et al 1999, **Level II**).

Opioids

Morphine either by IV infusion or oral sustained release preparation was effective in treating acute sickle cell pain (Jacobson et al 1997, **Level II**). IV opioid loading improved the analgesic efficacy of subsequent oral and PCA opioid therapy (Rees et al 2003, **Level II**) and continuous morphine infusion shortened pain duration compared with intermittent opioids (Robieux et al 1992, **Level II**). In children, the incidence of acute sickle chest syndrome, and plasma levels of morphine and morphine-6-glucuronide, was significantly higher with oral morphine compared with IV infusion (Kopecky et al 2004, **Level II**).

Inhaled nitrous oxide

Inhaled nitrous oxide in 50% oxygen used for limited periods may provide analgesia for acute sickle cell pain in the primary care setting (Rees et al 2003).

Inhaled nitric oxide

Nitric oxide (NO) deficiency or defective NO dependent mechanisms may underlie many of the processes leading to vaso-occlusion. Inhaled NO may be of benefit in painful acute vaso-occlusive crises in children; however, further studies are required (Weiner et al 2003, **Level II**).

Corticosteroids

In children, a short course of high dose IV methylprednisolone decreased the duration of severe pain associated with acute sickle cell crises but patients who received methylprednisolone had more rebound attacks after therapy was discontinued (Griffin et al 1994, **Level II**).

Epidural analgesia

In severe crises, where pain is unresponsive to other measures, epidural analgesia has been used effectively (Yaster et al 1994, **Level IV**).

Prevention of painful sickle cell crises

Hydroxyurea increases fetal haemoglobin levels, thereby reducing the frequency of acute crises, blood transfusions and life-threatening complications (including acute chest syndrome) in adults with severe disease who are homozygous for the sickle cell gene (Davies et al 2001, **Level I**).

NIPRISAN® (an anti-sickling agent), zinc and piracetam (which prevent red blood cell dehydration) may reduce the incidence of painful sickle cell crises (Wambebe et al 2001, **Level II**; Riddington & De Franceschi 2002, **Level II**).

Haemophilia

Deficiency of Factor VIII (haemophilia A) and deficiency of Factor IX (haemophilia B) are inherited disorders of coagulation characterised by spontaneous and post-traumatic haemorrhages, the frequency and severity of which are proportional to the degree of clotting factor deficiency. Bleeding into joints and muscle is common, although other sites such as abdominal organs may also be involved. In haemophilic arthropathy the most frequent sites of pain are the ankle joints (45%), knee joints (39%) spine (14%) and elbow joints (7%) (Wallny et al 2001, **Level IV**). Haemophilia patients may also have pain syndromes associated with HIV/AIDS (see Section 9.6.8). Recurrent acute pain may have a significant adverse impact on mood, mobility and quality of life in haemophilia patients; biopsychosocial assessment and treatment should be considered (Wallny et al 2001, **Level IV**).

Many haemophilia patients use Factor VIII to decrease pain associated with a bleeding episode (Wallny et al 2001, **Level IV**). Higher-dose Factor VIII replacement reduced the number of patients with restricted joint movement after an acute haemarthrosis (Aronstam et al 1983, **Level II**). Joint aspiration may reduce pain and improve joint function (Baker 1992).

Although there is no good evidence available, opioids, simple analgesics, cold therapy and bandaging have been used in treating acute pain associated with haemophilia. NSAIDS have been used to provide analgesia in haemophilic arthropathy, but there are no data on their use in acute haemarthrosis. COX-2-specific inhibitors may be of benefit due to a lack of platelet inhibitory effects (see Section 4.2). Intramuscular analgesics should be avoided due to the risk of bleeding.

Key messages

1. Hydroxyurea is effective in decreasing the frequency of acute crises, life-threatening complications and transfusion requirements in sickle cell disease (**Level I**).
2. IV opioid loading optimises analgesia in the early stages of an acute sickle cell crisis. Effective analgesia may be continued with intravenous (including PCA) opioids such as morphine, however pethidine should be avoided (**Level II**).
3. Methylprednisolone decreases acute pain in sickle cell crises (**Level II**).
4. Oxygen supplementation during a sickle cell crisis does not decrease pain (**Level II**).

9.6.5 Acute headache

Headaches are a common cause of acute pain. There are many causes of acute headache, some of which involve structures other than the head (eg the neck). Before treating acute headache, it is important to exclude serious cranial pathologies such as tumour, infection, cerebrovascular abnormalities, acute glaucoma and temporal arteritis (Silberstein 2000, Steiner & Fontebasso 2002).

The most frequent causes of acute headache are migraine and episodic tension type headache (TTH) (Headache Classification Subcommittee of the IHS 2004).

Less frequent causes include: trigemino-autonomic cephalalgias (episodic cluster headache, episodic paroxysmal hemicrania and Short-lasting Unilateral Neuralgiform headache attacks with Conjunctival injection and Tearing [SUNCT]); other primary headaches; acute post-traumatic headache; post dural puncture headache (PDPH); headache attributed to substance use or withdrawal; and cervicogenic headache (Headache Classification Subcommittee of the IHS 2004).

Migraine

Migraine is common, with a prevalence in Australia of 22% in women and 10% in men: up to 57% of patients do not seek medical attention for significant attacks (Mitchell 1998). Migraine headache is usually unilateral and is often severe, disabling and worsened by movement. Nausea, vomiting, photophobia and phonophobia are common and 20% of migraineurs experience an aura.

Patients presenting to the emergency department may represent a special group with approximately 80% having tried their usual medications including simple analgesics and triptans before presentation (Larkin & Prescott 1992; Shrestha et al 1996). The emergency department management of migraine is discussed in Section 9.9.2.

Treatment of acute migraine

Analgesia outcomes in migraine trials are usually listed as the proportion of patients who are either pain free at 2 hours, report pain relief at 2 hours (no headache or mild headache) or report a sustained response over 24 hours (migraine stays away for at least a day). Many trials fail to document associated outcomes such improvement in nausea, vomiting or disability (Moore et al 2003).

There are three major strategies for the use of analgesics in the treatment of acute migraine (Lipton et al 2000a):

- *stratified care* — where for each attack, the severity and disability caused by the migraine is assessed. The patient uses simple analgesia for a mild attack and a triptan for a severe attack;
- *step-up during an attack* — for each attack a simple analgesic is always tried first but the patient 'steps up' to a triptan if there is no relief in 2 hours; and
- *step-up across attacks* — a patient tries simple analgesics exclusively for the first three attacks: if there has been no benefit from simple analgesia over the trial period, then a triptan is used for all further attacks.

Stratified care was superior to 'step-up' strategies in producing pain relief and pain-free outcomes at 2 hours. The degree of disability predicted the type of treatment needed; a simple analgesic was effective with mild migraine-related disability, however a triptan was always required when there was severe disability (Lipton et al 2000b, **Level II**). The US Headache Consortium recommends a stratified care approach (Silberstein 2000).

Simple analgesics

Patients who experience mild migraine-related headache and disability may be effectively treated with simple analgesics, either alone or in combination with an anti-emetic. Soluble aspirin 900mg and metoclopramide 10mg was of similar analgesic efficacy to sumatriptan in mild acute migraine (Tfelt-Hanson et al 1995, **Level II**; Oldman et al 2002, **Level I**). Over the counter medications may be effective in migraine of mild to moderate severity with 21% to 76% of patients returning to normal function after 2 hours (Wenzel 2003, **Level IV**).

Table 9.2 Simple analgesics for the treatment of migraine

Analgesic regimen	NNT*	Source
Aspirin 600–900mg +metoclopramide 10mg	3.2	Oldman et al 2002, **Level I**
Paracetamol 1000mg	5.2	Lipton et al 2000b, **Level II**
Ibuprofen 200–400mg	7.5	Codispoti 2002, **Level II**

* Simple analgesics for the treatment of migraine: 2-hour pain response (nil or mild residual headache at 2 hours).

Triptans

Triptans are highly effective in the treatment of acute migraine, particularly in the presence of severe pain and disability, where simple analgesia has failed to provide adequate relief in the past. As there is considerable interindividual response to the different triptans, patients should trial a variety of drugs and doses until the most suitable regimen is found (Silberstein 2000, Oldman et al 2002, **Level I**).

The route of administration of a triptan may affect its efficacy, speed of onset and tolerability. Subcutaneous injections and nasal sprays provide fast onset of symptom relief and higher efficacy, particularly in the presence of nausea and vomiting, but are less well tolerated by patients: in contrast, oral triptans are well tolerated but have a slower onset of action and lower reliability due to gastric stasis associated with migraine (Dahlof 2002). Therefore, if the oral route is used, it should preferably be early in an attack: suppositories are well tolerated and avoid oral absorption problems (Dahlof 2002).

Table 9.3 Table of triptans

Drug	Route	NNT (95% Confidence intervals) *
Sumatriptan 6mg	SC	2.1 (1.9–2.4)
Rizatriptan 10mg	oral	3.1 (2.9–3.5)
Eletriptan 80mg	oral	3.7 (3.2–4.2)
Zolmitriptan 5mg	oral	3.9 (3.4–4.6)
Eletriptan 40mg	oral	4.5 (3.9–5.1)
Sumatriptan 20mg	IN	4.6 (3.6–6.1)
Sumatriptan 100mg	oral	4.7 (4.1–5.7)
Rizatriptan 2.5mg	oral	4.7 (4.0–5.7)
Zolmitriptan 2.5mg	oral	5.9 (4.5–8.7)
Sumatriptan 50mg	oral	7.8 (6.1–11)
Naratriptan 2.5mg	oral	8.2 (5.1–21)
Eletriptan 20mg	oral	10 (7–17)
Aspirin 900mg plus metoclopramide 10mg	oral	8.6 (6.2–14)

* NNTs to provide 2-hour pain-free response in migraine patient.

Source: Bandolier (www.jr2.ox.ac.uk/bandolier/); reproduced with permission.

The most frequent adverse events associated with triptans are dizziness, fatigue, sleepiness, nausea, chest tightness and paraesthesiae. Sensory side-effects, particularly allodynia (light touch) and thermal sensitivity, have been noted (Linde 2004). The average number of any adverse events reported using various triptans ranges from 18–50%. Sumatriptan has the greatest incidence and range of reported adverse events in placebo-controlled trials (Dahhof 2002a).

Concern about adverse cardiac events is the main reason why only 10% of patients with migraine receive a triptan for acute therapy (Dahlof 2002, Kelly 1995). A sensation of chest tightness occurred in 0.1–0.2% of patients who received almotriptan compared with 3–5% of patients on sumatriptan (Dahlof et al 2002). However, chest tightness may not always be due to a cardiac cause (Dahlof in IASP 2002). There is no association between a lifetime history of migraine with or without aura and coronary artery disease related angina (Rose 2004). In a positron emission tomography study, sumatriptan did not affect myocardial perfusion or the electrocardiogram in migraine patients who had no history of ischaemic heart disease (Lewis et al 1997).

Frequent use of triptans may lead to triptan induced rebound headaches (Silberstein & Welch 2002, Limmroth et al 2002).

Ergot derivatives

Ergotamine and dihydroergotamine preparations have been used for many years to treat migraine. Intranasal dihydroergotamine (2mg) has a NNT of 2.5 for 2-hour headache response in migraine (Oldman 2002, **Level I**). Despite previous wide usage, these preparations are rapidly being superseded by the triptans.

Opioids

Opioids have limited benefit in the treatment of acute migraine and their use is not recommended. Morphine without an antiemetic was no more effective than placebo (Elenbaas et al 1991, **Level II**; Nicolodi 1996, **Level II**). Pethidine resulted in no better analgesia than dihydroergotamine, antihistamines or NSAIDs (Lane et al 1989, **Level II**; Stiell et al 1991; Davis 1995; Scherl & Wilson 1995). Butorphanol was effective when given by the intranasal or IM route (Diamond et al 1992, **Level II**; Hoffert et al 1995, **Level II**).

Other medications

The efficacy of lignocaine (lidocaine) in the treatment of acute migraine is unclear. Analgesia provided by IV lignocaine was similar to dihydroergotamine, but not as effective as chlorpromazine (Bell et al 1990, **Level II**) and in one trial no better than placebo (Reutens et al 1991, **Level II**). Results for intranasal lignocaine are conflicting (Maizels et al 1996, **Level II**, Blanda et al 2001, **Level II**).

IV sodium valproate was ineffective in treating acute migraine (Tanen et al 2003, **Level II**). The efficacy of IV magnesium sulphate remains unclear (Corbo et al 2001, **Level II**; Demirkaya et al 2001, **Level II**).

Parenteral metoclopramide (Colman et al 2004, **Level I**), chlorpromazine (Bigal et al 2002, **Level II**) and prochlorperazine (Jones et al 1989, **Level II**) are effective treatments for acute migraine, particularly in the emergency department setting. Low dose IM droperidol was moderately effective but was associated with a 13% incidence of akathisia (Richman et al 2002, **Level II**; Silberstein et al 2003, **Level II**). Parenteral prochlorperazine was more effective than metoclopramide and placebo (Coppola 1995, **Level II**; Jones et al 1996, **Level II**) and led to better analgesia than IV ketorolac in adults and children (Seim et al 1998, **Level II**; Brousseau et al 2004, **Level II**). A combination of prochlorperazine, indomethacin and caffeine was more effective than sumatriptan alone (DiMonda et al 2003, **Level II**) and buccal prochlorperazine was superior to oral ergotamine-caffeine combination and placebo (Sharma et al 2002, **Level II**).

Paediatric migraine

Migraine headaches are common in children (3% in children aged 3 to 6 years) and increase in frequency up to adolescence (up to 23% in those aged 11 to 16 years). Guidelines for evaluation of children and adolescents with headache were published by the American Academies of Neurology and Paediatrics and the American Headache Society (Lewis et al 2002).

General principles of treatment are similar to adults but require consideration of paediatric pharmacological issues including efficacy and safety. Paracetamol and ibuprofen are appropriate for initial management and sumatriptan nasal spray is effective in children over 12 years of age; there were no data to support or refute the use of any oral triptans preparation in children or adolescents (Lewis et al 2004).

Tension type headache

Tension type headache (TTH) may be episodic (frequent or infrequent) or chronic in nature. The lifetime prevalence of TTH in the general population is 30–78%. Episodic TTH is usually bilateral and is often described as a mild to moderate 'pressing' or 'tight pain' (sometimes with peri-cranial tenderness), not worsened by movement and not associated with nausea. Photophobia or phonophobia may occasionally be present (Headache Classification Subcommittee of the IHS 2004).

The symptoms and pathogenesis of TTH may overlap with migraine, chronic daily headache, medication overuse headache and cervicogenic headache (Goadsby 2003). Psychological, physical and environmental factors are important in TTH and should be addressed during assessment and treatment (Holroyd 2002).

Treatment

Simple analgesics such as NSAIDs, paracetamol (Prior et al 2002, **Level II**; Steiner et al 2003) or aspirin (Steiner et al 2003, **Level II**), either alone or in combination, provide effective analgesia in TTH. Ketoprofen, ibuprofen and naproxen were equally effective and better than paracetamol (Lange & Lentz 1995, **Level I**; Dahlof & Jacobs 1996) and the addition of caffeine to paracetamol, aspirin (Migliardi et al 1994, **Level I**) and ibuprofen (Diamond et al 2000, **Level II**) significantly improved analgesia.

Cluster headache and other trigeminovascular cephalalgias

Cluster headache presents almost exclusively in males with recurrent, acute episodes of brief, severe, unilateral, periorbital pain associated with autonomic phenomena such as conjunctival injection and tearing.

Triptans

Subcutaneous sumatriptan injection (Ekbom 1995, **Level II**) and intranasal sumatripan spray (Van Vliet et al 2003, **Level II**) are effective first-line treatments for acute cluster headache, with subcutaneous administration providing faster onset and greater reliability of analgesia (Hardebo & Dahlof 1998, **Level II**). Oral zolmitriptan was effective in treating episodic cluster headache but not chronic cluster headache (Bahra et al 2000, **Level II**).

Oxygen

Oxygen therapy is effective for patients with a contraindication to sumatriptan or who experience several cluster attacks per day (Dahlof 2002). Oxygen delivered by face mask at a flow rate of 7–10 l/min for 15 minutes provided symptomatic relief in approximately 70% of patients with acute cluster headache (Kudrow 1981; Fogan 1985, **Level II**).

Hyperbaric oxygen was no better than sham hyperbaric treatment in reducing cluster headache frequency or duration. However, 83% of patients with episodic cluster headache improved significantly with either treatment, suggesting a possible placebo effect or a therapeutic benefit of the hyperbaric process itself (Nilsson Remahl et al 2002, **Level II**).

Other treatments

Injectable and intranasal dihydroergotamine may be of benefit in relieving acute cluster headaches, but its use has been superseded by sumatriptan (Dodick et al 2000). Intranasal lignocaine (lidocaine) may also be effective (Dahlof 2002).

Paroxysmal hemicrania and SUNCT

Paroxysmal hemicrania and SUNCT are rarer forms of trigeminovascular cephalalgias. Paroxysmal hemicrania is similar to cluster headache except that it is more common in females, episodes are shorter but more frequent and diagnosis requires the complete abolition of symptoms with indomethacin (Headache Classification Subcommittee of the IHS 2004). There is no high level evidence to guide the treatment of SUNCT.

Post dural puncture headache

Headache following dural puncture may occur with an incidence of 0.4–24%. PDPH is classically postural in nature and is more common in patients under 50 years of age and in the parturient. Up to 90% of cases improve spontaneously within 10 days (Candido & Stevens 2003).

The incidence of PDPH may be reduced by using a 26 gauge (or smaller) sized needle (NNT= 13) or the use of a needle with a non-cutting bevel (NNT= 27) (Halpern & Preston 1994, **Level I**).

There is no evidence that bed rest is beneficial in the prevention of PDPH (Sudlow & Warlow 2001a, **Level I**). However, patients with PDPH may have difficulty mobilising and the headache may subside with bed rest. Non-opioid and opioid analgesics may provide temporary relief (Candido & Stevens 2003). The preventive role of fluid therapy remains unclear (Sudlow & Warlow 2004a, **Level I**).

There was no evidence to support the use of sumatriptan (Connelly et al 2000, **Level II**), adrenocorticotrophic hormone (Candido & Stevens 2003), epidurally administered saline, dextran or fibrin glue or neuraxial opioids (Turnbull & Shepherd 2003) in the management of PDPH.

Intravenous (Sechzer & Abel 1978, **Level II**) and oral caffeine (Camann et al 1990, **Level II**) were effective in treating PDPH but did not reduce the rate of blood patch administration (Candido & Stevens 2003).

Although common practice, further high quality trials are required to determine the efficacy of epidural blood patch administration in the treatment of PDPH (Sudlow & Warlow 2001b, **Level I**). However significant symptomatic relief was obtained in 75–95% of patients who received a 15mL blood patch (Safa-Tisseront et al 2001, **Level IV**; Wu et al 1994, **Level IV**; Abouleish et al 1975, **Level IV**). There is conflicting evidence for the benefit of prophylactic epidural blood patches, with one trial showing a decreased incidence of PDPH (Colonna-Romano & Shapiro 1989, **Level II**). The use of autologous blood patches may be contraindicated in patients with leukaemia, a coagulopathy or infection including HIV.

Other headaches

There is little evidence to guide the treatment of acute cervicogenic headache, post traumatic headache, other primary headaches or acute headaches associated with substance use or withdrawal although general principles of evaluation of headache and management of acute pain must apply (US Headache Consortium 2000).

Complementary and alternative medicines and therapies

There is no good evidence for efficiency for acupuncture, hypnotherapy, chiropractic, spinal manipulation or homeopathy in the treatment of acute migraine or TTH (Vernon et al 1999, **Level I**; Astin & Ernst 2002, **Level I**; Melchart et al 2001, **Level I**)

Opioids and acute headache

Although opioids are commonly used for the emergency treatment of headache (Vinson 2002) they cannot be recommended for use on a regular basis because of the risk of dependency and other opioid-related adverse effects. The Australian Association of Neurologists recommends that opioids should not be used for migraine unless the patient is unresponsive to all other measures or, where the use of ergot agents and triptans is contraindicated (Lance et al 1997).

Key messages

1. Triptans are effective in the treatment of severe migraine (**Level I**).
2. Aspirin-metoclopramide is effective in the treatment of mild to moderate migraine (**Level I**).
3. Parenteral metoclopramide is effective in the treatment of acute migraine (**Level I**).
4. Parenteral prochlorperazine, chlorpromazine and droperidol are effective in the treatment of acute migraine (**Level II**).
5. Addition of caffeine to aspirin or paracetamol improves analgesia in acute tension-type headache (TTH) (**Level I**).
6. The incidence of post dural puncture headache (PDPH) is reduced by using small gauge needles with a non-cutting edge (**Level I**).
7. There is no evidence that bed rest is beneficial in the prevention of PDPH (**Level I** [Cochrane Review]).
8. Ibuprofen and paracetamol are effective in the treatment of mild to moderate migraine (**Level II**)
9. A 'stratified care strategy' is effective in treating migraine (**Level II**).
10. Simple analgesics such as aspirin, paracetamol, NSAIDs, either alone or in combination, are effective in the treatment of episodic TTH (**Level II**).
11. Sumatriptan is effective in the treatment of cluster headache (**Level II**).
12. Oxygen is effective in the treatment of cluster headache (**Level II**).

13. Epidural blood patch administration may be effective in the treatment of PDPH (**Level IV**).

The following tick boxes ☑ represent conclusions based on clinical experience and expert opinion.

☑ Opioids should be used with caution in the treatment of headaches; pethidine should be avoided.

☑ Frequent use of analgesics, triptans and ergot derivatives in the treatment of recurrent acute headache may lead to medication overuse headache.

9.6.6 Acute pain associated with neurological disorders

Pain associated with neurological disorders is usually neuropathic in nature, although nociceptive pain (eg with muscle spasms) may also occur. Neuropathic pain may be acute or chronic and may be due to a lesion or dysfunction of the peripheral nervous system (eg painful peripheral neuropathy) or the central nervous system (central pain, for example multiple sclerosis and post-stroke pain) (Merskey & Bogduk 1994).

As there is no good evidence to guide the management of acute pain associated with neurological disease, treatment must largely be based on evidence from trials of pain relief for a variety of chronic neuropathic pain states; including tricyclic antidepressants (TCAs), anticonvulsants, membrane stabilisers, NMDA-receptor antagonists, opioids and tramadol (see Sections 4.3.2 to 4.3.6 and 4.1).

Associated psychosocial problems and physical disabilities must also be managed within a multidisciplinary framework.

Multiple sclerosis

Central pain is reported in over 28% of patients with multiple sclerosis; 20% reported musculoskeletal pain such as back pain or muscle spasms (Wall & Melzack 1999). These patients may experience acute pain with trigeminal neuralgia, which responds to carbamazepine (Wiffen et al 2000; **Level I**). Other anticonvulsants may also be effective but evidence specific to multiple sclerosis is lacking. There is also no evidence to guide prescribing of antispasticity agents including baclofen (Shakespeare et al 2003, **Level I**).

Stroke

Central pain develops in 8.4% of stroke patients (Wall & Melzack 1999) and may be treated with tricyclic antidepressants (McQuay et al 1996, **Level I**). Anticonvulsant agents may also be effective: small studies have indicated benefit from lamotrigine (Vestergaard et al 2001, **Level II**) and gabapentin (Nicholson 2004). Post-stroke patients may also develop a musculoskeletal shoulder pain syndrome which requires physical therapy and treatment based on simple analgesics, NSAIDs or COX-2 selective inhibitors.

Guillain-Barre syndrome

See Section 9.8.

Spinal cord injury

See Section 9.2.

Key messages

The following tick box ☑ represents conclusions based on clinical experience and expert opinion.

☑ Treatment of acute pain associated with neurological disorders is largely based on evidence from trials for the treatment of a variety of chronic neuropathic pain states.

9.6.7 Orofacial pain

Acute orofacial pain may be caused by infective, traumatic, neuropathic, vascular, neoplastic or other pathologies (Zakrzewska & Harrison 2003; Keith 2004; Ward & Levin 2004). Most commonly, acute orofacial pain is due to dental or sinus disease but it may also be associated with chronic facial pain syndromes (eg trigeminal neuralgia) or be referred from adjacent regions such as the cervical spine and the thorax. A thorough history (including dental) and examination (particularly of the oral cavity and cranial nerves) are essential components of the assessment of orofacial pain.

Recurrent or persistent orofacial pain requires a biopsychosocial assessment and appropriate multidisciplinary management (Vickers et al 2000). Neuropathic orofacial pain (atypical odontalgia, phantom pain) may be exacerbated by repeated dental procedures (eg extraction of teeth, root canal therapy, sectioning of nerves), incorrect drug therapy or psychological factors (Vickers et al 1998).

Acute postoperative dental pain

Acute pain after third molar extraction is the most extensively studied model for testing postoperative analgesics; ibuprofen, paracetamol and aspirin are effective in this setting. Interestingly, analgesic response to placebo was significantly lower in postdental extraction pain than in other acute pain models (Barden et al 2004, **Level I**).

Table 9.4 Efficacy of commonly prescribed analgesics for acute pain after dental extraction

Drug	NNT*
Aspirin 600/650mg	4.7 (4.2–5.4)
Paracetamol 600/650mg	4.2 (3.6–5.2)
Paracetamol 1000mg	3.7 (3.1–4.7)
Ibuprofen 400mg	2.2 (2.6–3.4)

* NNT for 50% max TOTPAR (half pain relief) at 4–6 hours.

Source: Adapted from Barden et al (2004).

NSAIDS were more effective than paracetamol or codeine (either alone or in combination) for treating pain after third molar extraction (Ahmad et al 1997, **Level I**). Ketorolac provided better analgesia with fewer adverse effects than pethidine (Fricke et al 1992, **Level II**) or tramadol (Ong & Tan 2004, **Level II**).

COX-2 selective inhibitors were of similar efficacy to NSAIDS in acute postoperative dental pain (Chen et al 2004, **Level I**; Cicconetti et al 2004, **Level I**). Rofecoxib (Chang et al 2001, **Level II**) and valdecoxib were more effective and produced less nausea than paracetamol/opioid combinations (Chen et al 2004, **Level I**). Rofecoxib demonstrated extended analgesia with a NNT of 2.8 (2.5–3.1) at 24 hours (Edwards et al 2004, **Level I**). Rofecoxib and ibuprofen were both effective in treating acute postendodontic pain, with rofecoxib again demonstrating an extended duration of analgesia (Gopikrishna & Parameswaran 2003, **Level II**).

Tramadol 100mg had a similar efficacy to aspirin/opioid or paracetamol/opioid combinations in treating acute dental pain (Moore & McQuay 1997, **Level I**). A tramadol/paracetamol combination was superior to tramadol alone with fewer adverse effects (Edwards et al 2002, **Level I**; Fricke et al 2004, **Level II**).

Perioperative dexamethasone administration reduced acute postoperative pain, nausea and swelling after third molar extraction (Baxendale et al 1993, **Level II**; Schmelzeisen & Frolich 1993, **Level II**).

NSAIDS and emergency pulpectomy but not antibiotics provided significant pain relief in patients with acute apical periodontitis (Sutherland & Matthews 2003, **Level I**).

Acupuncture may be of benefit in reducing post-procedural dental pain but further high quality trials are required (Ernst & Pittler 1998, **Level I**).

Acute pain associated with sinusitis and otitis media

There is no evidence to guide choice of analgesic for acute pain associated with sinusitis or otitis media. It may be appropriate to use NSAIDs, COX-2 selective inhibitors, paracetamol, weak opioids or tramadol, based on evidence for treatment of dental pain.

Nasal irrigation with physiological saline may provide symptomatic relief (Clement et al 1996; Low et al 1997). Administration of penicillin V decreased pain scores over 3 days in patients with severe sinus pain (Hansen et al 2000, **Level II**).

In children, antibiotics provided only a small improvement (NNT 15) in pain associated with acute otitis media after 2 days of treatment (Glasziou et al 2003, **Level I**).

Acute post-tonsillectomy pain

There is no evidence that perioperative local anaesthetic infiltration improves postoperative pain control after tonsillectomy (Hollis et al 1999, **Level I**).

NSAIDs were as effective as opioids and reduced the risk of emesis in post-tonsillectomy patients. However aspirin (Krishna et al 2003, **Level I**) and NSAIDs (number-needed-to-harm [NNH] 29–60) increased the risk of reoperation for post-tonsillectomy bleeding (Marret et al 2003, **Level I**; Møiniche et al 2003, **Level I**) (see also Sections 4.2.2 and 10.1.5).

Diclofenac (Rømsing et al 2000, **Level II**; Schmidt et al 2001, **Level II**) and ketorolac (Rusy et al 1995, **Level II**) were no more effective than paracetamol in providing analgesia in children post-tonsillectomy but were associated with a higher intraoperative blood loss.

Rofecoxib was effective in providing analgesia for up to 24 hours post surgery with decreased nausea and no increased blood loss (Joshi et al 2003, **Level II**).

In children, the administration of IV dexamethasone after tonsillectomy decreased postoperative vomiting and shortened time to starting a soft diet although there were no specific data on pain (Steward et al 2002, **Level I**). Further evidence for the treatment of post-tonsillectomy pain is listed in Section 10.1.

Acute pain associated with oral ulceration including acute mucositis

Acute oral ulceration due to trauma (physical, chemical, thermal), infection (eg herpes simplex), drugs, radiation or chemotherapy (mucositis – see Section 9.7) may be extremely painful and debilitating. Mucosal analgesia may be achieved by topical application of EMLA® cream and 5% Xylocaine (Vickers & Punnia-Moorthy 1992, **Level II**).

In treating the pain of cancer-related acute mucositis, there was no significant difference in analgesia between PCA and continuous opioid infusion except that PCA was associated with lower opioid requirements and reduced duration of pain (Worthington et al 2004, **Level I**). PCA morphine provided better analgesia and less rapid dose escalation than hydromorphone or sufentanil (Coda et al 1997, **Level II**).

Lignocaine (lidocaine) solutions, chlorhexidine and sulcrafate were of no more benefit that simple salt and soda water mixtures; allopurinol mouthwash, vitamin E, immunoglobulin and human placental extract may improve outcomes in acute mucositis but the evidence is inconclusive (Worthington et al 2004, **Level I**). Topical ketamine rinse provided analgesia in a patient with acute mucositis pain (Slatkin & Rhiner 2003).

Key messages

1. NSAIDs, COX-2 selective inhibitors, paracetamol, opioids and tramadol provide effective analgesia after dental extraction (**Level I**).
2. NSAIDS and COX-2 selective inhibitors provide better analgesia with less adverse effects than paracetamol, paracetamol/opioid, paracetamol/tramadol, tramadol or weaker opioids after dental extraction (**Level I**).
3. Perioperative local anaesthetic infiltration does not improve analgesia after tonsillectomy (**Level I** [Cochrane Review]).
4. Aspirin and NSAIDs increase the risk of reoperation for post-tonsillectomy bleeding (**Level I**).
5. PCA and continuous opioid infusions are equally effective in the treatment of pain in mucositis, but opioid consumption is less with PCA (**Level I** [Cochrane Review]).
6. Perioperative dexamethasone administration reduces acute pain, nausea and swelling after third molar extraction (**Level II**).
7. Topical treatments may provide analgesia in acute oral ulceration (**Level II**).

The following tick box ☑ represents conclusions based on clinical experience and expert opinion.

☑ Recurrent or persistent orofacial pain requires biopsychosocial assessment and appropriate multidisciplinary approaches. Neuropathic orofacial pain (atypical odontalgia, phantom pain) may be exacerbated by repeated dental procedures, incorrect drug therapy or psychological factors.

9.6.8 Acute pain in patients with HIV infection

Pain is a common problem in people infected with the human immunodeficiency virus (HIV), particularly when they develop the acquired immunodeficiency syndrome (AIDS). Pain may be due to the effects of the virus, which is neurotropic, or an infective or neoplastic process associated with immunodeficiency. Pain may also be a side effect of treatment or related to debilitation (in patients with end-stage AIDS) or may be due to an unrelated comorbidity (O'Neill & Sherrard 1993; Glare 2001).

In patients with HIV/AIDS pain is progressive, affecting approximately 25% with early stage disease, 50–75% with AIDS and almost all patients in the terminal phase (Singer et al 1993, **Level IV**; Breitbart et al 1996a, Kimball & McCormick 1996). CD4+ T-cell count does not predict number of symptoms or severity of distress (Vogl et al 1999, **Level IV**).

Pain occurs at multiple sites with the number of pains reported per patient increasing throughout the course of AIDS. The most frequent neurological diagnosis is a distal symmetrical polyneuropathy (DSP, 38%). Common clinical features of DSP include non-painful paresthesias (71%), abnormalities of pain and temperature perception (71%), and reduced or absent ankle reflexes (66%). Increased age, immunosuppression, poor nutritional status and the presence of chronic disease all contribute to distal peripheral nerve dysfunction associated with HIV infection (Tagliati et al 1999, **Level IV**).

Pain associated with HIV/AIDS is often undertreated due to patient and clinician-related barriers (Breitbart et al 1996b, **Level IV**; Larue et al 1997; Breitbart et al 1998; Breitbart et al 1999; Frich & Borgbjerg 2000). Undertreatment is more common in certain patient groups (non-Caucasians, women, those with a substance abuse disorder, less educated individuals, and those with higher levels of psychosocial distress (Breitbart et al 1998, **Level IV**).

Disease-specific therapy, psychosocial interventions and physical modalities should accompany standard analgesic treatment (Jacox et al 1994; Glare 2001). Disease-specific therapy may need to be ceased prematurely if pain is a side effect (eg peripheral neuropathy caused by some antiretrovirals).

Treatment of HIV/AIDS-related pain

A significant reduction in pain intensity was achievable with controlled-release opioids in a variety of painful conditions with limited or manageable side effects, supporting the usefulness of opioid analgesia for HIV-related severe pain (Kaplan et al 1996; Kaplan et al 2000 **Level IV**). Approximately 15–20% of patients need parenteral opioids in the terminal phase (Dixon & Higginson 1991, **Level IV**; Kimball & McCormick 1996, **Level IV**; Frich & Borgbjerg 2000, **Level IV**).

CHAPTER 9

Transdermal fentanyl provided better pain relief and improvement in daily functioning in patients with severe AIDS-related pain who were previously taking oral opioids (Newshan & Lefkowitz 2001, **Level IV**).

Several complex drug interactions may occur between opioids and other medications taken by patients with HIV/AIDS; however the clinical relevance of most of these interactions is still unclear.

The HIV-1 protease inhibitor ritonavir inhibits the metabolism of methadone and buprenorphine (Iribarne et al 1998) but this has no relevant clinical effect (McCance-Katz et al 2003, **Level III-2**). However, ritonavir results in a clinically relevant inhibition of fentanyl metabolism (Olkkola et al 1999, **Level II**) and leads to increased concentrations of the toxic metabolite norpethidine if used in combination with pethidine (Piscitelli et al 2000, **Level III-2**). Lopinavir induces metabolism of methadone leading to withdrawal symptoms in patients on maintenance doses (McCance-Katz et al 2003, **Level III-2**). Rifampicin and rifabutin may increase opioid metabolism (particularly methadone) (Finch et al 2002) and fluconazole may potentiate adverse effects of methadone (Tarumi et al 2002). Zidovudine metabolism is inhibited by methadone, thereby increasing its bioavailability and possibly toxicity (McCance-Katz et al 1998, **Level III-3**).

Painful peripheral neuropathy associated with HIV infection has been the subject of a number of treatment trials, including tricyclic antidepressants (Kieburtz 1998, **Level II**; Shlay 1998, **Level II**) anticonvulsants (Simpson et al 2000, **Level II**; La Spina et al 2001, **Level IV**), antiarrythymics (Kemper et al 1998, **Level II**; Kieburtz 1998, **Level II**), topical capsaicin (Paice et al 2000a, **Level IV**), Peptide T (Simpson et al 1996, **Level II**), vibratory counterstimulation (Paice et al 2000b, **Level III-1**) and acupuncture (Shlay 1998, **Level II**). Of these, the only treatments that have been demonstrated to be better than placebo are lamotrigine (Simpson et al 2000, **Level II**) and gabapentin (La Spina et al 2001, **Level IV**).

Patients with a history of substance abuse

HIV/AIDS patients with a history of substance abuse are more likely to receive inadequate analgesia, report more pain and suffer greater psychological distress (Breitbart et al 1997, **Level III-2**). The principles of pain management in these patients are outlined in Section 10.9.

Key messages

The following tick boxes ☑ represent conclusions based on clinical experience and expert opinion.

☑ Neuropathic pain is common in patients with HIV/AIDS.

☑ In the absence of specific evidence, the treatment of pain in patients with HIV/AIDS should be based on similar principles to those for the management of cancer and chronic pain.

☑ Interaction between anti-retroviral and antibiotic medications and opioids should be considered in this population.

9.7 ACUTE CANCER PAIN

Acute pain in cancer patients is common, in particular as breakthrough pain in patients with chronic cancer pain (Fine & Busch 1998). Breakthrough pain is defined as pain that breaks through an existing analgesic regimen; this includes incident pain (McQuay & Jadad 1994).

Such acute pain requires urgent provision of analgesia. Normal breakthrough doses of analgesic agents may be insufficient (see Section 10.8) and retitration of opioid analgesia might become necessary. In an emergency situation, IV titration with fentanyl (Soares et al 2003, **Level II**) or use of transmucosal fentanyl (Farrar et al 1998, **Level II**; Coluzzi et al 2001) has been successful.

The management of cancer pain has been assessed in an evidence-based manner by the Scottish Cancer Therapy Network and a national clinical guideline on *Control of Pain in Patients with Cancer* has been published by the Scottish Intercollegiate Guidelines Network (SIGN 2000). These guidelines can be found at www.sign.ac.uk/pdf/sign44.pdf.

Overall there is a deficit of evidence for a number of practices in cancer pain management. Where evidence exists the specific issues related to acute pain in cancer patients have been extracted and condensed from these guidelines.

For the management of acute pain in children with cancer see Section 10.1.8; for the management of pain associated with mucositis see Section 9.6.7.

Key messages

1. Oral transmucosal fentanyl is effective in treating acute breakthrough pain in cancer patients (**Level II**).
2. Analgesic medications prescribed for cancer pain should be adjusted to alterations of pain intensity (**Level III**).
3. Opioid doses for individual patients with cancer pain should be titrated to achieve maximum analgesic benefit with minimal adverse effects (**Level III**).

The following tick boxes ☑ represent conclusions based on clinical experience and expert opinion.

☑ Acute pain in patients with cancer often signals disease progression; sudden severe pain in patients with cancer should be recognised as a medical emergency and immediately assessed and treated.

☑ Cancer patients receiving controlled-release opioids need access to immediate-release opioids for breakthrough pain; if the response is insufficient after 30–60 minutes, administration should be repeated.

☑ Breakthrough analgesia should be one-sixth of the total regular daily opioid dose in patients with cancer pain (except when methadone is used, because of its long and variable half life).

☑ If nausea and vomiting accompany acute cancer pain, parenteral opioids are needed.

CHAPTER 9

9.8 Acute pain management in intensive care

The management of pain in intensive care requires the application of many principles detailed elsewhere in these guidelines. Analgesia may be required for a range of painful conditions, for example after surgery and trauma, in association with invasive devices and procedures and acute neuropathic pain. There may also be a need for the intensivist to provide palliative care (Hawryluck et al 2002).

Updated consensus guidelines have been published in the USA for the provision of analgesia and sedation in adult intensive care (Jacobi et al 2002), but there remains a dearth of sufficient large-scale randomised intensive care unit (ICU) pain studies from which to form evidence-based guidelines. Some of the key consensus findings regarding IV analgesia and sedation in the ICU setting were (Jacobi et al 2002):

- a therapeutic plan and goal of analgesia should be established and communicated to caregivers;
- pain assessment and response to therapy should be performed regularly;
- the level of pain reported by the patient is the standard for assessment but subjective observation and physiological indicators may be used when the patient cannot communicate; and
- sedation of agitated critically ill patients should only be started after providing adequate analgesia and treating reversible physiological causes.

It is difficult to separate pain management from sedation in this context and intensive care sedation algorithms usually address both aspects. Probably the most useful intervention during sedation and analgesia in ICU is the provision of a daily drug 'holiday' to reassess the need for sedation and analgesia. This simple step is associated with significantly shorter periods of mechanical ventilation and shorter stays in the ICU (Kress et al 2000, **Level II**), but does not cause adverse psychological outcomes and reduces symptoms of post-traumatic stress disorder (Kress et al 2003, **Level III-2**).

9.8.1 Pain assessment in the ICU

Assessment of pain in the ICU is difficult. The most important index of pain is the patient's own subjective experience, but it is frequently impossible to quantify this because of the presence of an endotracheal tube, or decreased conscious state due to illness or co-administered sedative agents. In 17 trauma patients admitted to an ICU, 95% of doctors and 81% of nurses felt that the patients had adequate analgesia whereas 74% of patients rated their pain as moderate or severe (Whipple et al 1995, **Level IV**).

Traditional subjective scales including the visual analogue scale (VAS) or numeric rating scale (NRS) are not applicable to the unresponsive patient. Instead, the observation of behavioural and physiological responses may be the only information available to modify pain management (Puntillo et al 1997, **Level IV**; Puntillo et al 2002, **Level IV**; Chong & Burchett 2003).

9.8.2 Non-pharmacological measures

Much of the discomfort associated with a prolonged admission to intensive care can be alleviated by holistic nursing care. Attention to detail with positioning, pressure care, comfortable fixation of invasive devices, care in the management of secretions and excretions, minimisation of noise from spurious alarms and unnecessary equipment (such as the uncritical application of high-flow mask oxygen) can substantially lessen the burden of discomfort for the patient (Aaron et al 1996; Chong & Burchett 2003, **Level IV**; Puntillo et al 2004, **Level III-3**). Maintenance of a day/night routine (lighting and activity) is thought to aid sleep quality (Horsburgh 1995). A flexible and liberal visiting policy should decrease the pain of separation from family and friends. Physiotherapy maintains range of movement of joints and slows deconditioning while massage can trigger a relaxation response leading to improved sleep.

9.8.3 Pharmacological treatment

The mainstay of treatment of acute pain in the ICU remains parenteral opioid analgesia (Shapiro et al 1995; Hawryluck et al 2002). Partial agonists are contraindicated because of the possibility of precipitation of withdrawal in patients exposed to opioids for long periods. Morphine is usually the first choice, but it is relatively contraindicated in the presence of renal impairment because of possible accumulation of its active metabolites. Pethidine is rarely used in the ICU because of concerns about accumulation of norpethidine, especially in the presence of renal dysfunction or prolonged exposure, and because of its potential interaction with several drugs (eg tramadol, MAOIs and selective serotonin re-uptake inhibitors). Fentanyl is emerging as a useful alternative to morphine, with a lesser tendency to cause haemodynamic instability (Shapiro et al 1995). It has a short duration of action after a single dose due to redistribution, but its long elimination half-life suggests that it may be accumulative when given in high doses for long periods.

The newer opioids, alfentanil and remifentanil, have potentially favourable kinetics for use in patients with organ dysfunction. Alfentanil combined with propofol led to shorter time to extubation and ICU discharge compared with a morphine and midazolam combination (Manley et al 1997, **Level II**). Remifentanil exhibits rapid clearance that is independent of renal function (Cohen & Royston 2001; Breen et al 2004); while remifentanil acid, a weak active metabolite, may accumulate in the presence of renal impairment (Pitsiu et al 2004, **Level IV**). This has no clinical consequences (Breen et al 2004, **Level IV**). When titrated carefully against a sedation scale, remifentanil did not reduce the need for supplementary sedation or the time to extubation after cessation compared with fentanyl (Muellejans et al 2004, **Level II**).

For analgesia-based sedation in the ICU, adherence to a clear protocol might be more important than the choice of medication (Kuhlen & Putensen 2004).

Dexmedetomidine is a highly selective alpha-2 agonist sedative, with anxiolytic and analgesic properties. It has the advantage of providing titratable sedation with minimal respiratory depression (Martin et al 2003, **Level II**). It can cause a temporary increase in blood pressure during administration, but the subsequent reductions in heart rate and blood pressure are more noticeable, especially in haemodynamically labile individuals. It has been introduced into intensive care practice as an aid to increase tolerance of intubation and mechanical ventilation and to smooth the transition to spontaneous respiration and extubation. After coronary artery surgery, dexmedetomidine was associated with similar ventilation times to propofol-based sedation but significantly lower morphine requirements and fewer ventricular arrhythmias (Herr et al 2003, **Level II**).

9.8.4 Guillain-Barre syndrome

Patients with Guillain-Barre syndrome commonly need treatment in an ICU. They may report significant pain including painful paraesthesiae, backache, sciatica, meningism, muscle and joint pain. The distal to proximal distribution of pain that characterises peripheral neuropathies is not usually seen (Khatri & Pearlstein 1997).

Early treatment of pain with carbamazepine improved analgesia and reduced requirements for pethidine and sedation in patients with Guillain-Barre syndrome (Tripathi & Kaushik 2000; **Level II**). Gabapentin (Pandey et al 2002, **Level II**) and ketamine infusions (Parisod 2002) also improved pain relief. IV lignocaine (lidocaine) may be useful in the treatment of acute neuropathic pain in Guillain-Barre syndrome based on evidence of benefit in other neuropathic pain disorders (Kalso et al 1998, **Level I**).

Plasma exchange in acute Guillain-Barre syndrome was associated with a shortened duration of disease and improved outcomes, including pain (The Guillain-Barre Syndrome Study Group 1985, **Level II**).

While steroid therapy is not advocated as primary management in post-infectious polyneuropathy, it may provide rapid resolution of the severe backache associated with the acute phase of the neuropathy (Kabore 2004, **Level IV**).

9.8.5 Procedure-related pain

There is often an assumption that patients who are intubated and sedated in intensive care will not recall or perceive pain during procedures. Lines and catheters are sometimes inserted without supplementary anaesthesia. Some patients have specific recollection of painful procedures in an ICU. Therefore, adequate local and/or parenteral anaesthesia should be provided during any noxious procedure (Puntillo et al 2004, **Level III**).

Key messages

1. Daily interruptions of sedative infusions reduce duration of ventilation and ICU stay without causing adverse psychological outcomes (**Level II**).

2. Gabapentin and carbamazepine are effective in reducing the pain associated with Guillain-Barre syndrome (**Level II**).

3. Patients should be provided with appropriate sedation and analgesia during potentially painful procedures (**Level III**).

The following tick box ☑ represents conclusions based on clinical experience and expert opinion.

☑ Observation of behavioural and physiological responses permits assessment of pain in unconscious patients.

9.9 Acute pain management in emergency departments

Pain is the single most common reason for presentation to emergency departments (EDs). However the aetiologies of pain are diverse and include both medical and surgical causes.

There is evidence that, as in many other areas of health care, patients in EDs around the world receive suboptimal pain management (Rupp & Delaney 2004). Systems should be adopted to ensure adequate pain assessment, timely and appropriate analgesia, frequent monitoring and reassessment of pain and additional analgesia as required. In the ED setting, analgesia should be simple to administer, condition-specific and where possible based on local-regional rather than systemic techniques.

9.9.1 Systemic analgesics

Opioids and tramadol

In the ED, opioids are frequently prescribed for the treatment of severe pain and should preferably be administered via the IV route given the wide interindividual variability in dose response and the delayed absorption via the intramuscular or subcutaneous routes. Doses should be adjusted for age (see Section 4.1) and titrated to effect. Patients require close observation for sedation, respiratory depression and occasionally hypotension (Coman & Kelly 1999, **Level IV**).

Intranasal opioids such as fentanyl may be effective analgesics in the ED and prehospital setting (Borland et al 2002, **Level IV**). The role of opioid PCA in the ED is yet to be defined, although it was found to be safe in patients with definite pathology (Brana et al 2004, **Level IV**).

In the management of severe trauma pain, IV tramadol had similar analgesic efficacy to morphine (Vergnion et al 2001, **Level II**). For renal colic, tramadol was of less benefit than pethidine (Eray 2002, **Level II**) but as effective as ketorolac 30mg (Nicolas-Torralba 1999, **Level II**).

Opioid-tolerant patients pose a special challenge in the ED and their management is discussed in Section 10.8.

Non-steroidal anti-inflammatory agents

Oral NSAIDs including aspirin, are useful for treating mild to moderate trauma pain, musculoskeletal pain and renal and biliary colic as discussed elsewhere in this document (see also Section 4.2).

Inhalational

Nitrous oxide in oxygen (see Sections 4.3.1 and 10.1.5) provided effective analgesia and anxiolysis for minor procedures in both adults and children (Gamis et al 1989, **Level II**; Gregory & Sullivan 1996, **Level II**; Burton et al 1998, **Level II**; Gerhardt et al 2001, **Level II**; Burnweit et al 2004, **Level IV**) and may be useful as a temporising measure while more definitive analgesia is instituted (eg insertion of a digital nerve block for finger injury).

Methoxyflurane is used to provide analgesia, most commonly in prehospital emergency care. However, the evidence to support its use is limited (Chin et al 2002, **Level II**).

Ketamine

Although there is no evidence from the ED setting, ketamine may be useful in the management of acute severe pain such as in burns injury (see Section 4.3.2).

9.9.2 Analgesia in specific conditions

Abdominal pain

Previous dogma suggested that analgesia should be withheld from patients with abdominal pain until a diagnosis is made. However there is good evidence showing that provision of early analgesia does not affect diagnostic accuracy in adults or children (McHale & LoVecchio 2001, **Level I**; Kim et al 2002, **Level II**; Thomas & Silen 2003, **Level II**; Thomas et al 2003, **Level II**).

If pain is severe, opioids may be required. Although it has previously been recommended that pethidine be used in preference to morphine, particularly for renal and biliary colic due to the theoretical risk of smooth muscle spasm, there is no evidence to support this position (see Section 9.6.1).

Renal colic

NSAIDS produced clinically significant reductions in pain scores, less vomiting and a decreased requirement for rescue analgesia when compared with opioids (Holdgate & Pollock 2004, **Level I**). NSAIDs also provided better analgesia than hyoscine-N-butylbromide (al-Waili & Saloom 1998, **Level II**). NSAIDs reduced the incidence of recurrent renal colic after an ED visit (Kapoor et al 1989, **Level II**; Laerum et al 1995, **Level II**). There was no difference in analgesic efficacy between morphine and pethidine in renal colic (O'Connor et al 2000, **Level II**).

Biliary colic

Parenteral NSAIDs such as ketorolac, tenoxicam and diclofenac were at least as effective as parenteral opioids and more effective than hyoscine-N-butylbromide in providing analgesia for biliary colic (Goldman et al 1989, **Level II**; Al-Waili & Saloom 1998, **Level II**; Dula et al 2001, **Level II**; Henderson et al 2002, **Level II**; Kumar et al 2004, **Level II**) and may also prevent progression to cholecystitis (Goldman et al 1989, **Level II**; Akriviadis et al 1997, **Level II**; Al-Waili & Saloom 1998, **Level II**; Kumar et al 2004, **Level II**).

Migraine

Most migraine headaches are successfully managed by the patient and their GP. However a small number of patients fail to respond and present for treatment at EDs.

Approximately 80% of patients have tried their usual medications including simple analgesics and triptans before presentation (Larkin & Prescott 1992; Shrestha et al 1996).

Triptans, phenothiazines (chlorpromazine and prochlorperazine) metoclopramide and ketorolac are effective agents for treating acute migraine in the ED (Level II; see Table 9.5).

Table 9.5 Pooled effectiveness data from ED studies of the treatment of migraine

Agent	No. of studies	Total patients	Clinical success rate	NNT: Clinical success# (95% CI)	Level of evidence
Chlorpromazine	6	189	85%	1.67 (1.53–1.85)	II
Sumatriptan	1	88	75%	2 (1.72–2.5)	II
Prochlorperazine	3	70	76%	2 (1.67–2.5)	II
Metoclopramide	4	121	59%	2.9 (2.38–4)	II
Ketorolac	4	75	57%	3.11 (2.27–4.76)	II

Notes: Only agents with an aggregate of 50 patients or more have been included.

= calculated as 1% success of active agent – % success placebo (assumes placebo success of 25%).

Source: Adapted from Kelly (in press).

In the ED setting, parenteral triptans are usually required. However there are a number of contraindications to their use including ischaemic heart disease, uncontrolled hypertension or the concomitant use of ergot preparations. Clinical trials of sumitriptan in the ED setting have reported clinical success rates of approximately 75%, but there are also a significant number of non-responders (up to 25%)(Akpunonu et al 1995, **Level II**).

The effectiveness of dihydroergotamine in acute migraine is difficult to interpret because it is often administered in combination with other agents (eg metoclopramide). However, it was less effective than chlorpromazine (Bell et al 1990, **Level II**) and sumatriptan (Winner et al 1996, **Level II**) and has a high rate of unpleasant side effects (Bell et al 1990, **Level II**).

Opioids, in particular pethidine, are not recommended in the treatment of migraine due to lack of evidence of efficacy and the risk of developing dependency (see Section 9.5.5).

IV lignocaine (lidocaine) (Reutens et al 1991, **Level II**) and IV sodium valproate (Tanen et al 2003, **Level II**) are ineffective in acute migraine. The efficacy of IV magnesium sulphate (1or 2mg) remains unclear. It was shown to be effective in a small placebo-controlled trial (Demirkaya et al 2001, **Level II**). However in another study, the combination of magnesium with metoclopramide was less effective than metoclopramide and placebo (Corbo et al 2001, **Level II**). IM droperidol 2.5mg was moderately effective in acute migraine, although with a 13% incidence of akathisia (Richman et al 2002, **Level II**). Further research would be required before these agents could be recommended.

Fractured neck of femur

In patients with a fractured neck of femur, a '3 in 1' femoral nerve block using bupivacaine plus IV morphine was more effective than IV morphine alone with a faster onset of analgesia (Fletcher et al 2003, **Level II**) although ropivacaine or levobupivacaine may be preferred to bupivacaine (see Section 5.1).

Wounds

Local anaesthesia is frequently required for the treatment of wounds. Agents most commonly used for infiltration are lignocaine (lidocaine) and bupivacaine depending on the duration of anaesthesia required and whether analgesia post-procedure is desirable.

Topical anaesthetic preparations such as ALA (adrenaline [epinephrine], lignocaine [lidocaine], amethocaine) are effective alternatives to infiltration with local anaesthesia for selected simple lacerations (Smith et al 1997, **Level II**;: Singer & Stark 2000, **Level II**) and may reduce the pain of infiltration when injectable local anaesthetics are required (Singer & Stark 2000, **Level II**). There is conflicting data on whether buffering of lignocaine (lidocaine) reduces the pain of infiltration (Boyd 2001, **Level II**). In patients with sensitivity to local anaesthetic agents, infiltration with diphenhydramine may provide adequate analgesia (Pollack & Swindle 1989).

9.9.3 Non-pharmacological management of pain

Although analgesic agents may be required to treat pain in the ED setting, the importance of non-pharmacological treatments should not be forgotten. These include ice, elevation and splintage for injuries and explanation of the cause of pain and its likely outcome to allay anxiety. Psychological techniques such as distraction, imagery or hypnosis may also be of value.

Key messages

1. Provision of analgesia does not interfere with the diagnostic process in acute abdominal pain (**Level I**).
2. In patients with renal colic, NSAIDs provide better pain relief with fewer adverse effects compared with opioids (**Level I** [Cochrane Review]).
3. Pethidine does not provide better pain relief than morphine in the treatment of renal colic (**Level II**).
4. Parenteral NSAIDs provide pain relief in biliary colic that is comparable to opioids and superior to hyoscine-N-butylbromide (**Level II**).
5. Triptan and phenothiazines (prochlorperazine, chlorpromazine) are effective in at least 75% of patients presenting to the emergency department with migraine (**Level II**).
6. Femoral nerve blocks in combination with IV opioids are superior to IV opioids alone in the treatment of pain from a fractured neck of femur (**Level II**).

The following tick box ☑ represents conclusions based on clinical experience and expert opinion.

☑ To ensure optimal management of acute pain, emergency departments should adopt systems to ensure adequate assessment of pain, provision of timely and appropriate analgesia, frequent monitoring and reassessment of pain.

REFERENCES

Aaron JN, Carlisle CC, Carskadon MA et al (1996) Environmental noise as a cause of sleep disruption in an intermediate respiratory care unit. *Sleep* 19: 707–10.

Abouleish E, Vega S, Blender I et al (1975) Long term follow up of epidural blood patch. *Anesth Analg* 54: 459–63.

Ahmad N, Grad HA, Haas DA et al (1997) The efficacy of non opioid analgesics for post operative dental pain: a meta-analysis. *Anesth Prog* 44: 119–26.

Akpunonu BE, Mutgi AB, Federman DJ et al (1995) Subcutaneous sumatriptan for the treatment of acute migraine in patients admitted to the emergency department. *Ann Emerg Med* 25: 464–69.

Akriviadis EA, Hatzigavriel M, Kapnias D et al (1997) Treatment of biliary colic with diclofenac: a randomised, double-blind, placebo-controlled study. *Gastroenterol* 113: 225–31.

Al-Waili N & Saloom KY (1998) The analgesic effect of intravenous tenoxicam in symptomatic treatment of biliary colic: a Comparison with hyoscine-N-butylbromide. *Eur J Med Res* 14: 475–79.

Aronstam A, Wassef M, Hamad Z et al (1983) A double-blind controlled trial of two dose levels of factor VIII in the treatment of high risk haemarthroses in haemophilia A. *Clin Lab Haematol* 5: 157–63.

Ashburn MA (1995) Burn pain: the management of procedure-related pain. *J Burn Care Rehabil* 16: 365–71.

Astin JA & Ernst E (2002) The effectiveness of spinal manipulation for the treatment of headache disorders: a systematic review of randomised controlled trials. *Cephalalgia* 22: 617–23.

Attal N, Gaude V, Brasseur L et al (2000) Intravenous lignocaine in central pain; a double blind, placebo controlled, psychophysical study. *Neurology* 54: 564–74.

Attal N, Guirimand F, Brasseur L et al (2002) Effects of IV morphine in central pain - A randomized placebo-controlled study. *Neurology* 58: 554–63.

Australian Acute Musculoskeletal Pain Guidelines Group (2003) *Evidence-based Management of Acute Musculoskeletal Pain*. Brisbane: NHMRC Australian Academic Press. (www.health.gov.au/nhmrc/publications/pdf/cp94.pdf)

Bahra A, Gawel MJ, Hardebo JE et al (2000) Oral zolmitriptan is effective in the acute treatment of cluster headache. *Neurology* 54 1832–39.

Baker CL (1992) Acute Haemarthrosis of the knee. *J Med Assoc Ga* 81: 301–05.

Balakrishnan S, Bhushan K, Bhargava VK et al (2001) A randomised parallel trial of topical aspirin-moisturiser solution vs oral aspirin for acute herpetic neuralgia. *Int J Dermatol* 40: 535–38.

Ballas SK & Delengowski A (1993) Pain measurement in hospitalized adults with sickle cell painful episodes. *Ann Clin Lab Sci* 23: 358–61.

Barber FA, McGuire DA, Click S (1998) Continuous-flow cold therapy for outpatient anterior cruciate ligament reconstruction. *Arthroscopy* 14: 130–35.

Barden J, Edwards JE, McQuay HJ et al (2004) Pain and analgesic response after third molar extraction and other postsurgical pain. *Pain* 107: 86–90.

Bates RE Jr & Stewart CM (1991) Atypical odontalgia: Phantom tooth pain. *Oral Surg Oral Med Oral Pathol* 72: 479–83.

Baumann BM, Perrone J, Hornig SE et al (2000) Randomized, double blind, placebo controlled trial of diazepam, nitroglycerin or both for the treatment of patients with potential cocaine-associated acute coronary syndromes. *Acad Emerg Med* 7: 878–85.

Baxendale BR, Vater M, Lavery KM (1993) Dexamethasone reduces pain and swelling following extraction of third molar teeth. *Anaesthesia* 48: 961–64.

Beauregard L, Pomp A, Choinière M (1998) Severity and impact of pain after day-surgery. *Can J Anesth* 45: 304–11.

Bell R, Montoya D, Shuaib A et al (1990) A comparative trial of three agents in the treatment of migraine headache. *Ann Emerg Med* 19: 1079–82.

Bigal ME, Bordini CA, Speciali JG. (2002) Intravenous chlorpromazine in the emergency department treatment of migraines: A randomised controlled trial. *J Emerg Med* 23:141–48.

Blanda M, Rench T, Gerson LW et al (2001) Intranasal lignocaine for the treatment of migraine headache: a randomized controlled trial. *Acad Emerg Med* 8: 337–42.

Boas RA, Schug SA, Acland RH (1993) Perineal pain after rectal amputation: A 5-year follow-up. *Pain* 52: 67–70.

Bone M, Critchley P, Buggy DJ (2002) Gabapentin in postamputation phantom limb pain: A randomized, double-blind, placebo-controlled, cross-over study. *Reg Anesth Pain Med* 27: 481–86.

Borland ML, Jacobs I, Geelhoed G (2002) Intranasal fentanyl reduces acute pain in children in the emergency department: a safety and efficacy study. *Emerg Med (Fremantle)* 14: 275–80.

Bowsher D (1997) The effects of pre-emptive treatment of postherpetic neuralgia with amitriptyline: A randomised, double-blind, placebo-controlled trial. *J Pain Sympt Manage* 13: 327–31.

Boyd R (2001) Plain or buffered lignocaine for local anaesthetic. (www.bestbets.org).

Brana A, Getti R, Mezaib K et al (2004) Self-administered morphine algorithm in an emergency department observation unit. *Acad Emerg Med* 11: 495.

Braunwald E (2002) ACC/AHA Committee on the Management of Patients with Unstable Angina: ACC/AHA 2002 guideline update for the management of patients with unstable angina and non-ST-segment elevation myocardial infarction. *J Am Coll Cardiol* 40: 1366–74.

Breen D, Wilmer A, Bodenham A et al (2004) Offset of pharmacodynamic effects and safety of remifentanil in intensive care unit patients with various degrees of renal impairment. *Crit Care* 8: R21–30.

Breitbart W, McDonald MV, Rosenfeld B et al (1996a) Pain in ambulatory AIDS patients. I. Pain characteristics and medical correlates. *Pain* 68: 315–21.

Breitbart W, Rosenfeld BD, Passik SD et al (1996b) The undertreatment of pain in ambulatory AIDS patients. *Pain* 65: 243–49.

Breitbart W, Rosenfeld B, Passik S et al (1997) A comparison of pain report and adequacy of analgesic therapy in ambulatory AIDS patients with and without a history of substance abuse. *Pain* 72: 235–43.

Breitbart W, Passik S, McDonald MV et al (1998) Patient-related barriers to pain management in ambulatory AIDS patients. *Pain* 76: 9–16.

Breitbart W, Kaim M, Rosenfeld B (1999) Clinicians' perceptions of barriers to pain management in AIDS. *J Pain Sympt Manage* 18: 203–12.

Brofeldt BT, Cornwell P, Doherty D et al (1989) Topical lidocaine in the treatment of partial-thickness burns. *J Burn Care Rehabil* 10: 63–68.

Brousseau DC, Duffy SJ, Anderson AC et al (2004) Treatment of pediatric migraine headaches: a randomised, double-blind trial of prochlorperazine versus ketorolac *Ann Emerg Med* 53: 256–62.

Buerkle H, Huge V, Wolfgart M et al (2000) Intra-articular clonidine analgesia after knee arthroscopy. *Eur J Anaesthesiol* 17: 295–99.

Burduk P, Guzik P, Piechocka M et al (2000) Comparison of fentanyl and droperidol mixture (neuroleptanalgesia II) with morphine on clinical outcomes in unstable angina patients. *Cardiovasc Drugs Ther* 14: 259–69.

Burnweit C, Diana-Zerpa JA, Nahmad MH et al (2004) Nitrous oxide analgesia for minor pediatric surgical procedures: an effective alternative to conscious sedation. *J Pediatr Surg* 39: 495–9.

Burton JH, Auble TE, Fuchs SM (1998) Effectiveness of 50% nitrous oxide /50% oxygen during laceration repair in children. *Acad Emerg Med* 5: 112–17.

Camann WR, Murray RS, Mushlin PS et al (1990) Effects of oral caffeine on post dural puncture headache: a double blind placebo controlled trial. *Anesth Analg* 70: 181–84.

Campbell JK,Penzien DB, Wall EM (2000) *US Headache Consortium: Evidence Based Guidelines for Migraine Headache: Behavioural and Physical Treatments.* (www.aan.com/public/practice guidelines)

Candido K & Stevens R (2003) Post-dural puncture headache: pathophysiology, prevention and treatment. *Best Pract Res Clin Anaesthesiol* 17: 451–69.

Capdevila X, Barthelet Y, Biboulet P et al (1999) Effects of perioperative analgesic technique on the surgical outcome and duration of rehabilitation after major knee surgery. *Anesthesiology* 91: 8–15.

Cardenas DD, Warms CA, Turner JA et al (2002) Efficacy of amitriptyline for relief of pain in spinal cord injury: results of a randomised controlled trial. *Pain* 96: 365–73.

Chang DJ, Fricke JR, Bird SR et al (2001) Rofecoxib versus codeine/acetaminophen in post-operative dental pain: a double blind, randomised placebo and active comparator-controlled clinical trial. *Clin Ther* 23: 1446–55.

Charters A (1998) Topical anaesthesia before suturing children's minor lacerations: a critical review. *Accid Emerg Nurs* 6: 180–83.

Chen LC, Elliott RA, Ashcroft DM (2004) Systematic review of the analgesic efficacy and tolerability of COX -2 inhibitors in post operative pain control. *J Clin Pharm Ther* 29: 215–29.

Chin R et al (2002) A randomised control trial of inhaled methoxyflurane pain relief, in children with upper limb fracture. *J Paediatr Child Health* 38: A13–A14.

Chiou Tan FY, Tuel SM, Johnson JC et al (1996) Effect of mexiletine on spinal cord injury dysesthetic pain. *Am J Phys Med Rehabil* 75: 84–87.

Choinière M, Melzack R, Rondeau J et al (1989) The pain of burns: characteristics and correlates. *J Trauma* 29: 1531–39.

Choinière M, Grenier R, Paquette C (1992) Patient-controlled analgesia: a double-blind study in burn patients. *Anaesthesia* 47: 467–72.

Choinière M (2001) Burn pain: a unique challenge. In: *Pain Clinical Updates*. Seattle: IASP.

Chong C & Burchett K (2003) Pain management in critical care. *Br J Anaesth CEPD Reviews* 3: 183–86.

Choyce A & Peng P (2002) A systematic review of adjuncts for intravenous regional anesthesia for surgical procedures. *Can J Anesth* 49: 32–45.

Chung F, Ritchie E, Su J (1997) Postoperative pain in ambulatory surgery. *Anesth Analg* 85: 808–16.

Cicconetti A, Bartoli A, Ripari F et al (2004) COX-2 selective inhibitors: a literature review of analgesic efficacy and safety in oro-maxillofacial surgery. *Oral Surg Oral Med Oral Path Oral Radiol Endod* 97: 139–46.

Clement PA, Bluestone CD, Gordts F et al (1998) Management of rhinosinusitis in children: consensus meeting, Brussels, Belgium, September 13, 1996. *Arch Otolaryngol Head Neck Surg* 124: 31–34.

Coda BA, O'Sullivan B, Donaldson G et al (1997) Comparative efficacy of patient controlled administration of morphine, hydromorphone or sufentanil for the treatment of oral mucositis pain following bone marrow transplantation. *Pain* 72: 333–46.

Codispoti JR (2002) Efficacy of non prescription doses of ibuprofen for treating migraine headache. A randomised controlled trial. *Headache* 41: 665–79.

Cohen J & Royston D (2001) Remifentanil. *Curr Opin Crit Care* 7: 227–31.

Colman I, Brown MD, Innes GD et al (2004) Parenteral metoclopramide for acute migraine: meta-analysis of randomised controlled trials. *BMJ* 329: 1369–73.

Coimbra C, Choinière M, Hemmerling TM (2003) Patient-controlled sedation using propofol for dressing changes in burns patients: a dose finding study. *Anesth Analg* 97: 839–42.

Colbert ST, Curran E, O'Hanlon DM et al (1999) Intra-articular tenoxicam improves postoperative analgesia in knee arthroscopy. *Can J Anesth* 46: 653–57.

Collins JJ, Geake J, Grier HE et al (1996) Patient-controlled analgesia for mucositis pain in children: a three-period crossover study comparing morphine and hydromorphone. *J Pediatr* 129: 722–28.

Colonna-Romano P & Shapiro BE (1989) Unintentional dural puncture headache and prophylactic epidural blood patch in obstetrics *Anesth Analg* 69: 522–23.

Coluzzi P H, Schwartzberg L, Conroy J D et al (2001) Breakthrough cancer pain: a randomized trial comparing oral transmucosal fentanyl citrate(OTFC) and morphine sulfate immediate release(MSIR) *Pain* 91: 123–30.

Coman M & Kelly AM (1999) Safety of a nurse-manage, titrated intravenous analgesia policy on the management of severe pain in the emergency department. *Emerg Med* 11: 128–32.

Connelly NR, Parker RK, Rahimi A et al (2000) Sumatriptan in patients with post dural puncture headache. *Headache* 40: 316–19.

Convery PN, Milligan KR, Quinn P et al (1998) Low-dose intra-articular ketorolac for pain relief following arthroscopy of the knee joint. *Anaesthesia* 53: 1125–29.

Cook TM, Tuckey JP, Nolan JP (1997) Analgesia after day-case knee arthroscopy: double-blind study of intra-articular tenoxicam, intra-articular bupivacaine and placebo. *Br J Anaesth* 78: 163–68.

Coppola M, Yearly DM, Leibold RA (1995) Randomised, placebo-controlled evaluation of prochlorperazine versus metoclopramide for emergency department treatment of migraine headache. *Ann Emerg Med* 26: 541–46.

Corbo J, Esses D, Bijur PE et al (2001) Randomised clinical trial of intravenous magnesium sulphate as an adjunctive medication in the emergency department treatment of migraine. *Ann Emerg Med* 38: 621–27.

Dahlof CG & Jacobs LD (1996) Ketoprofen, paracetamol and placebo in the treatment of episodic tension type headache. *Cephalalgia* 16: 117–23.

Dahlof CGH (2002) In: Giamberardino MA (Ed) *Pain 2002- An Updated Review: Refresher Course Syllabus*. Seattle: IASP Press.

Dahlof CGH, Dodick D, Dowson AI et al (2002) How does almotriptan compare with other triptans? A review of data from placebo controlled clinical trials. *Headache* 2: 99–113.

Dauber A, Osgood P, Breslau A et al (2002) Chronic persistent pain after severe burns: a survey of 358 burn survivors. *Pain Med* 3: 6–17.

Davies JW (1982) Prompt cooling of burn areas: a review of benefits and the effector mechanisms. *Burns INCL Therm Inj* 9: 1–6.

Davies S, Olujohungbe A, Jones AP (2001) Hydroxyurea for sickle cell disease. *The Cochrane Database of Systematic Review*, Issue 2. Art. No.: CD002202. DOI: 10.1002/14651858.CD002202.

Davis CP (1995) Ketorolac versus meperidine plus promethazine treatment of migraine headache-evaluation by patients. *Am J Emerg Med* 13: 146–50.

De Benedittis G & Lorenzetti A (1996) Topical aspirin/ diethyl ether mixture versus indomethacin and diclofenac/ diethyl ether mixtures for acute herpetic neuralgia and postherpetic neuralgia: a double-blind crossover placebo-controlled study. *Pain* 65: 45–51.

Demirkaya S, Vural O, Dora B et al (2001) Efficacy of intravenous magnesium sulphate in the treatment of acute migraine attacks. *Headache* 41: 171–77.

Dertwinkel R, Heinrichs C, Senne I et al (2002) Prevention of severe phantom limb pain by perioperative administration of ketamine - an observational study. *Acute Pain* 4: 9–13.

Diamond S, Frietag FG, Diamond ML et al (1992) Transnasal butorphanol in the treatment of migraine headache pain. *Headache Quarterly Curr Treat Res* 3: 2 164–70.

Diamond S, Balm TK, Frietag FG (2000) Ibuprofen plus caffeine in the treatment of tension type headache. *Clin Pharmacol Ther* 68: 312–19.

Di Monda V, Nicolodi M, Aloisio I et al (2003) efficacy of a fixed combination of indomethacin, prochlorperazine and caffeine versus sumaptriptan in acute treatment of multiple migraine attacks: a multicentre, randomised, crossover trial. *Headache* 43: 835–44.

Ding Y &White PF (1995) Post-herniorrhaphy pain in outpatients after pre-incision ilioinguinal-hypogastric nerve block during monitored anaesthesia care. *Can J Anesth* 42: 12–15.

Dixon P & Higginson I (1991) AIDS and cancer pain treated with slow release morphine. *Postgrad Med J* 67: S92–94.

Dodick DW, Rozen TD, Goadsby PJ et al (2000) Cluster headache. *Cephalalgia* 20: 787–803.

Drewes AM, Andreasen A, Poulsen LH (1994) Valproate for the treatment of chronic central pain after spinal cord injury. A double blind cross over study. *Paraplegia* 32: 565–69.

Dula DJ, Anderson R, Wood GC (2001) A prospective study comparing IM ketorolac with IM meperidine in the treatment of acute biliary colic. *J Emerg Med* 20: 121–24.

Dworkin RH, Boon RJ et al (1998) Postherpetic neuralgia: impact of famciclovir, age, rash severity, and acute pain in herpes zoster patients *J Infect Dis* 178 Suppl 1: S76-80

Edwards JE, Mc Quay HJ, Moore RA (2002) Combination analgesic efficacy; individual patient data meta-analysis of single dose oral tramadol plus acetaminophen in acute post operative pain. *J Pain Sympt Manage* 23: 121–30.

Edwards JE, Moore RA, McQuay HJ (2004) Individual patient meta-analysis of single dose rofecoxib in post operative pain. *BMC Anaesthesiol* 4: 3.

Eide PK, Stubhaug A, Stenehjem AE (1995) Central dysesthesia pain after traumatic spinal cord injury is dependent on N-methyl-D-aspartate receptor activation. *Neurosurgery* 37: 1080–87.

Ekbom K (1995) Treatment of cluster headache: clinical trials, design and results. *Cephalalgia* 15: 33–36.

Elenbaas RM, Iacono CU, Koellner KJ et al (1991) Dose effectiveness and safety of butorphanol in acute migraine headache. *Pharmacother* 11: 56–63.

Elhakim M, Fathy A, Elkott M etal (1996) Intra-articular tenoxicam relieves post-arthroscopy pain. *Acta Anaesthesiol Scand* 40: 1223–26.

Eray O, Cete Y, Oktay C et al (2002) Intravenous single-dose tramadol versus meperidine for pain relief in renal colic. *Eur J Anaesthesiol* 19: 368–70.

Eriksson H, Tenhunen A, Korttila K (1996) Balanced analgesia improves recovery and outcome after outpatient tubal ligation. *Acta Anaesthesiol Scand* 40: 151–55.

Ernst E & Pittler MH (1998) The effectiveness of acupuncture in treating acute dental pain. *Br Dent J* 184: 443–47.

Ernst ME, Santee JA, Klepser TB (1998) Oral corticosteroids for pain associated with herpes zoster. *Annals Pharmacother* 32: 1099–03.

Everts B, Karlson BW, Herlitz J et al (1998) Morphine use and pharmacokinetics in patients with chest pain due to suspected or definite acute myocardial infarction. *Eur J Pain* 2: 115–25.

Everts B, Karlson B, Abdon NJ et al (1999) A comparison of metoprolol and morphine in the treatment of chest pain in patients with suspected acute myocardial infarction- the MEMO study. *J Intern Med* 245: 133–41.

Farrar J, Cleary J, Rauck R et al (1998) Oral transmucosal fentanyl citrate: randomised, double-blinded, placebo-controlled trial for treatment of breakthrough pain in cancer patients. *J Nat Cancer Inst* 0: 611–16.

Felhendler D & Lisander B (1996) Pressure on acupoints decreases postoperative pain. *Clin J Pain* 12: 326–29.

Finch CK, Chrisman CR, Baciewicz AM et al (2002) Rifampin and rifabutin drug interactions: an update. *Arch Intern Me* 162: 985–92.

Fine PG & Busch MA (1998) Characterization of breakthrough pain by hospice patients and their caregivers. *J Pain Sympt Manage* 16: 179–83.

Finnerup NB, Sindrup SH, Bach FW et al (2002) Lamotrigine in spinal cord injury pain: a randomised controlled trial. *Pain* 96: 375–83.

Fletcher AK, Rigby AS, Heyes FL (2003) Three-in-one femoral nerve block as analgesia for fractured neck of femur in the emergency department: a randomised, controlled trial. *Ann Emerg Med* 41: 227–33.

Flor H, Denke C, Schaefer M et al (2001) Effect of sensory discrimination training on cortical reorganisation and phantom limb pain. *Lancet* 357: 1763–64.

Fogan L (1985) Treatment of cluster headache. A double blind comparison of oxygen air inhalation. *Arch Neurol* 42: 362–63.

Frenay MC, Faymonville ME, Devlieger S et al (2001) Psychological approaches during dressing changes of burned patients: a prospective randomised study comparing hypnosis against stress reducing strategy. *Burns* 27: 793–99.

Frich LM & Borgbjerg FM (2000) Pain and pain treatment in AIDS: a longitudinal study. *J Pain Sympy Manage* 19: 339–47.

Fricke JR, Angelocci D, Fox K et al (1992) Comparison of the efficacy and safety of ketorolac and meperidine in the relief of dental pain. *J Clin Pharm* 2: 376–84.

Fricke JR, Hewitt DJ, Jordan DM et al (2004) A double blind placebo controlled comparison of tramadol / acetaminophen and tramadol in patients with post operative dental pain. *Pain* 109: 250–57.

Gallagher G, Rae CP, Kinsella J (2000a) Treatment of pain in severe burns. *Am J Clin Dermatol* 1: 329–35.

Gallagher G, Rae CP, Kenny GN et al (2000b) The use of a target-controlled infusion of alfentanil to provide analgesia for burn dressing changes. A dose finding study. *Anaesthesia* 55: 1159–63.

Gamis AS, Knapp JF, Genski JA (1989) Nitrous oxide analgesia in a pediatric emergency department. *Ann Emerg Med* 18: 177–81.

Gehling M, Tryba M (2003) Prophylaxis of phantom pain: is regional analgesia ineffective? *Schmerz* 17: 11–19.

Gentili M, Juhel A, Bonnet F (1996) Peripheral analgesic effect of intra-articular clonidine. *Pain* 64: 593–96.

Gentili M, Enel D, Szymskiewicz O et al (2001) Postoperative analgesia by intraarticular clonidine and neostigmine in patients undergoing knee arthroscopy. *Reg Anesth Pain Med* 26: 342–47.

Gerhardt RT, King KM, Wiegert RS (2001) Inhaled nitrous oxide versus placebo as an analgesic and anxiolytic adjunct to peripheral IV cannulation. *Am J Emerg Med* 19: 492–94.

Gilbert MS (1993) Haemophilia: the changing role of the surgeon in the era of HIV infection. *SE Asian J Trop Med Public Health* 24 30–33.

Glare P (2001) Pain in patients with HIV infection: issues for the new millennium. *Eur J Pain* 5 (suppl A): 43–48.

Glasziou PP, Del Mar CB, Sanders SL et al (2003) Hayem M. Antibiotics for acute otitis media in children. *The Cochrane Database of Systematic Reviews* Issue 4. Art. No.: CD000219. DOI: 10.1002/14651858.CD000219.pub2.

Goadsby PJ (2003) Headache (chronic tension type). *Clin Evid* Jun: 1432–40.

Gold BS, Kitz DS, LeckyJH et al (1989) Unanticipated admissions to the hospital following ambulatory surgery. *JAMA* 262: 3008–10.

Goldman G, Kahn PJ, Alon R et al (1989) Biliary colic treatment and acute cholecystitis prevention by prostaglandin inhibitor. *Dig Dis Sci* 34: 809–11.

Gopikrishna V & Parameswaran A (2003) Effectiveness of prophylactic use of rofecoxib in comparison with ibuprofen on post endodontic pain. *J Endod* 29: 62–64.

Gregory PR & Sullivan JA (1996) Nitrous oxide compared with intravenous regional anesthesia in pediatric forearm fracture manipulation. *J Pediatr Orthop* 16: 187–91.

Griffin TC, McIntire D, Buchanan GR (1994) High-dose intravenous methylprednisolone therapy for pain in children and adolescents with sickle cell disease. *N Engl J Med* 330: 733–37.

Gupta A, Axelsson K, Allvin R et al (1999) Postoperative pain following knee arthroscopy: the effects of intra-articular ketorolac and/or morphine. *Reg Anesth Pain Med*. 1999;24: 225–30.

Gupta A, Bodin L, Holmstrom B et al (2001) A systematic review of the peripheral analgesic effects of intraarticular morphine. *Anesth Analg* 2001;93: 761–70.

Halbert J, Crotty M, Cameron ID (2002) Evidence for the optimal management of acute and chronic phantom pain: a systematic review. *Clin J Pain* 18: 84–92.

Halpern S & Preston R (1994) Postdural puncture headache and spinal needle design. Metaanalyses. *Anesthesiology*. 81: 1376–83.

Hansen JG, Schmidt H, Grinsted P (2000) Randomised double blind placebo controlled trial of penicillin V in the treatment of acute maxillary sinusitis in adults in general practice. *Scand J Prim Health Care* 18: 44–47.

Hardebo JE & Dahlof C (1998) Sumatriptan nasal spray (20mg/dose) in the acute treatment of cluster headache *Cephalalgia* 18: 487–89.

Hardwick WE Jr, Givens TG, Monroe KW et al (1999) Effect of ketorolac in pediatric sickle cell vaso-occlusive pain crisis. *Pediatr Emerg Care* 15: 179–82.

Hargrave DR, Wade A, Evans JPM et al Nocturnal oxygen saturation and painful sickle cell crises in children. *Blood* 101: 846–48.

Hawryluck LA, Harvey WL et al (2002) Consensus guidelines on analgesia and sedation in dying intensive care unit patients. *BMC Med Ethics* 3: E3.

Hayes C, Browne S, Lantry G et al (2002) Neuropathic pain in the acute pain service: a prospective survey. *Acute Pain* 4: 45–48.

Hayes C, Armstrong-Brown A, Burstal R (2004) Perioperative intravenous ketamine infusion for the prevention of persistent post-amputation pain: a randomized, controlled trial. *Anaesth Intensive Care*. 32: 330–38.

Headache Classification Subcommittee of the IHS (2004) The International Classification of Headache Disorders: 2nd edition. *Cephalalgia* 24 (Suppl 1): 9–160.

Henderson SO, Swadron S, Newton E (2002) Comparison of intravenous ketorolac and meperidine in the treatment of biliary colic. *J Emerg Med* 23: 237–41.

Henrikson CA, Howell EE, Bush DE et al (2003) Chest pain relief by nitroglycerin does not predict active coronary artery disease. *Ann Intern Med* 139: 979–86.

Herr DL, Sum-Ping ST, England M et al (2003) ICU sedation after coronary artery bypass graft surgery: dexmedetomidine-based versus propofol-based sedation regimens. *J Cardiothorac Vasc Anesth* 17: 576–84.

Hoffert MJ, Couch JR, Diamond S et al (1995) Transnasal butorphanol in the treatment of acute migraine. *Headache* 35: 65–69.

Holdgate A & Pollock T (2004) Systematic review of the relative efficacy of non-steroidal anti-inflammatory drugs and opioids in the treatment of acute renal colic. *BMJ* 328: 1401.

Hollis LJ, Burton MJ, Millar JM. (1999)Perioperative local anaesthesia for reducing pain following tonsillectomy. *The Cochrane Database of Systematic Reviews*. Issue 3. Art. No.: CD001874. DOI: 10.1002/14651858.CD001874.

Holroyd KA (2002) Behavioural and psychologic aspects of the pathophysiology and management of tension-type headache. *Curr Pain Headache Rep* 6: 401–07.

Honderick T, Williams D, Seaberg D et al (2003) A prospective randomised, controlled trial of benzodiazepine and nitroglyerine or nitroglycerine alone in the treatment of cocaine-associated acute coronary syndromes. *Am J Emerg Med* 21: 39–42.

Horsburgh CR Jr (1995) Healing by design. *N Engl J Med* 333: 735–40.

Huse E, Larbig W, Flor H et al (2001) The effect of opioids on phantom limb pain and cortical reorganization. *Pain* 90: 47–55.

Hwang SM, Kang YC, Lee YB et al (1999) The effects of epidural blockade on the acute pain in herpes zoster. *Arch Dermatol* 135: 1359–64.

Ilfeld BM, Morey TE, Wang RD et al (2002a) Continuous popliteal sciatic nerve block for postoperative pain control at home: a randomized, double-blinded, placebo-controlled study. *Anesthesiology* 97: 959–65.

Ilfeld BM, Morey TE, Enneking FK (2002b) Continuous infraclavicular brachial plexus block for postoperative pain control at home: a randomized, double-blinded, placebo-controlled study. *Anesthesiology* 96: 1297–304.

Ilfeld BM, Morey TE, Wright TW et al (2004) Interscalene perineural ropivacaine infusion: a comparison of two dosing regimens for postoperative analgesia. *Reg Anesth Pain Med* 29: 9–16.

Ilkjaer S, Petersen KL, Brennum J et al (1996) Effect of systemic NMDA receptor antagonist (ketamine) on primary and secondary hyperalgesia in humans. *Br J Anaesth* 76: 829–34.

Ilkjaer S, Dirks J, Brennum J et al (1997) Effect of systemic NMDA receptor antagonist (dextromethorphan) on primary and secondary hyperalgesia in humans. *Br J Anaesth* 79: 600–05.

Iribarne C, Berthou F, Carlhant D et al (1998) Inhibition of methadone and buprenorphine N-dealkylations by three HIV-1 protease inhibitors. *Drug Metab Dispos* 26: 257–60.

Iqbal J, Wig J, Bhardwaj N et al (2000) Intra-articular clonidine vs. morphine for post-operative analgesia following arthroscopic knee surgery (a comparative evaluation). *Knee* 7: 109–13.

Jackson JL, Gibbons R, Meyer G et al (1997) The effect of treating herpes zoster with oral acyclovir in preventing postherpetic neuralgia. A meta-analysis. *Arch Intern Med* 157: 909–12.

Jacobi J, Fraser L, Coursin DB et al (2002) Clinical practice guidelines for the sustained use of sedatives and analgesics in the critically ill adult. *Crit Care Med* 30: 119–41.

Jacobson SJ, Kopecky EA, Joshi P et al (1997) Randomised trial of oral morphine for painful episodes of sickle cell disease in children. *Lancet* 350: 1358–61.

Jacox A, Carr D, Payne R (1994) *Clinical Practice Guideline No. 9: Management of Cancer Pain.* US Dept of Health and Human Services, Agency of Health Care Policy and Research. Publication No. 94-0592, pp139–141.

Jaeger H & Maier C (1992) Calcitonin in phantom limb pain: A double-blind study. *Pain* 48: 21–27.

Jensen TS, Krebs B, Nielsen J et al (1983) Phantom limb, phantom pain and stump pain in amputees during the first 6 months following limb amputation. *Pain* 17: 243–56.

Jensen TS, Krebs B, Nielsen J et al (1985) Immediate and long-term phantom limb pain in amputees: Incidence, clinical characteristics and relationship to pre-amputation limb pain. *Pain* 21: 267–78.

Johnson RW & Whitton TL (2004) Management of herpes zoster (shingles) and postherpetic neuralgia. *Expert Opin Pharmacother* 5: 551–59.

Jones JB, Giles BK, Brizendine EJ et al (2001) Sublingual hyoscyamine sulfate in combination with ketorolac tromethamine for ureteral colic: a randomised double-blind, controlled trial. *Ann Emerg Med* 37: 141–46.

Jonsson A, Cassuto J, Hanson B (1991) Inhibition of burn pain by intravenous lignocaine infusion. *Lancet* 338: 151–52.

Joshi W, Reuben SS, Kilaru PR et al (2000) Postoperative analgesia for outpatient arthroscopic knee surgery with intraarticular clonidine and/or morphine. *Anesth Analg* 90: 1102–06.

Joshi W, Connelly NR, Reuben SS et al (2003) An evaluation of the safety and efficacy of administering rofecoxib for post operative pain management. *Anesth Analg* 97: 35–38.

Kabore R, Magy L, ,Boukhris , et al (2004) contribution of corticosteroid to the treatment of pain in the acute phase of Guillain-Barre syndrome. *Rev Neurol [Paris]* 160: 821–23.

Kalso E, Tramèr MR, Moore RA et al (1998) Systemic local anaesthetic type drugs in chronic pain: a qualitative systematic review. *Eur J Pain* 2: 3–14.

Kalso E, Smith L, McQuay HJ et al (2002) No pain, no gain: clinical excellence and scientific rigour--lessons learned from IA morphine. *Pain* 98: 269–75.

Kaplan R, Conant M, Cundiff D et al (1996) Sustained-release morphine sulfate in the management of pain associated with acquired immunodeficiency syndrome. *J Pain Sympt Manage* 12: 150–60.

Kaplan R, Slywka J, Slagle S et al (2000) A titrated morphine analgesic regimen comparing substance users and non- users with AIDS-related pain *J Pain Sympt Manage* 19: 265–73.

Kapoor DA, Weitzel S, Mowad JJ et al (1989) Use of indomethacin suppositories in the prophylaxis of recurrent ureteric colic. *J Urol* 142: 1428–30.

Katz J & Melzack R (1990) Pain 'memories' in phantom limbs: Review and clinical observations. *Pain* 43: 319–36.

Keith DA (2004) Orofacial pain. In: Warfield DA & Bajwa ZH (Eds) *Principles and Practice of Pain Medicine*. 2nd Edn, McGraw-Hill, pp252–59.

Kelly AM (in press) Specific pain syndromes: Headache. In: Mace S, Ducharme J, Murphy M (Eds) *Pain Management and Procedural Sedation in the Emergency Department*. McGraw-Hill.

Kelly KM (1995) Cardiac arrest following use of sumaptriptan. *Neurology* 45: 1211–13.

Kemper CA, Kent G, Burton S et al (1998) Mexiletine for HIV-infected patients with painful peripheral neuropathy: a double-blind, placebo-controlled, crossover treatment trial. *J Acquir Immune Defic Syndr Hum Retrovirol* 19: 367–72.

Khatri A & Pearlstein L (1997) Pain in Guillain-Barre syndrome. *Neurology* 49: 1474.

Kieburtz K, Simpson D, Yiannoutsos C et al (1998) A randomized trial of amitriptyline and mexiletine for painful neuropathy in HIV infection. AIDS Clinical Trial Group 242 Protocol Team. *Neurology* 51: 1682–88.

Kim MK, Strait RT, Sato TT et al (2002) A randomised clinical trial of analgesia in children with acute abdominal pain. *Acad Emerg Med* 9: 281–87.

Kimball LR & McCormick WC (1996) The pharmacologic management of pain and discomfort in persons with AIDS near the end of life: use of opioid analgesia in the hospice setting. *J Pain Sympt Manage* 11: 88–94.

Kinsella J & Booth MG (1991) Pain relief in burns: James Laing memorial essay 1990. *Burns* 17: 391–95.

Kinsella J & Rae CP (2003) Burns. In: Rowbotham DJ & Macintyre PE (Eds) *Clinical Pain Management: Acute Pain*. London: Arnold Publishers.

Klein SM, Bergh A, Steele SM et al (2000) Thoracic paravertebral block for breast surgery. *Anesth Analg* 0: 1402–05.

Klein SM, Nielsen KC, Greengrass RA et al (2002a) Ambulatory discharge after long-acting peripheral nerve blockade: 2382 blocks with ropivacaine. *Anesth Analg* 94: 65–70.

Klein SM, Pietrobon R, Nielsen KC et al (2002b) Paravertebral somatic nerve block compared with peripheral nerve blocks for outpatient inguinal herniorrhaphy. *Reg Anesth Pain Med* 27: 476–80.

Kooijman CM, Dijkstra PU, Geertzen JH et al (2000) Phantom pain and phantom sensations in upper limb amputees: An epidemiological study. *Pain* 87: 33–41.

Kopecky EA, Jacobson S, Joshi P et al (2004) Systemic exposure to morphine and the risk of acute chest syndrome in sickle cell disease. *Clin Pharm Ther* 75: 140–46.

Kost RG & Straus SE (1996) Postherpetic neuralgia- pathogenesis, treatment, and prevention. *New Engl J Med* 4: 32–42.

Kress JP, Pohlman AS, O'Connor MF et al (2000) Daily interruption of sedative infusions in critically ill patients undergoing mechanical ventilation. *N Engl J Med* 342: 1471–77.

Kress JP, Gehlbach B, Lacy M et al (2003) The long-term psychological effects of daily sedative interruption on critically ill patients. *Am J Respir Crit Care Med* 168: 1457–61.

Krishna S, Hughes LF, Lin SY (2003) Post operative haemorrhage with non steroidal anti-inflammatory drug use after tonsillectomy: a meta-analysis. *Arch Otolaryngol Head Neck Surg* 129: 1086–89.

Kroner K, Knudsen UB, Lundby L et al (1994) [Phantom breast syndrome]. *Ugeskr Laeger* 156: 977–80.

Kudrow L (1981) Response of cluster headache attacks to oxygen inhalation. *Headache* 21: 1–4.

Kuhlen R & Putensen C (2004) Remifentanil for analgesia-based sedation in the intensive care unit. *Crit Care* 8: 13–14.

Kumar A, Deed JS, Bhasin B et al (2004) Comparison of the effect of diclofenac with hyoscine-N-butylbromide in the symptomatic treatment of acute biliary colic. *ANZ J Surg* 74: 573–76.

Kumar V, Krone K, Mathieu A (2004) neuraxial and sympathetic blocks in herpes zoster and post-herpetic neuralgia: an appraisal for current evidence. *Reg Anesth Pain Med* 29: 454–61.

CHAPTER 9

La Spina I, Porazzi D, Maggiolo F et al (2001) Gabapentin in painful HIV-related neuropathy: a report of 19 patients, preliminary observations. *Eur J Neurol* 8: 71–75.

Labrecque M, Dostaler LP, Rousselle R et al (1994) Efficacy of non steroidal anti-inflammatory drugs in the treatment of acute renal colic. A meta-analysis. *Arch Intern Med* 154: 1381–87.

Laerum E, Ommundsen OE, Gronseth JE et al (1995) Oral diclofenac in the prophylactic treatment of recurrent renal colic. A double-blind comparison with placebo. *Eur Urol* 28: 108–11.

Lambert A, Dashfield A, Cosgrove C et al (2001) Randomized prospective study comparing preoperative epidural and intraoperative perineural analgesia for the prevention of postoperative stump and phantom limb pain following major amputation. *Reg Anesth Pain Med* 26: 316–21.

Lance JW, Anthony M, Spira PJ et al (1997) *Report of the Australian Association of Neurologists Ad Hoc Committee on the use of Opioids in the Management of Migraine*. Sydney: AAN.

Lane PL, Mc Lennan BA, Baggoley CJ (1989) Comparative efficacy of chlorpromazine and meperidine with dimenhydrinate in migraine headache. *Ann Emerg Med* 18: 360–65.

Lange R & Lentz R (1995) Comparison ketoprofen, ibuprofen and naproxen sodium in the treatment of tension-type headache. *Drugs Exp Clin Res* 21: 89–96.

Larkin GL & Prescott JE (1992) A randomized, double-blind, comparative study of the efficacy of ketorolac tromethamine versus meperidine in the treatment of severe migraine. *Ann Emerg Med* 21: 919–24.

Larue F, Fonatine A, Colleau SM (1997) Underestimation and undertreatment of pain in HIV disease: multicenter study. *BMJ* 314: 23–28.

Levendoglu F, Ogun CO, Ozerbil et al (2004) Gabapentin is a first line drug for the treatment of neuropathic pain in spinal cord injury. *Spine* 29: 743–51.

Lewis DW, Ashwal S, Dahl G et al (2002) Practice Parameter: evaluation of children and adolescents with recurrent headache. *Neurology* 59: 490–98.

Lewis DW, Ashwal S, Hershey A et al (2004) Practice Parameter: pharmacological treatment of migraine headache in children and adolescents [report of the American Academy of Neurology Quality Standards Subcommittee and Practice Committee of the Child neurology Society. *Neurology* 63: 2215–24.

Limmroth V, Katsarava Z, Fritsche G et al (2002) Features of medication overuse headache following overuse of different acute headache drugs *Neurology* 59: 1011–14.

Linde M, Elam M, Lundblad L et al (2004) Sumaptriptan (5HT 1B/1D-agonist) causes a transient allodynia. *Cephalalgia* 24: 1057–66.

Lewis PJ, Barrington SF, Marsden PK et al (1997) A study of the effects of sumatriptan on myocardial perfusion in healthy female migraineurs using 13NH3 positron emission tomography. *Neurology* 48: 1542–50.

Linneman PK, Terry BE, Burd RS (2000) The efficacy and safety of fentanyl for the management of severe procedural pain in patients with burn injuries. *J Burn Care Rehabil* 21: 519–22.

Lipton RB, Stewart WF, Stone AM, et al (2000a) Stratified care vs step care strategies for migraine: The Disability in Strategies of Care (DISC) Study group: A randomised trial. *JAMA* 284: 2599–605.

Lipton RB, Baggish JS, Stewart WF et al (2000b) Efficacy and safety of acetaminophen in the treatment of migraine: results of a randomised, double blind, placebo controlled population based study. *Arch Intern Med* 160: 3486–92.

Long TD, Cathers TA, Twillman R et al (2001) Morphine-Infused silver sulfadiazine (MISS) cream for burn analgesia: a pilot study. *J Burn Care Rehabil* 22: 118–23.

Low DE, Desrosiers M, McSharry J, et al (1997) A practical guide for the diagnosis and treatment of acute sinusitis. *CMAJ* 156 (Suppl 6): S1–14.

Matchar D, Young W, Rosenberg J et al (2000) *US Headache Consortium: Evidence Based Guidelines for Migraine Headache in the Primary Care Setting: Pharmacological Management of Acute Attacks.* (www.aan.com/public/practiceguidelines/03)

Maizels M, Scott B, Cohen W et al (1996) Intranasal lignocaine for the treatment of migraine *JAMA* 276: 319–21.

Manley NM, Fitzpatrick RW, Long T et al (1997) A cost analysis of alfentanil+propofol vs morphine+ midazolam for the sedation of critically ill patients. *Pharmacoeconomics* 12: 247–55.

Marjoribanks J, Proctor ML, Farquhar C. Nonsteroidal anti-inflammatory drugs for primary dysmenorrhoea. *The Cochrane Database of Systematic Reviews* 2003, Issue 4. Art. No.: CD001751. DOI: 10.1002/14651858.CD001751.

Marret E, Flahault A, Samama CM et al (2003) Effects of postoperative, nonsteroidal, antiinflammatory drugs on bleeding risk after tonsillectomy: meta-analysis of randomized, controlled trials. *Anesthesiology* 98: 1497–502.

Martin E, Ramsay G, Mantz J et al (2003) The role of the alpha2-adrenoceptor agonist dexmedetomidine in postsurgical sedation in the intensive care unit. *J Intensive Care Med* 18: 29–41.

McCance-Katz EF, Rainey PM, Jatlow P et al (1998) Methadone effects on zidovudine disposition (AIDS Clinical Trials Group 262). *J Acquir Immune Defic Syndr Hum Retrovirol* 18: 35–43.

McCance-Katz EF, Rainey PM, Friedland G et al (2003) The protease inhibitor lopinavir-ritonavir may produce opiate withdrawal in methadone-maintained patients. *Clin Infect Dis* 37: 476–82.

McHale PM & LoVecchio F (2001) Narcotic analgesia in the acute abdomen: a review of prospective trials. *Eur J Emerg Med* 8: 131–36.

McQuay HJ & Jadad AR (1994) Incident pain. *Cancer Surv* 21: 17–24.

McQuay HJ, Tramèr M, Nye BA et al (1996) A systematic review of antidepressants in neuropathic pain. *Pain* 68: 212–27.

Melchart D, Linde K, Fischer P et al (2001)Acupuncture for idiopathic headache. *The Cochrane Database of Systematic Reviews*. Issue 1. Art. No.: CD001218. DOI: 10.1002/14651858.CD001218.

Memis D, Turan A, Karamanlioglu B et al (2004) Adding dexmedetomidine to lidocaine for intravenous regional anesthesia. *Anesth Analg* 98: 835–40.

Merskey H & Bogduk N (Eds) (1994) *Classification of Chronic Pain*. 2nd Edition, IASP Task Force on Taxonomy. Seattle: IASP Press, pp209–14.

Michaloliakou C, Chung F, Sharma S(1996) Preoperative multimodal analgesia facilitates recovery after ambulatory laparoscopic cholecystectomy. *Anesth Analg* 82: 44–51.

Migliardi JR, Armellino JJ, Friedman M et al (1994) Caffeine as an analgesic adjuvant in tension headache. *Clin Pharmacol Ther* 56: 576–86.

Mitchell P, Wang JJ, Cumming RG et al (1998) Prevalence and vascular associations with migraine in the older Australians: *Aust NZ J Med*, 28: 627–32

Møiniche S, Mikkelsen S, Wetterslev J et al (1999) A systematic review of intra-articular local anesthesia for postoperative pain relief after arthroscopic knee surgery. *Reg Anesth Pain Med* 24: 430–37.

Møiniche S, Rømsing J, Dahl JB et al (2003) Non steroidal antiinflammatory drugs and the risk of operative site bleeding after tonsillectomy: a quantitative systematic review. *Anesth Analg* 96: 68–77.

Moore RA & McQuay HJ (1997) Single patient data meta-analysis of 3453 post operative patients: oral tramadol versus placebo, codeine and combination analgesics. *Pain* 69: 287–94.

Moore A, Edwards J, Barden J et al (2003) *Bandolier's Little Book of Pain*. Oxford: Oxford University Press.

Muellejans B, Lopez A, Cross MH et al (2004) Remifentanil versus fentanyl for analgesia based sedation to provide patient comfort in the intensive care unit: a randomized, double-blind controlled trial (ISRCTN43755713). *Crit Care* 8: R1–R11.

Mulroy MF, Larkin KL, Batra MS et al (2001) Femoral nerve block with 0.25% or 0.5% bupivacaine improves postoperative analgesia following outpatient arthroscopic anterior cruciate ligament repair. *Reg Anesth Pain Med* 26: 24–29.

Namavar Jahromi B, Tartifizadeh A, Khabnadideh S (2003) Comparison of fennel and mefenamic acid for the treatment of primary dysmenorrhoea. *Int J Gynaecol Obstet* 80: 153–57.

Newshan G & Lefkowitz M (2001) Transdermal fentanyl for chronic pain in AIDS: a pilot study. *J Pain Sympt Manage* 21: 69–77.

Nicolas Torralba JA, Rigabert Monteil M, Banon Perez V et al (1999) Intramuscular ketorolac compared to subcutaneous tramadol in the initial emergency treatment of renal colic. *Arch Esp Urol* 52: 435–37.

Nicolodi M (1996) Differential sensitivity to morphine challenge in migraine sufferers and headache exempt subjects. *Cephalalgia* 16: 297–304.

Nicholson BD (2004) Evaluation and treatment of central pain syndromes. *Neurology* 62: S30–36

Nielsen JR, Pedersen KE, Dahlstrom CG et al (1984) Analgetic treatment in acute myocardial infarction. A controlled clinical comparison of morphine, nicomorphine and pethidine. *Acta Med Scand* 215: 349–54.

Nikolajsen L, Hansen CL, Nielsen J et al (1996) The effect of ketamine on phantom pain: A central neuropathic disorder maintained by peripheral input. *Pain* 67: 69–77.

Nikolajsen L, Ilkjaer S, Kroner K et al (1997) The influence of preamputation pain on postamputation stump and phantom pain. *Pain* 72: 393–405.

Nikolajsen L & Jensen TS (2001) Phantom limb pain. *Br J Anaesth* 87: 107–16.

Nilsson Remahl AI, Ansjon R, Lind F et al (2002) Hyperbaric oxygen treatment of active cluster headache: a double-blind placebo-controlled cross-over study. *Cephalalgia* 22: 730–39.

O'Connor A, Schug SA, Cardwell H. (2000) A comparison of the efficacy and safety of morphine and pethidine for suspected renal colic in the emergency setting. *J Accid Emerg Med* 17: 261–64.

O'Leary U, Puglia C, Friehling TD et al (1987) Nitrous oxide anaesthesia in patients with ischaemic chest discomfort: effect on beta endorphin levels. *J Clin Pharmacol* 27: 957–61.

Olkkola KT, Palkama VJ, Neuvonen PJ et al (1999) Ritonavir's role in reducing fentanyl clearance and prolonging its half-life. *Anesthesiology* 91: 681–85.

O'Neill WM & Sherrard JS (1993) Pain in human immunodeficiency virus disease: a review. *Pain* 54: 3–14.

Oldman AD, Smith LA, McQuay HJ et al (2002) Pharmacological treatments for acute migraine: quantitative systematic review. *Pain* 97: 247–57.

Ong KS & Tan JM (2004) Preoperative intravenous tramadol versus ketorolac for preventing post operative pain after third molar surgery. *Int J Oral Maxillofac Surg* 33: 274–78.

Ornato JP (2003) Management of patients with unstable angina and non-ST-segment elevation myocardial infarction: update ACC/AHA guidelines. *Am J Emerg Med* 21: 346–51.

Paice JA, Ferrans CE, Lashley FR et al (2000a) Topical capsaicin in the management of HIV-associated peripheral neuropathy. *J Pain Sympt Manage* 1: 45–52.

Paice JA, Shott S, Oldenburg FP et al (2000b) Efficacy of a vibratory stimulus for the relief of HIV-associated neuropathic pain. *Pain* 84: 291–96.

Pandey CK, Bose N, Garg G et al (2002) Gabapentin for the treatment of pain in Guillain-Barre syndrome: a double-blinded, placebo-controlled, crossover study. *Anesth Analg* 95: 1719–23.

Parisod E (2002) Management of pain in a patient with Guillain-Barre syndrome. *ANZCA Bull* 11: 53–61.

Patterson DR, Ptacek JT, Carrougher JG et al (1997) Lorazepam as an adjunct to opioid analgesics in the treatment of burn pain. *Pain* 72: 367–74.

Pavlin JD, Chen C, Penaloza DA et al (2002) Pain as a factor complicating recovery and discharge after ambulatory surgery. *Anesth Analg* 95: 627–34.

Perkins F & Kehlet H (2000) Chronic pain as an outcome of surgery. *Anaesthesiology* 93: 1123–33.

Perreault S, Choinière M, du Souich PB et al (2001) Pharmacokinetics of morphine and its glucuronidated metabolites in burn injuries. *Ann Pharmacother* 35: 1588–92.

Pinzur MS, Garla PG, Pluth T et al (1996) Continuous postoperative infusion of a regional anesthetic after an amputation of the lower extremity. A randomized clinical trial. *J Bone Joint Surg Am* 78: 1501–05.

Piscitelli SC, Kress DR, Bertz RJ et al (2000) The effect of ritonavir on the pharmacokinetics of meperidine and normeperidine. *Pharmacotherapy* 20: 549–53.

Pitsiu M, Wilmer A, Bodenham A et al (2004) Pharmacokinetics of remifentanil and its major metabolite, remifentanil acid, in ICU patients with renal impairment. *Br J Anaesth* 92: 493–503.

Pittler MH & Ernst E (1998) Peppermint oil for irritable bowel syndrome; a critical review and metaanalysis. *Am J Gastroenterol* 93: 1131–35.

Pollack CV Jr & Swindle GM (1989) Use of diphenhydramine for local anesthesia in '-caine' sensitive patients. *J Emerg Med* 7: 611–14.

Pollack CV Jr, Roe MT, Peterson ED (2003) 2002 update to the ACC/AHA guidelines for the management of patients with unstable angina and non-ST-segment elevation myocardial infarction: implications for emergency department practice. *Ann Emerg Med* 41: 355–69.

Poynard T, Regimbeau C, Benhamou Y (2001) Meta-analysis of smooth muscle relaxants in the treatment of irritable bowel syndrome. *Ailiment Pharmacol Ther* 15: 355–61.

Prakash S, Fatima T, Pawar M (2004) Patient-controlled analgesia with fentanyl for burn dressing changes. *Anesth Analg* 99: 552–55.

Prior MJ, Cooper KM, May LG et al (2002) Efficacy and safety of acetaminophen and naproxen in the treatment of tension type headache. A randomised, double blind placebo controlled trial. *Cephalalgia* 22: 740–48.

Proctor ML, Smith CA, Farquhar CM et al (2002) Transcutaneous electrical nerve stimulation and acupuncture for primary dysmenorrhoea. *The Cochrane Database of Systematic Reviews*. Issue 1. Art. No.: CD002123. DOI: 10.1002/14651858.CD002123.

Puntillo K, Miaskowski C, Kehrle K et al (1997) Relationship between behavioral and physiological indicators of pain, critical care patients' self-reports of pain, and opioid administration. *Crit Care Med* 25: 1159–66.

Puntillo K, Stannard D, Miakowski C et al (2002) Use of a pain assessment and intervention notation (P.A.I.N.) tool in critical care nursing practice: nurses' evaluations. *Heart Lung* 31: 303–14.

Puntillo KA, Morris AB, Thompson CL et al (2004) Pain behaviors observed during six common procedures: results from Thunder Project II. *Crit Care Med* 32: 421–27.

Rapaport E (2002) Guidelines for the acute coronary syndromes. ACC/AHA American College of Cardiology/American Heart Association. *Curr Cardiol Rep* 3: 289–98.

Rasmussen PV, Sindrup SH, Jensen TS et al (2004) Symptoms and signs in patients with suspected neuropathic pain. *Pain* 110: 461–69.

Rawal N, Allvin R, Axelsson K et al (2002) Patient-controlled regional analgesia (PCRA) at home: controlled comparison between bupivacaine and ropivacaine brachial plexus analgesia. *Anesthesiology* 96: 1290–96.

Rees DC, Olujohungbe AD, Parker NE et al (2003) Guidelines for the management of the acute painful crisis in sickle cell disease. *Br J Haematol* 120: 744–52.

Rettig G & Kropp J (1980) [Analgesic effect of tramadol in acute myocardial infarct] *Ther Ggw* 119: 705–07.

Reuben SS & Connelly NR (1995) Postoperative analgesia for outpatient arthroscopic knee sugery with intraarticular bupivacaine and ketorolac. *Anesth Analg* 80: 1154–57.

Reuben SS & Connelly NR (1996) Postarthroscopic meniscus repair analgesia with intraarticular ketorolac or morphine. *Anesth Analg* 82: 1036–39.

Reuben SS & Connelly NR (1999) Postoperative analgesia for outpatient arthroscopic knee surgery with intraarticular clonidine. *Anesth Analg* 88: 729–33.

Reutens DC, Fatovich DM, Stewart-Wynne EG et al (1991) Is intravenous lidocaine clinically effective in acute migraine? *Cephalalgia* 11: 245–47.

Richman PB, Allegra J, Eskin B et al (2002) A randomised clinical trial to assess the efficacy of intramuscular droperidol for the treatment of acute migraine headache. *Am J Emerg Med* 20: 39–42.

Riddington C, De Franceschi L. Drugs for preventing red blood cell dehydration in people with sickle cell disease. *The Cochrane Database of Systematic Reviews* 2002, Issue 4. Art. No.: CD003426. DOI: 10.1002/14651858.CD003426.

Robieux IC, Kellner JD, Coppes MJ et al (1992) Analgesia in children with sickle cell crisis: comparison of intermittent opioids vs. continuous intravenous infusion of morphine and placebo controlled study of oxygen inhalation. *Pediatr Hematol Oncol* 9: 317–26.

Rømsing J, Ostergaard D, Drozdziewicz D et al (2000) Diclofenac or acetaminophen for analgesia in paediatric tonsillectomy outpatients. *Acta Anaesthesiol Scand* 44: 291–95.

Rose K M, Carson AP, Sanford CP et al (2004) Migraine and other headaches - associations with Rose angina and coronary heart disease. *Neurology* 63: 2233–39.

Rupp T & Delaney KA (2004) Inadequate analgesia in emergency medicine. *Ann Emerg Med* 43: 494–503.

Rusy LM, Houck CS, Sullivan LJ et al (1995) A double blind evaluation of ketorolac tromethamine versus acetaminophen in paediatric tonsillectomy: analgesia and bleeding. *Anesth Analg* 80: 226–29.

Safa-Tisseront V et al (2001) Effectiveness of epidural blood patch in the management of post-dural puncture headache. *Anesthesiology* 95: 334–39.

Savoie FH, Field LD, Jenkins RN et al (2000) The pain control infusion pump for postoperative pain control in shoulder surgery. *Arthroscopy* 16: 339–42.

Scherl ER & Wilson JF (1995) Comparison of dihydroergotamine with metoclopramide versus meperidine with promethazine in the treatment of migraine. *Headache* 35: 256–59.

Schifferdecker B & Spodick DH (2003) Nonsteroidal anti-inflammatory drugs in the treatment of pericarditis. *Cardiol Rev* 11: 211–17.

Schmelzeisen R & Frolich JC (1993) Prevention of post operative swelling and pain by dexamethasone after operative removal of impacted third molar teeth. *Eur J Clin Pharmacol* 44: 275–77.

Schmidt A, Bjorkman S, Akeson J (2001) Preoperative rectal diclofenac versus paracetamol for tonsillectomy: effects on pain and blood loss. *Acta Anaesthesiol Scand* 45: 48–52.

Sechzer P & Abel L (1978) Post spinal anesthesia headache treated with caffeine evaluation with demand method. *Curr Ther Res* 24: 307–12.

Shakespeare DT, Boggild M, Young C (2003) Anti-spasticity agents for multiple sclerosis. *The Cochrane Database of Systematic Reviews* 2003, Issue 4. Art. No.: CD001332. DOI: 10.1002/14651858.CD001332.

Shapiro BA, Warren J, Egol AB et al (1995) Practice parameters for intravenous analgesia and sedation for adult patients in the intensive care unit: an executive summary. Society of Critical Care Medicine. *Crit Care Med* 23: 1596–600.

Sharma S, Prasad A, Nehru R et al (2002) Efficacy and tolerabilty of prochlorperazine buccal tablets in treatment of acute migraine. *Headache*42: 896–902.

Sherman RA, Sherman CJ, Gall NG (1980) A survey of current phantom limb pain treatment in the United States. *Pain* 8: 85–99.

Shlay JC, Chaloner K, Max MB et al (1998) Acupuncture and amitriptyline for pain due to HIV-related peripheral neuropathy: a randomized controlled trial. Terry Beirn Community Programs for Clinical Research on AIDS. *JAMA* 280: 1590–95.

Shrestha M, Singh R, Moreden J et al (1996) Ketorolac vs chlorpromazine in the treatment of acute migraine without aura: A prospective, randomised, double-blind trial. *Arch Int Med* 156: 1725–28.

Siddall PJ, Taylor DA, McClelland JM et al (1999) Pain report and the relationship of pain to physical factors in the first six months following spinal cord injury. *Pain* 81: 187–97.

Siddall PJ, Yezierski RP, Loeser JD (2002) Taxonomy and epidemiology of spinal cord injury pain. In: Burchiel KJ & Yezierski RP (Eds) *Spinal Cord Injury Pain: Assessment, Mechanisms, Management. Progress in Pain Research and Management*, Vol. 23. Seattle: IASP Press.

SIGN (2000) *Control of Pain in Patients with Cancer.* SIGN Publication Number 44. Edinburgh: Scottish Intercollegiate Guidelines Network. (www.sign.ac.uk/pdf/sign44.pdf)

Silberstein S D (2000) US Headache Consortium: Practice Parameter: Evidence Based Guidelines for Migraine Headache. *Neurology* 55: 754–63.

Silberstein SD, Welch KMA (2002) Painkiller Headache. *Neurology*: 59: 972–74.

Silberstein SD, Young WB, Mendizabal JE et al (2003) Acute migraine treatment with droperidol: A randomised, double-blind, placebo-controlled trial. *Neurology* 60: 315–21.

Silvast T & Saarnivaara L (2001) Comparison of alfentanil and morphine in the pre hospital treatment of patients with acute ischaemic-type chest pain. *Eur J Emerg Med* 8: 275–78.

Sim KM, Hwang NC, Chan YW et al (1996) Use of patient-controlled analgesia with alfentanil for burns dressing procedures: a preliminary report of five patients. *Burns* 22: 238–41.

Simpson DM, Dorfman D, Olney RK et al (1996) Peptide T in the treatment of painful distal neuropathy associated with AIDS: results of a placebo-controlled trial. The Peptide T Neuropathy Study Group. *Neurology* 47: 1254–59.

Simpson DM, Olney R, McArthur JC et al (2000) A placebo-controlled trial of lamotrigine for painful HIV-associated neuropathy. *Neurology* 54: 2115–19.

Sindrup SH & Jensen TS (1999) Efficacy of pharmacological treatment of neuropathic pain: an update and effect related mechanism of drug action. *Pain* 83: 389–400.

Singer EJ, Zorilla C, Fahy-Chandon B et al (1993) Painful symptoms reported by ambulatory HIV-infected men in a longitudinal study. *Pain* 54: 15–19.

Singer AJ & Stark MJ (2000) Pretreatment of lacerations with lidocaine, epinephrine and tetracaine at triage: a randomised double blind trial. *Acad Emerg Med* 7: 751–56.

Slatkin NE & Rhiner M (2003) Topical ketamine in the treatment of mucositis pain. *Pain Med* 4: 298–303.

Smith GA, Strausbaugh SD, Harbeck-Weber C et al (1997) Comparison of topical anesthetics with lidocaine infiltration during laceration repair in children. *Clin Pediatr* (*Phila*) 36: 17–23.

Soares LG, Martins M, Uchoa R (2003) Intravenous fentanyl for cancer pain: a fast titration protocol for the emergency room. *J Pain Sympt Manage* 26: 876–81.

Stankov S (1995) Haemodynamic effects of tramadol and morphine in patients with acute myocardial infarction (abstract). In: *7th World Congress on Pain 1993 Aug 22–27 Paris*. Seattle: IASP, p293.

Steiner TJ, Stewart WF, Kolodner K et al (1999) Epidemiology of migraine in England. *Cephalalgia* 19: 305–06.

Steiner TJ, Fontebasso M (2002) Headaches not to be missed. *BMJ* 325: 881–86.

Steiner TJ, Lange R, Voelker M (2003) Aspirin in episodic tension-type headache: placebo controlled dose ranging comparison with paracetamol. *Cephalalgia* 23: 59–66.

Steward DL, Welge JA, Myer CM. Steroids for improving recovery following tonsillectomy in children. *The Cochrane Database of Systematic Reviews* 2002, Issue 3. Art. No.: CD003997. DOI: 10.1002/14651858.CD003997.

Stiell IG, Dufour DG, Moher D et al (1991) Methotrimeprazine versus meperidine and dimenhydrinate in the treatment of severe migraine, a randomised, controlled trial. *Ann Emerg Med* 20: 1201–05.

Strassels SA, Chen C, Carr DB (2002) Postoperative analgesia: economics, resource use, and patient satisfaction in an urban teaching hospital. *Anesth Analg* 4: 130–37.

Sudlow C, Warlow C. Posture and fluids for preventing post-dural puncture headache. *The Cochrane Database of Systematic Reviews* 2001a, Issue 2. Art. No.: CD001790. DOI: 10.1002/14651858.CD001790.

Sudlow C, Warlow C. Epidural blood patching for preventing and treating post-dural puncture headache. *The Cochrane Database of Systematic Reviews* 2001b, Issue 2. Art. No.: CD001791. DOI: 10.1002/14651858.CD001791.

Sutherland S & Matthews DC (2003) Emergency management of acute apical periodontitis in the permanent dentition: a systematic review of the literature. *J Can Dent Assoc* 69: 160.

Tagliati M, Grinnell J, Godbold J et al (1999) Peripheral nerve function in HIV infection: clinical, electrophysiologic, and laboratory findings. *Arch Neurol* 56: 84–89.

Tanen DA, Miller S, French T et al (2003) Intravenous valproate versus prochlorperazine for the emergency department treatment of acute migraine headache: A prospective, randomised, double-blind trial. *Ann Emerg Med* 41: 847–53.

Tarumi Y, Pereira J, Watanabe S et al (2002) Methadone and fluconazole: respiratory depression by drug interaction. *J Pain Symptom Manage* 23: 48–53.

Tfelt-Hansen P, Mulder H, Scheldewaert TG et al (1996) The combination of oral lysine-acetylsalicylate and metoclopramide compared with sumatriptan in the treatment of migraine attacks. A randomised, double blind, placebo controlled clinical trail. *Ugeskrift for Lager* 158: 6435–39.

The Guillain-Barre Syndrome Study Group (1985) Plasmapheresis and acute Guillain-Barre syndrome. *Neurol* 35 1096–104.

Thomas SH & Silen W (2003) Effect on diagnostic efficiency of analgesia for undifferentiated abdominal pain. *Br J Surg* 90: 5–9.

Thomas SH, Sien W, Cheema F et al (2003) Effects of morphine analgesia in diagnostic accuracy in emergency department patients with abdominal pain: a prospective, randomised trial. *J Am Coll Surg* 196: 18–31.

Thompson DR (2001) Narcotic analgesia effects on the sphincter of Oddi: a review of data and the therapeutic implications in treating pancreatitis. *Am J Gastroenterol* 96: 1266–72.

Thune A, Baker RA, Saccone GT et al (1990) Differing effects of pethidine and morphine on sphincter of Oddi motility. *Br J Surg* 77: 992–95.

Tramèr MR, Williams JE, Carroll D et al (1998) Comparing analgesic efficacy of non-steroidal anti-inflammatory drugs given by different routes in acute and chronic pain: a quantitative systematic review. *Acta Anaesthesiol Scand* 42: 71–79.

Tripathi M & Kaushik S (2000) Carbamezapine for pain management in Guillain-Barre syndrome patients in the intensive care unit. *Crit Care Med* 28: 655–58.

Turnbull DK & Shepherd DB (2003) Post–dural puncture headache: pathogenesis, prevention and treatment. *Br J Anaesth* 91: 718–29.

Tyring S, Beutner KR, Tucker BA et al (2000) Antiviral therapy for herpes zoster: randomized, controlled clinical trial of valacyclovir and famciclovir therapy in immunocompetent patients 50 years and older. *Arch Fam Med* 9: 863–69.

Vakharia SB, Tomas PS, Rosenbaum AP et al (1997) Magnetic resonance imaging of cerebrospinal fluid leak and tamponade effect of blood patch in post-dural puncture headache. *Anesth Analg* 84: 585–90.

Van Vliet JA, Bahra A Martin V et al (2003) Intranasal sumatriptan in cluster headache: randomised placebo controlled double blind study. *Neurology* 60: 630–32.

Vergnion M, Degesves S, Gareet L et al (2001) Tramadol, an alternative to morphine for treating posttraumatic pain in the prehospital situation. *Anesth Analg* 92: 1543–6.

Vernon H, McDermaid CS, Hagino C (1999) Systematic review of randomised clinical trials of complementary/alternative therapies in the treatment of tension-type and cervicogenic headache. *Comp Ther Med* 7: 142–55.

Vickers ER & Punnia-Moorthy A (1992) A clinical evaluation of three topical anaesthetic agents. *Aust Dent J* 37: 266–70.

Vickers ER, Cousins M, Walker S et al (1998) Analysis of 50 patients with atypical odontalgia: a preliminary report on pharmacological procedures for diagnosis and treatment. *Oral Surg Oral Med Oral Pathol Oral Radiol Endod* 85: 24–32.

Vickers ER, Cousins M, Nicholas M (2000) Facial pain – a biopsychosocial problem. *Med Today* 11: 42–48.

Viggiano M, Badetti C, Roux JF et al (1998) Controlled analgesia in a burn patient: fentanyl sparing effect of clonidine. *Ann Fr Anesth Reanim* 17: 19–26.

Vinson DR (2002) Treatment patterns of isolated benign headache in US emergency departments. *Ann Emerg Med* 39: 215–22.

Vogl D, Rosenfeld B, Breitbart W et al (1999) Symptom prevalence, characteristics and distress in AIDS outpatients. *J Pain Sympt Manage* 18: 253–62.

Wall GC & Heyneman CA (1999) Calcitonin in phantom limb pain. *Ann Pharmacother* 33: 499–501.

Wall PD & Melzack R (Eds) (1999) *Textbook of Pain*. 4th ed, Edinburgh: Churchill Livingstone, p905.

Wallny T, Hess L, Seuser A et al (2001) Pain status of patients with severe haemophilic arthropathy. *Haemophilia* 7: 453–58.

Wambebe C, Khamofu H, Momoh JA et al (2001) Double blind, placebo-controlled, randomised cross-over clinical trial of NIPRISAN® in patients with sickle cell disorder. *Phytomed* 8: 252–61.

Ward TN & Levin M (2004) Facial pain. In: Warfield DA & Bajwa ZH (Eds) *Principles and Practice of Pain Medicine*. 2nd Edition, McGraw-Hill, pp246–51.

Watson CP & Babul N (1998) Efficacy of oxycodone in neuropathic pain: a randomised controlled trial in post herpetic neuralgia. *Neurology* 50: 1837–41.

Weiner DL, Hibberd PL, Betit P et al (2003) Preliminary assessment of inhaled nitric oxide for acute vaso-occlusive crisis in pediatric patients with sickle cell disease. *JAMA* 289: 1136–42.

Weiss P & Ritz R (1988) Analgesic effect and side effects of buprenorphine in acute coronary heart disease. A randomised double blind comparison with morphine. *Anasth Intensivether Notfallmed* 23: 309–12.

Wenzel RG, Sarvis CA, Krause ML (2003) Over-The-Counter Drugs for Acute Migraine Attacks: Literature review and recommendations. *Pharmacotherapy* 23: 494–505.

Whipple JK, Lewis KS, Quebbeman EJ et al (1995) Analysis of pain management in critically ill patients. *Pharmacotherapy* 15: 592–99.

Wiffen P, Collins S, McQuay H, Carroll D et al (2000) Anticonvulsant drugs for acute and chronic pain. *The Cochrane Database of Systematic Reviews*, Issue 3. Art. No.: CD001133. DOI: 10.1002/14651858.CD001133.

Williams BA, Kentor ML, Vogt MT et al (2004) Economics of nerve block pain management after anterior cruciate ligament reconstruction: potential hospital cost savings via associated postanesthesia care unit bypass and same-day discharge. *Anesthesiology* 100: 697–706.

Winner P, Ricalde O, Le Force B et al (1996) A double-blind study of subcutaneous dihydroergotamine vs subcutaneous sumatriptan in the treatment of acute migraine. *Arch Neurol* 53: 180–84.

Wood MJ, Kay R, Dworkin RH et al (1996) Oral acyclovir therapy accelerates pain resolution in patients with herpes zoster: a meta-analysis of placebo-controlled trials. *Clin Infect Dis* 22: 341–47.

Worthington HV, Clarkson JE, Eden OB. Interventions for treating oral mucositis for patients with cancer receiving treatment. *The Cochrane Database of Systematic Reviews* 2004, Issue 2. Art. No.: CD001973. DOI: 10.1002/14651858.CD001973.pub2.

Wright SW, Norris RL, Mitchell TR (1992) Ketorolac for sickle cell vaso-occlusive crisis pain in the emergency department; lack of narcotic sparing effect. *Ann Emerg Med* 21: 925–28.

Wu CL, Tella P, Staats PS et al (2002) Analgesic effects of intravenous lidocaine and morphine on postamputation pain: A randomized double-blind, active placebo-controlled, crossover trial. *Anesthesiology* 96: 841–48.

Wu YW, Hui YL, Tan PP(1994) Experience of epidural blood patch for post-dural puncture headache. Acta *Anesthesiology Sinica* 32: 137–40.

Yaster M, Tobin JR, Billett C et al (1994) Epidural analgesia in the management of severe vaso-occlusive sickle cell crisis. *Pediatrics* 93: 310–15.

Zakrzewska JM, Harrison SH (2003) Facial pain. In: Jensen TS, Wilson PR, Rice ASC (Eds) *Clinical Pain Management, Chronic Pain*. London: Arnold, pp481–504.

Zhang WY, LI Wan Po A (1998) Efficacy of minor analgesics in primary dysmenorrhoea: a systematic review. *Br J Obstet Gynaecol* 105: 780–89.

Zipursky A, Robieux IC, Brown EJ et al (1992) Oxygen therapy in sickle cell disease. *Am J Pediatr Hematol Oncol* 14: 222–28.

10. SPECIFIC PATIENT GROUPS

10.1 THE PAEDIATRIC PATIENT

10.1.1 Developmental neurobiology of pain

Even the most premature neonate has the neural pathways required for nociception and responds to potentially tissue damaging stimuli. However, significant functional and structural changes occur during the first months of life as the expression of a number of molecules and channels involved in nociception are developmentally regulated. There are changes in the distribution and density of many important receptors and the levels and effects of several neurotransmitters alter significantly during the postnatal period.

Although C-fibre polymodal nociceptors are mature in their pattern of firing at birth and are capable of being activated in the periphery by exogenous stimuli, their central synaptic connections in the dorsal horn are initially immature. However, 'wind up' can be produced by relatively low intensity A-fibre (rather than C-fibre) stimulation, as A-beta fibres initially extend up into laminae I and II and only withdraw once C-fibres have matured. This overlap is likely to contribute to the larger receptive fields of dorsal horn neurones observed in early development. The N-methyl-D-aspartate (NMDA) receptor, which is important for central sensitisation, is present in a higher concentration and more generalised distribution in the dorsal horn early in development, and activation results in a greater influx of calcium ions. In addition, descending inhibitory pathways, diffuse noxious inhibitory controls and local interneuronal inhibitory mechanisms in the dorsal horn are not fully mature in early development. Therefore, rather than neonates being less sensitive to painful stimuli as was once thought, the relative excess of excitatory mechanisms and delayed maturation of inhibitory mechanisms produce more generalised and exaggerated reflex responses to lower intensity stimuli during early development (Fitzgerald & Howard 2002).

Factors affecting the pharmacokinetic profile of analgesic drugs (body water and fat composition, plasma protein binding, hepatic metabolism and renal function) change rapidly during the first weeks of life. The developmental pharmacokinetic profiles of a number of analgesic drugs (eg morphine and paracetamol) (Kart et al 1997; Anderson et al 2002) have been determined, but are often based on single dose administration and the effects of repeated or prolonged administration are unknown. In addition to changes in pharmacokinetic factors, developmental changes in nociceptive processing may have significant effects on the pharmacodynamics and dose requirement of commonly utilised analgesics. Therefore, size changes that can be predicted by weight need to be considered along with developmental changes predicted by age. Laboratory studies have found reduced dose requirements for opioids and local anaesthetics in early development (Marsh et al 1999; Howard et al 2001), but further clinical data are required to fully evaluate the developmental pharmacodynamics of analgesic drugs.

10.1.2 Long-term consequences of early pain and injury

Significant reorganisation of synaptic connections occurs in the postnatal period. Activity within sensory pathways is required for normal development, but abnormal or excessive activity related to pain and injury during the neonatal period may alter normal development and produce persistent changes (Fitzgerald & Walker 2003).

In laboratory studies, the degree of long-term change varies with the type and severity of injury. Neonatal full thickness skin wounds produce prolonged increases in sensitivity in the absence of any visible persistent peripheral injury. The anatomical distribution of peripheral nerve terminals in the spinal cord can be permanently altered by nerve injury or chronic inflammation induced during the first postnatal week in rat pups. Although less severe inflammation does not produce long-term structural effects, an acute reversible change is seen in neonates but not in adult animals subjected to a similar stimulus, thus emphasising the plasticity of the nervous system early in development (Walker et al 2003). These findings are of considerable importance as pain and injury in neonates may have effects on nociceptive processing that differ in mechanism and duration from that experienced by older children and adults. Clinical studies also suggest that early pain related to surgery and clinical procedures in premature and term neonates may have long-term effects upon pain-related behaviour and the perception of pain (Grunau 2000).

Importantly, analgesia at the time of the initial painful stimulus may modulate long-term effects. Male neonates circumcised without analgesia show an increased behavioural pain response to immunisation several months later, but this is reduced if local anaesthetic is used prior to surgery (Taddio et al 1997). Infants who had undergone surgery in the neonatal period with perioperative morphine did not show any increase in later response to immunisation when compared with infants without significant previous pain experience (Peters et al 2003a).

CHAPTER 10

Key messages

The following tick boxes ☑ represent conclusions based on clinical experience and expert opinion.

☑ Even the most premature neonate responds to nociceptive stimuli.

☑ In early development more generalised reflex nociceptive responses occur in response to lower intensity stimuli.

☑ Due to the increased plasticity of the developing nervous system, pain and injury in early life may have adverse long-term consequences.

10.1.3 Paediatric pain assessment

Pain assessment is a prerequisite to optimal pain management in children (Howard 2003a) and should involve a clinical interview with the child (and/or their parent/carer), physical assessment and use of an age- and context-appropriate pain measurement tool. As in adults (see Chapter 2) other domains of pain (eg location, quality) and the multidimensional nature of the pain experience (eg concomitant emotional distress, coping style of the child, previous pain experience) should be incorporated into overall assessment. Regular assessment and measurement of pain may improve pain management and increase patient, parent and staff satisfaction (Treadwell et al 2002).

Pain measurement scales

Verbal self-report is considered to be the best measure of pain in adults. However, although it should be used in children whenever possible, children's understanding of pain and their ability to describe it changes with age. Therefore measurement tools must be appropriate to the different stages of their development. A large number of scales have been developed for neonates and infants, encompassing a number of surrogate measures (eg physical signs such as increased heart rate) or behavioural responses (eg facial characteristics and cry). Choice of the most appropriate tool depends on the age of the infant, the stimulus (eg procedural or postoperative pain) and the purpose of the measurement (eg clinical care or research).

In older children, age-appropriate scales for self-report need to consider the child's ability to differentiate levels of intensity and separate the emotional from the physical components of pain. It is important that a measurement tool be used regularly and uniformly within each centre as staff familiarity and ease of use are major factors in the successful implementation of a pain management strategy.

Examples of acute pain measurement tools are listed in Tables 10.1, 10.2 and 10.3.

Physiological measures

Changes in physiological parameters associated with procedural interventions and assumed to indicate the presence of pain include: increases in heart rate, respiratory rate, blood pressure, intracranial pressure, cerebral blood flow and palmar sweating; and decreases in oxygen saturation, transcutaneous carbon dioxide tension and vagal tone (Sweet & McGrath 1998). As these changes are reduced by analgesia, they are useful surrogate outcome measures of pain, but their sensitivity and specificity will also be influenced by concurrent clinical conditions (eg increased heart rate due to sepsis)and other factors (eg distress, environment, movement).

Behavioural measures

Noxious stimuli produce a series of behavioural responses in infants that can be used as surrogate measures of pain (McGrath 1998; Gaffney et al 2003) including crying, changes in facial activity, movement of torso and limbs, consolability and sleep state. Crying can be described in terms of its presence or absence, duration and amplitude or pitch.

The reliability and validity of behavioural measures are best established for short sharp pain associated with procedural interventions such as heel stick. The specificity and sensitivity of the response can be influenced by habituation, motor development, previous handling and manifestations of other states of distress (eg hunger and fatigue).

Ten facial actions are included in the Neonatal Facial Coding Scale (NFCS) which was originally validated for procedural pain in neonates and infants (see Table 10.1) (Grunau & Craig 1987). A reduced scale with 5 items (brow bulge, eye squeeze, nasolabial furrow, horizontal mouth stretch and taut tongue) has been found to be a sensitive and valid measure of postoperative pain in infants ages 0–18 months (Peters et al 2003b).

In infants and young children, behavioural items that predict analgesic demand in the postoperative period are crying, facial expression, posture of the trunk, posture of the legs and motor restlessness (Buttner & Finke 2000).

Composite measures

Many scales incorporate both physiological and behavioural parameters to determine an overall pain score and may result in more comprehensive measurement (Franck et al 2000). Some examples are included in Table 10.2 but a wider range of measures, their strengths and limitations, and issues of testing reliability and validity are discussed in recent reviews (Johnston 1998; Stevens 1998; Franck et al 2000; Stevens et al 2000; Johnston et al 2003). No single scale has been shown to be clearly superior or been universally adopted (Franck et al 2000).

Self-report

Self-report of pain is usually possible by 4 years of age but will depend on the cognitive and emotional maturity of the child. At 4–5 years of age, children can differentiate 'more', 'less' or 'the same', and can use a *Faces Pain Scale* (Figure 10.1) if it is explained appropriately and is a relatively simple scale with a limited number of options. At this age, children have some capacity to appraise current pain and match it to previous experience and they are more likely to choose the extremes of the scale (Hicks et al 2001). In scales anchored with smiling or tearful faces, pain may be confused with other emotional states such as happiness, sadness or anxiety (Champion et al 1998).

Between 7 and 10 years of age children develop skills with measurement, classification and seriation (ie putting things in ascending or descending order). The upper end of the scale is less static than in adults as it will change with the individual child's ability to objectify, label and remember previous pain experiences (Gaffney et al 2003). It is not until 10–12 years of age that children can clearly discriminate the sensory intensity and the affective emotional components of pain and report them independently (McGrath et al 1996). Verbally competent children aged 12 years and above can understand and use the McGill Pain Questionnaire (Gaffney et al 2003).

As with adults, there can be disagreement between the child's ratings of pain and the rating given by nurses and medical staff, with the latter groups often underestimating the severity of the pain (Rømsing et al 1996, **Level III-3**; LaMontagne et al 1991, **Level III-3**).

Children with cognitive impairment

In children with cognitive impairment and/or communication problems, assessment of pain is difficult and can contribute to inadequate analgesia. Neonates at risk of neurological impairment required more procedural interventions in intensive care, but received less analgesia (Stevens et al 2003). A retrospective chart review of children who had undergone spine fusion surgery found that pain was assessed less frequently in cognitively impaired children and that they received less analgesia (Malviya et al 2001). Another group found that while cognitively impaired children received less analgesia during surgery, they received comparable amounts and types of analgesics as cognitively intact children in the postoperative period (Koh et al 2004, **Level III-2**).

Behaviours reported by caregivers to be associated with potentially painful stimuli and that discriminate these from distressful or calm events, have been compiled in the revised Non-Communicating Children's Pain Checklist (NCCPC-R) (Breau et al 2002a) and a postoperative version has also been developed (NCCPC-PV)(Breau et al 2002b). In the assessment of postoperative pain in children with cognitive impairment, scores on the FLACC scale (see Table 10.2) correlated with parental pain report and were reduced after analgesia (Voepel-Lewis et al 2002).

Key messages

The following tick boxes ☑ represent conclusions based on clinical experience and expert opinion.

☑ Pain assessment and measurement are important components of paediatric pain management.

☑ Pain measurement tools are available for children of all ages.

☑ Pain measurement tools must be matched to the age and development of the child, be appropriate for the clinical context and be explained and used consistently.

Figure 10.1 Faces Pain Scale — revised

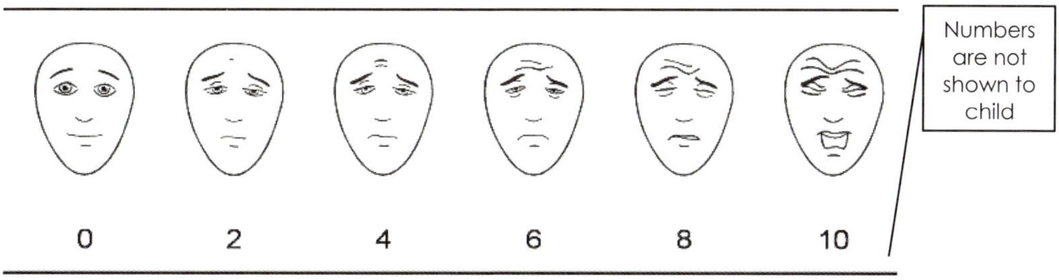

Note: The full-size version of the Faces Pain Scale (FPS-R), together with instructions for administration (available in many languages), are freely available for non-commercial clinical and research use from www.painsourcebook.ca.

Source: FPS-R; Hicks et al 2001; adapted from Bieri et al (1990).
Copyright ©2001 International Association for the Study of Pain (IASP). Reproduced by permission.

CHAPTER 10

Table 10.1 Acute pain intensity measurement tools — neonates

Scale	Indicators	Score	Utility
Premature Infant Pain Profile (PIPP) (Stevens et al 1996)	gestational age behavioural state heart rate oxygen saturation brow bulge eye squeeze nasolabial furrow	each scored on 4 point scale (0,1,2,3) 6 or less = minimal pain; >12 = moderate to severe pain	procedural pain preterm and term neonates; postoperative pain in term neonates
Neonatal Infant Pain Scale (NIPS) (Lawrence et al 1993)	facial expression cry breathing patterns arms legs state of arousal	each scored on 2 (0,1) or 3-point (0,1,2) scale; total score: 0-7	preterm and term neonates; procedural pain
Neonatal Facial Coding Scale (NFCS) (Grunau & Craig 1987; Johnston et al 1993)	brow bulge deep nasolabial fold eyes squeezed shut open mouth taut tongue horizontal mouth stretch vertical mouth stretch pursing of lips chin quiver tongue protrusion	presence or absence of action during discrete time intervals scored	preterm to 4 months; procedural pain
CRIES (Krechel & Bildner 1995)	cries requires oxygen increased vital signs (heart rate/blood pressure) expression sleeplessness	each scored 3-point scale (0,1,2); total score: 0–10	32–60 weeks postoperative pain

Source: Adapted from Finley & McGrath (1998), Franck et al (2000), Stevens et al (2000), Gaffney et al (2003) and Howard (2003b). Further examples and details are available in these reviews.

Table 10.2 Composite scales for infants and children

Scale	Indicators	Score	Utility
Children's Hospital of Eastern Ontario Pain Scale (CHEOPS) (McGrath et al 1985)	cry facial expression verbal expression torso position touch leg position	each scored as 0, 1, 2 or 3; total 4–18	1–7 years postoperative pain procedural pain
FLACC (Merkel et al 1997)	face legs activity cry consolability	each scored on 3 point scale (0,1,2); total 0–10	young children postoperative pain
COMFORT scale (Ambuel et al 1992)	alertness calmness/agitation respiratory response physical movement muscle tone facial expression mean arterial pressure heart rate	score 8–40	newborn to adolescent distress in PICU; postoperative pain 0–3 year olds (Van Dijk et al 2000)

Source: Adapted from Finley & McGrath (1998), Franck et al (2000), Stevens et al (2000), Gaffney et al (2003) and Howard (2003b). Further examples and details are available in these reviews.

Table 10.3 Self-report tools for children

Scale	Components	Anchors	Utility
Poker Chip Tool (Hester 1979)	4 chips = pieces of 'hurt'	± white 'no pain' chip; 1 chip = 'a little hurt'; 4 chips = 'most hurt you could ever have'	4–8 years
Faces Pain Scale - Revised (Hicks et al 2001)	6 faces		> 4 years
Wong-Baker Faces Pain Rating Scale (Wong & Baker 1988)	6 cartoon faces	faces graded from smiling to tears	3–8 years postoperative and procedural pain
Coloured Analogue Scale (McGrath et al 1996)	modification of 10 cm horizontal VAS; scored 0–10 in 0.25 increments	gradations in colour (white to dark red) and area (progressively wider tetragon); labels 'no pain' to 'most pain'	5 years and above

Source: Adapted from Finley & McGrath (1998), Franck et al (2000), Stevens et al (2000), Gaffney et al (2003) and Howard (2003b). Further examples and details are available in these reviews.

10.1.4 Management of procedural pain

Procedure-related pain is a frequent and distressing component of medical care for children (Cummings et al 1996, **Level IV**; Ljungmanet al 1996, **Level IV**). Repeated interventions are often required (eg bone marrow aspirates and lumbar punctures for cancer treatment) and the level of pain and memory of the first procedure affect the pain (Weisman et al 1998) and distress (Chen et al 2000) associated with subsequent procedures.

The aim of procedural pain management is to minimise physical discomfort or pain, movement and psychological disturbance without compromising patient safety. Management can include analgesic agents via different routes of administration, concurrent sedation or general anaesthesia, and non-pharmacological methods. The choice of technique will depend on the age and previous experience of the child, the type of procedure, the expected intensity and duration of pain, the treatment environment and available resources (Murat et al 2003). Sedation alone must not be seen as an alternative to appropriate analgesia.

Types of procedures

The level of pain and/or discomfort associated with different procedures affects choice of treatment. For *minor* procedures (eg venipuncture, intravenous [IV] cannulation, minor laceration repair), inhalation of nitrous oxide (50%) and/or topical local anaesthetic application have established efficacy and safety (Murat et al 2003, **Level I**).

Common *moderate* severity procedures include lumbar puncture and bone marrow aspiration. The combination of nitrous oxide with local anaesthetic agents (both topically and infiltrated) is effective in the majority of children and has a wide safety margin (Murat et al 2003, **Level I**). Combinations of hypnotic and analgesic agents are also effective but are associated with a relatively high incidence of side effects, and there are few randomised trials to evaluate comparative efficacy (Murat et al 2003).

Closed fracture reduction is a *major* procedure which may be performed with a number of analgesic techniques in emergency departments (Kennedy et al 2004). IV regional block with local anaesthetic is safe and effective in 90–98% of cases (Murat et al 2003), but complications may arise with faulty equipment, inappropriate use of local anaesthetic, or inadequate monitoring and training of staff. Inhalation of nitrous oxide was as effective as IV regional anaesthesia using lignocaine (lidocaine) (Gregory et al 1996, **Level III-1**) and better than intramuscular (IM) analgesia and sedation with pethidine and promethazine (Evans et al 1995, **Level III-1**). IV ketamine plus midazolam was more effective than IV fentanyl plus midazolam (Kennedy et al 1998, **Level II**). As there is a potential for complications and a high incidence of side effects, general anaesthesia may be more appropriate than sedation or local anaesthesia in some clinical settings (Murat et al 2003).

Pharmacological management

Topical local anaesthetics

The topical preparations EMLA® cream and amethocaine (tetracaine) 4% gel or cream have comparable efficacy for procedural pain relief in children, but EMLA® requires a longer application time (60 vs 30 mins) (Murat et al 2003, **Level I**). In neonates, EMLA® reduces the behavioural pain response to venipuncture but not heel lance; single doses have not been associated with methaemoglobinaemia (Taddio et al 1998, **Level I**). Although EMLA® reduces the behavioural response to circumcision in neonates, more effective analgesic interventions are recommended (Brady-Fryer et al 2004, **Level I**).

Nitrous oxide

Nitrous oxide can be delivered in a variable concentration of 30–70% by a continuous flow device or as premixed 50:50 oxygen to nitrous oxide (Section 4.3.1). Delivery systems that do not require a tight mask seal and activation of a demand valve may be more acceptable to young children.

For a variety of minor procedures, nitrous oxide alone or in combination with local anaesthesia (in 63%) or oral premedication (in 17.9%) was effective in 88% of children: behavioural responses, including crying, were more common during the procedures in children under 3 years of age, but may in part relate to intolerance of the face mask (Annequin et al 2000, **Level IV**). Nitrous oxide is as effective or superior to topical local anaesthesia for IV cannulation (Murat et al 2003, **Level I**) but the combination may be better than either alone (Hee et al 2003, **Level III-1**).

Minor transient side effects are common (37%) but major adverse events are rare (0.3%) and resolve within minutes of discontinuation (Gall et al 2001, **Level IV**). See Section 4.3.1 for possible complications of nitrous oxide, including neuropathy.

Opioids

Opioids can be titrated to effective analgesic levels and delivered by a number of routes. Lipid soluble opioids such as fentanyl, alfentanil and remifentanil may be preferable for brief procedures because of a more rapid onset and offset. The incidence of side effects is high with IV or oral transmucosal fentanyl (Murat et al 2003) and remifentanil can be associated with significant respiratory depression (Litman 1999, **Level IV**). Intranasal preparations have a rapid onset, are effective for emergency room procedures (Borl et al 2002, **Level IV**) and may be more acceptable to children than IM injection, but comparative trials are required.

Ketamine

Ketamine is an analgesic and sedative agent and low doses are safe and effective for procedural pain (Green et al 1999, **Level IV**; Murat et al 2003, **Level I**). Adverse effects such as unpleasant hallucinations, salivation and hypertension are uncommon with low doses (Marx et al 1997, **Level II**) and side effects may be less with ketamine than opioid-based techniques (Murat et al 2003, **Level I**). Unintentional deep sedation and complications can occur with large or repeated doses (Murat et al 2003).

Midazolam

Midazolam is a short-acting benzodiazepine that produces sedation, amnesia and anxiolysis, and therefore may be used in conjunction with analgesics for the management of procedure-associated distress. Combinations of midazolam with opioids, ketamine and nitrous oxide (Litman et al 1996, **Level III-3**; Parker et al 1997, **Level IV**; Kennedy et al 1998, **Level II**; Litman 1999, **Level IV**) are reported to be effective, but excessive sedation and side effects may occur (Murat et al 2003). Progression to deep sedation occurs with midazolam and the higher concentrations of nitrous oxide (Litman et al 1996, **Level III-3**) and is associated with partial airway obstruction in children with enlarged tonsils (Litman et al 1998, **Level III-2**). Addition of midazolam to ketamine reduced the incidence of vomiting but increased episodes of oxygen desaturation (Wathen et al 2000, **Level II**).

Adverse events

Combinations of analgesic and sedative agents are effective for procedural pain management, but are associated with a relatively high incidence of side effects (Murat et al 2003). No single drug or route of administration is clearly associated with greater risk, but the use of combinations of drugs (particularly when three or more drugs are given) increases negative outcomes (Cote et al 2000a, **Level IV**). Inadequate resuscitation and monitoring are associated with major adverse outcomes, and inadequate presedation medical evaluation, lack of an independent observer, medication errors, and inadequate recovery procedures are contributory factors (Cote et al 2000b). Adherence to guidelines and regular assessment of sedation score in order to avoid inadvertent deep sedation reduce the risk of adverse events (Hoffman et al 2002, **Level III-3**).

Non-pharmacological management

Oral sucrose decreases the physiological and behavioural responses to heel stick and venipuncture in term and preterm neonates (Stevens et al 2004, **Level I**). However, the optimal dose, efficacy and safety of repeated doses, and comparison with pharmacologic interventions have not been determined.

Non-pharmacological techniques, good psychological preparation and carer education and involvement may obviate or reduce the need for drug sedation, but interventions need to be matched to the specific characteristics of the child (Kuppenheimer & Brown 2002, **Level IV**). Cognitive-behavioural techniques (such as imagery, slow-breathing and relaxation) and hypnosis (see Section 8.1) improve coping and reduce distress (Chen et al 2000, **Level IV**; Murat et al 2003, **Level I**; Powers 1999, **Level IV**). Combinations of pharmacological and psychological interventions may be more effective for reducing distress than psychological strategies alone (Kazak et al 1998, **Level II**).

Key messages

1. Sucrose reduces the behavioural response to heel stick in neonates (**Level I** [Cochrane Review]).
2. Topical local anaesthetic application, inhalation of nitrous oxide (50%) or the combination of both provides effective and safe analgesia for minor procedures (**Level I**).
3. Psychological interventions (cognitive-behavioural techniques, hypnosis) reduce procedure-related distress (**Level II**).
4. A combination of pharmacological and psychological interventions reduces pain and distress (**Level II**).
5. Combinations of hypnotic and analgesic agents are effective for procedures of moderate and major severity (**Level II**).

The following tick box ☑ represents conclusions based on clinical experience and expert opinion.

☑ Inadequate monitoring of the child, lack of adequate resuscitation skills and equipment, and use of multiple drug combinations (particularly three or more) have been associated with major adverse outcomes.

10.1.5 Analgesic agents

Non-steroidal anti-inflammatory drugs

Non-steroidal anti-inflammatory drugs (NSAIDs) are effective analgesic agents for mild to moderate pain. Ibuprofen, diclofenac and ketorolac are effective in children and the choice mainly depends on the available formulation and convenience of administration. Clinical studies suggest similar efficacy of NSAIDs and paracetamol (Rømsing et al 2000, **Level II**; Tay & Tan 2002, **Level II**; Koki 2003, **Level III-2**), but assume that equi-effective doses are being given (Anderson 2004). Combining an NSAID and paracetamol has been shown to improve early (Pickering et al 2002, **Level II**) and late (Viitanen et al 2003, **Level II**) analgesia after tonsillectomy. As a component of multimodal analgesia, NSAIDs decrease opioid consumption (Morton & O'Brien 1999, **Level III-1**; Pickering et al 2002, **Level II**; Viitanen et al 2003, **Level II**) and improve the quality of analgesia (Morton & O'Brien 1999, **Level III-1**).

The elimination half-life for ketorolac (Dsida et al 2002), ibuprofen and diclofenac (Litalien et al 2001) are similar in children and adults. Rectal bioavailability of diclofenac is high in children (van der Marel et al 2004) but target concentrations required for analgesia and developmental changes in pharmacodynamics have not yet been determined (Anderson 2004).

Adverse effects

In large series of children with febrile illnesses, the risk of serious adverse events following short-term use of ibuprofen was low, and similar to that following the use of paracetamol (Lesko & Mitchell 1995, **Level II**; Lesko & Mitchell 1999, **Level II**). Aspirin should be avoided in children with a febrile illness, as it has been associated with Reye's syndrome (encephalopathy and liver dysfunction) (Kokki 2003).

NSAIDs should be avoided in children with a sensitivity reaction to aspirin or other NSAIDs. NSAIDs may be safe in children with mild asthma (Kokki 2003, **Level IV**) as single dose diclofenac had no significant effect on respiratory function tests (spirometry) in children with asthma (Short et al 2000, **Level III-3**) and short-term use of ibuprofen did not increase outpatient visits for asthma (Lesko et al 2002, **Level II**).

The use of NSAIDs in children undergoing tonsillectomy remains controversial. Three meta-analyses included different trials, defined the primary outcome in different ways, used different methodology, and reported different results and recommendations.

The risk of post-tonsillectomy haemorrhage with aspirin was significantly higher than in the ibuprofen and diclofenac group (Krishna et al 2003, **Level I**) and it was concluded that these NSAIDS but not aspirin were safe. Although the rate of postoperative bleeding was not significantly increased (Møiniche et al 2003) the risk of reoperation for post-tonsillectomy bleeding (number-needed-to-harm [NNH] 29–60) was increased by NSAIDs (Marret et al 2003, **Level I**; Møiniche et al 2003, **Level I**) and it was concluded that NSAIDs should be used cautiously until further evidence is available (Møiniche et al 2003) (see also Sections 4.2.2 and 9.6.7).

NSAID use has been restricted in infants less than 6 months of age due to an increased risk of pulmonary hypertension and alterations in cerebral and renal blood flow following bolus doses (Morris et al 2003).

At present, there is little clinical experience with COX-2-specific inhibitors in children.

Paracetamol

Paracetamol is effective for mild pain in children and is a useful adjunct to other treatments for more severe pain. Paracetamol has similar analgesic efficacy to NSAIDs (see above). The dose required for analgesia is greater than for an anti-pyretic effect (Anderson 2004). Supplemental opioid requirements were reduced after day case surgery by 40mg/kg but not 20mg/kg rectal paracetamol (Korpela et al 1999, **Level II**) and after tonsillectomy by 40mg/kg oral paracetamol (Anderson et al 1996, **Level II**).

Pharmacokinetics

Paracetamol's bioavailability is dependent on the route of administration. Oral doses are subject to first pass hepatic metabolism of 10–40% and peak plasma concentrations are reached in 30 minutes (Arana et al 2001). Rectal administration is associated with slower and more erratic absorption and bioavailability varies from 50–98% (Anderson et al 1996; Coulthard et al 1998; Hansen et al 1999; Anderson et al 2002). Rectal loading doses of 30–40mg/kg paracetamol may be required to achieve therapeutic plasma concentrations (Birmingham et al 1997, **Level II**; Howell & Patel 2003, **Level II**).

Dose regimens that target a steady state plasma concentration of 10–20mg/L have been determined. There is some evidence for analgesic efficacy at this concentration in children (Anderson 1999, **Level III-3**) but a relationship between plasma concentration and analgesia has not been confirmed in infants (van Lingen et al 1999). The volume of distribution of paracetamol decreases and clearance increases from 28 weeks postconceptional age resulting in a gradual fall in elimination half-life. Suggested maximum doses are: 25mg/kg/day at 30 weeks postconceptional age; 45mg/kg/day at 34 weeks postconceptional age; 60mg/kg/day in term neonates and infants; and 90mg/kg/day in children aged between 6 months and 12 years. These doses are suitable for acute administration for 2–3 days (Anderson et al 2002).

Adverse effects

Paracetamol is metabolised in the liver, predominantly via glucuronidation and sulphation. Increased production of a reactive oxidative product N-acetyl-p-benzoquinoneimine occurs if the usual metabolic enzyme systems become saturated (eg acute overdose) or if glutathione is depleted (eg with prolonged fasting). An increased contribution of sulphation to metabolism and reduced production of oxidative metabolites may reduce the risk of toxicity in neonates (van der Marel 2003), but as overall clearance is reduced a lower dose is appropriate. Risk factors for paracetamol hepatotoxicity may include fasting, vomiting, dehydration, systemic sepsis, pre-existing liver disease and prior paracetamol intake, however the situation remains unclear (Kaplowitz 2004).

Opioids and tramadol

As there are significant developmental changes in the pharmacokinetic handling (Kart et al 1997a) and pharmacodynamic response to opioids, doses must be adjusted according to age and individual response. The clearance of morphine is reduced and half-life prolonged in neonates and infants (Kart et al 1997a). Within age groups, individual variability in kinetics results in 2–3 fold differences in plasma concentration with the same rate of infusion (Lynn et al 1998). In neonates, infants and children up to 3 years, age was the most important factor affecting morphine requirements and plasma morphine concentrations (Bouwmeester et al 2003, **Level II**), and in older children average patient-controlled morphine requirements also changed with age (Hansen et al 1996, **Level IV**).

The risk of respiratory depression is reduced when infusions are targeted to plasma morphine concentrations less than 20ng/mL. However, no minimum effective concentration for analgesia has been determined (Kart et al 1997b). A wide range of concentrations has been associated with analgesia due to variability in individual requirements, the clinical state of the child, the type of surgery, the assessment measure used and the small sample size in many studies (Tyler et al 1996, **Level IV**; Olkkola & Hamunen 2000). Routine and regular assessment of pain severity, the analgesic response to opioids and the incidence of side effects (particularly nausea and vomiting and sedation) is essential so that treatment can be adjusted according to individual needs. As with adult patients, appropriate dose regimens, guidelines for monitoring, documentation, management of side effects, and education of staff and carers are required (see Section 7.1)(Morton 1993, **Level IV**).

Codeine is a weak opioid and conversion to morphine (by CYP2D6) is required for analgesia. Intermediate or poor metabolisers (46% of children undergoing tonsillectomy in a UK population) may have reduced or minimal effect from codeine. In addition, the activity of the enzyme is low in neonates. Perceived advantages of codeine include less respiratory depression in neonates and reduced nausea and vomiting compared with morphine (Semple et al 1999, **Level II**; Williams et al 2002, **Level II**), but may relate to low levels of active metabolites and be associated with reduced efficacy.

Codeine is effective orally. It has a similar time to peak effect but decreased total absorption compared with rectal and IM delivery (McEwen et al 2000, **Level II**). IV administration should be avoided as severe hypotension may result (Shanahan et al 1983, **Level IV**).

There are conflicting reports of efficacy for postoperative pain. Addition of codeine to paracetamol has been reported to improve analgesia (Tobias et al 1995, **Level II**; Pappas et al 2003, **Level II**) or have no effect following myringotomy (Ragg & Davidson 1997, **Level II**). No difference in post-tonsillectomy analgesia was detected between paracetamol alone or combined with codeine (Moir et al 2000, **Level II**). Comparison of codeine and morphine for tonsillectomy has shown both no difference (Semple et al 1999, **Level II**), and an increased requirement for rescue analgesia following codeine (Williams et al 2002, **Level II**).

Evidence for the use of tramadol in paediatric acute pain is currently limited by studies of small sample size and difficulty determining comparative analgesic doses. Oral, rectal and IV preparations have been utilised (Finkel et al 2002; Engelhardt et al 2003; Zwaveling et al 2004). Tramadol reduced supplemental analgesic requirement when added to rectal ibuprofen (Viitanen & Annila 2001, **Level II**). Tramadol was more effective for control of post-tonsillectomy pain compared with low dose paracetamol (Pendeville et al 2000, **Level II**). Following cessation of PCA, oral tramadol 2mg/kg was more effective than 1mg/kg (Finkel et al 2002, **Level III-3**). Tramadol 1mg/kg was less effective than pethidine following tonsillectomy (Ozer et al 2003, **Level II**) but in another tonsillectomy study no difference between morphine and 1 or 2mg/kg tramadol could be detected (Engelhardt et al 2003, **Level II**). Further controlled trials are required to determine the role and optimum dose of tramadol in children.

Key messages

1. Aspirin and NSAIDs increase the risk of reoperation for post-tonsillectomy bleeding (**Level I**).
2. Paracetamol and NSAIDs are effective for moderately severe pain and decrease opioid requirements after major surgery (**Level II**).
3. The efficacy of oral codeine in children is variable, particularly in individuals with a reduced ability to generate active metabolites (**Level II**).

The following tick boxes ☑ represent conclusions based on clinical experience and expert opinion.

☑ Safe dosing of paracetamol requires consideration of the age and body weight of the child, and the duration of therapy.

☑ Aspirin should be avoided in children, but serious adverse events after NSAIDs are rare in children over 6 months of age. Evidence for safety of NSAIDs following tonsillectomy is inconclusive.

10.1.6 Opioid infusions and PCA

Opioid infusions

The safety and efficacy of IV opioid infusion for the management of acute pain is well established for children of all ages (Beasley & Tibballs 1987, **Level IV**; Esmail et al 1999, **Level IV**). An IV infusion of morphine provides superior analgesia compared with intermittent IM injections of opioids (Bray 1983, **Level III-1**). This may relate to a lower total dose of morphine in the IM group (Hendrickson et al 1990, **Level III-2**), but as intermittent IM injections are distressing for children, the IV route is preferred. If peripheral perfusion is normal, the subcutaneous route can be used for continuous infusion (McNicol 1993, **Level IV**) or for PCA, with similar safety and efficacy to the IV route (Doyle et al 1994a, **Level II**).

Differences between intermittent bolus doses and continuous infusions of opioid relate more to the total dose given than to the method of administration. Comparison of age-adjusted infusions targeted to 20ng/mL plasma morphine versus intermittent boluses (50 micrograms/kg every 1–2 hours) found improved pain scores in the infusion group, but this group also received significantly higher total doses of morphine (Lynn et al 2000, **Level III-2**). Comparison of the same total dose of morphine given via infusion (10 micrograms/kg/hr) or bolus (30 micrograms/kg every 3 hours) found no difference in pain scores (COMFORT scale and observer visual analogue scale) (van Dijk et al 2002, **Level II**) or stress response to surgery (Bouwmeester et al 2001, **Level II**) in neonates and young infants. However, these doses were inadequate in older children (1–3 years of age) who required additional bolus doses and the 3-hourly interval was less effective (possibly due to more rapid clearance) (van Dijk et al 2002, **Level II**). Similar levels of analgesia were achieved with intermittent boluses of morphine via the epidural or IV route; side effects were common and individual dose adjustments were required in all groups, but a lower total dose and less frequent dosing was required in the epidural group (Haberken et al 1996, **Level III-2**).

Initial infusion rates based on pharmacokinetic parameters and doses that minimise respiratory effects have been suggested (Kart 1997b; Lynn et al 1998). These include: neonates 10 micrograms/kg/hr; infants 1–3 months 20 micrograms/kg/hr; infants 3–6 months 25 micrograms/kg/hr (Lynn et al 1998). As clearance is reduced after cardiac surgery, lower doses should be used (Lynn et al 1993).

In older children, initial infusion rates often range from 20-40 micrograms/kg/hr. Early postoperative analgesia was most often associated with infusion rates of >20 micrograms/kg/hr (Esmail et al 1999, **Level IV**) and PCA use in children averaged 40 micrograms/kg/hr (Gaukroger et al 1989, **Level IV**). These doses are suggested initial rates only, and must be titrated against the individual's response in terms of efficacy and side effects.

PCA

PCA can provide safe and effective analgesia for children as young as 5 years old (Gaukroger et al 1991, **Level IV**). Patient selection depends on the ability of the child and carers to understand the concepts of PCA and the availability of suitable equipment and trained staff.

Efficacy

Compared with continuous infusions or IM administration of opioids, PCA provides greater dosing flexibility and can be more effective for managing incident pain (Berde et al 1991, **Level III-1**; Bray et al 1996a, **Level II**). Compared with intermittent IM administration, PCA was associated with lower pain scores, improved satisfaction and less sedation (Berde et al 1991, **Level III-1**). Compared with IV infusion, similar analgesia, increased opioid consumption and increased side effects have been reported with PCA (Bray 1996a, **Level II**; Bray 1996b, **Level II**) but results vary depending on the PCA parameters and the degree of titration of continuous infusions. Comparison of continuous infusion 20–40 microgram/kg/hr and PCA with a high background infusion (bolus 15 microgram/kg and background 15 microgram/kg/hr) found higher opioid consumption in the PCA group but no difference in pain scores or side effects (Peters et al 1999, **Level II**).

The PCA prescription

Morphine is the drug used most frequently in PCA. Fentanyl is a useful alternative, particularly for patients with renal impairment or those experiencing morphine-related side effects (Tobias & Baker 1992, **Level IV**). Pethidine does not have any advantage over other opioids and neurotoxicity from norpethidine accumulation has been reported in a healthy adolescent (Kussman & Sethna 1998, **Level IV**).

A bolus dose of morphine 20 microgram/kg is a suitable starting dose and is associated with improved pain scores during movement compared with 10 microgram/kg (Doyle 1994b, **Level II**).

The addition of a background infusion is more common in children than adults and efficacy and side effects vary with the dose. The addition of a background infusion of 20 microgram/kg/hr to a bolus dose of 20 microgram/kg increased opioid consumption, nausea, sedation and hypoxaemia when compared with bolus only PCA (Doyle et al 1993a, **Level II**). A night time background infusion of 15 microgram/kg/hr added to a bolus of 25 microgram/kg with a 10-minute lock-out was associated with increased hypoxaemia and no additional benefit (McNeely & Trentadue 1997, **Level III-2**). Comparison of 10 microgram/kg/hr and 4 microgram/kg/hr background infusions found hypoxaemia and nausea and vomiting were increased with the higher dose, whereas the lower dose improved the sleep pattern compared with a no-background group without increasing side effects (Doyle et al 1993b, **Level II**).

Nausea and vomiting occurs in 30–45% of children using morphine PCA and can be reduced by prophylactic antiemetics (Doyle 1994c, **Level II**; Kokinsky et al 1999, **Level II**; Allen et al 1999, **Level II**).

Adding anti-emetics directly to PCA solutions for children has not been shown to be useful (Habre et al 1999, **Level IV**; Munro et al 2002, **Level II**).

Nurse-controlled analgesia

In younger children and infants, PCA pumps have been used to allow administration of a background infusion and intermittent bolus doses by nurses (ie nurse-controlled analgesia). This technique increases ease of administration particularly prior to movement or procedural interventions, increases dose flexibility, and increases parent and nurse satisfaction (Lloyd-Thomas & Howard 1994, **Level IV**). Effective analgesia was achieved in 81–95% of patients; 25% required supplemental oxygen, and 4% required naloxone for respiratory depression (Monitto et al 2000, **Level IV**). In this series, dosing by parents and nurses was allowed, although the parameters for giving a bolus and the differentiation of the parent and nurse roles are unclear. Administration by a nurse trained in pain assessment, rather than parents, is recommended in most centres (Howard 2003a, **Level IV**). Nurse-controlled analgesia has also been used in older children in intensive care who are unable to activate a conventional PCA device. Adequate analgesia comparable to PCA was reported, but efficacy is dependent on accurate nurse assessment of pain (Weldon et al 1993, **Level III-2**).

Key messages

1. Effective PCA prescription in children incorporates a bolus that is adequate for control of movement-related pain, and may include a low dose background infusion to improve efficacy and sleep (**Level II**).
2. Intermittent intramuscular injections are distressing for children and are less effective for pain control than intravenous infusions (**Level III-1**).

The following tick boxes ☑ represent conclusions based on clinical experience and expert opinion.

☑ Intravenous opioids can be used safely and effectively in children of all ages.

☑ Initial doses of opioid should be based on the age and weight of the child and then titrated against the individual's response.

10.1.7 Regional analgesia

Peripheral nerve blocks

Peripheral local anaesthetic techniques are an effective and safe adjunct for the management of procedural, perioperative, and injury-related acute pain (Giaufre et al 1996, **Level IV;** Brown et al 1999, **Level IV**) (see also Section 10.1.3). As placebos are rarely used in children, many current studies compare two active treatments and differences between groups can be difficult to detect if the sample size is small or the outcome measure is relatively insensitive (eg supplemental analgesic requirements following procedures with low ongoing pain).

The efficacy of different local anaesthetic techniques has been compared for common paediatric surgical conditions.

Circumcision

A dorsal penile nerve block provides similar analgesia to caudal block (Gauntlett 2003, **Level II**) and is more effective than application of topical local anaesthetic cream (EMLA®)(Choi et al 2003, **Level II**). Subcutaneous ring block of the penis is less effective than dorsal penile nerve block (Holder et al 1997, **Level II**) and has a higher failure rate than caudal analgesia, but potentially fewer complications (Yeoman et al 1983, **Level III-2**; Irwin & Chen 1996, **Level II**). There are insufficient controlled trials to adequately rank the efficacy of all local anaesthetic techniques for circumcision (Cyna et al 2003, **Level I**) but as topical local anaesthetic cream only partially attenuates the pain response to circumcision in awake neonates, more effective analgesic techniques such as dorsal penile nerve block are recommended (Brady-Fryer et al 2004, **Level I**). A recent policy statement (RACP 2002) emphasises the need for adequate analgesia for infant circumcision.

Inguinal hernia repair

Similar levels of efficacy for reducing pain following inguinal hernia repair have been found following wound infiltration, ilioinguinal / iliohypogastric nerve block or caudal analgesia (Reid et al 1987, **Level III-2**; Fell et al 1988, **Level III-1**; Casey et al 1990, **Level II**; Splinter et al 1995, **Level II**; Machotta et al 2003, **Level II**).

Tonsillectomy

Although the number of suitably designed studies is limited, local anaesthetic applied to the tonsillar bed does not reduce pain following tonsillectomy (Hollis et al 1999, **Level I**). The effect of dexamethasone on pain following tonsillectomy could not be assessed from current studies, but a reduction in vomiting and earlier return to diet was confirmed (Steward et al 2003, **Level I**).

Plexus blocks

Femoral nerve or fascia iliaca compartment blocks provide analgesia for surgery on the anterior aspect of the thigh and reduce pain associated with femoral fractures (Paut et al 2001, **Level IV**). Axillary brachial plexus blocks provide satisfactory analgesia for hand and forearm surgery in 75–94% of cases (Fisher et al 1999, **Level IV**; Tobias 2001, **Level IV**). Descriptive studies of the efficacy and safety of continuous peripheral nerve block infusions in children are encouraging (Johnson 1994, **Level IV**; Semsroth et al 1996, **Level IV**; Paut et al 2001, **Level IV**; Sciard et al 2001; Dadure et al 2003, **Level III-3**) but controlled comparisons with other analgesic techniques are required.

Central neural blockade

The use of regional analgesia in children is well established but patient selection, technique, choice of drugs, availability of experienced staff for performing blocks, acute pain service resources and adequacy of follow-up vary between different centres (Williams & Howard 2003). This is compounded by limited evidence to guide clinical decision-making.

Caudal epidural analgesia

Single-shot caudal analgesia is one of the most widely used regional techniques in children. Injection of local anaesthetic through the sacrococcygeal ligament into the caudal epidural space provides intra and postoperative analgesia for surgery on the lower abdomen, perineum and lower limbs (Howard 2003b). Large series have reported a high success rate (particularly in children under 7 years), and a low incidence of serious complications (Dalens & Hasnaoui 1989, **Level IV**; Veyckemans et al 1992, **Level IV**). The duration of postoperative analgesia after caudal local anaesthetic varies with the type of procedure, timing of administration, and the concentration and volume of local anaesthetic used.

Following circumcision, the need for rescue analgesia and the incidence of nausea and vomiting were lower with caudal analgesia compared with parenteral analgesia (Cyna et al 2003, **Level I**). Ilioinguinal nerve block and caudal local anaesthetic were equally effective for day-case herniotomy and orchidopexy (Cross & Barrett 1987, **Level III-2**; Fisher et al 1993, **Level II**; Splinter et al 1995, **Level II**) but caudal analgesia was more effective when a combination of ketamine and local anaesthetic was used following orchidopexy (Findlow et al 1997, **Level II**).

Bupivacaine, ropivacaine and levobupivacaine (see Section 5.1) have all been successfully used for paediatric caudal analgesia (de Beer & Thomas 2003). Addition of adrenaline (epinephrine) to bupivacaine has minimal effect on the duration of analgesia, particularly in older children (Ansermino et al 2003, **Level II**). Opioid and non-opioid adjuvants have been added to caudal local anaesthetic with the aim of improving the efficacy or duration of analgesia.

Addition of morphine to caudal local anaesthetic prolongs analgesia (Wolf et al 1991, **Level II**) and decreases supplemental analgesic requirements (Wolf et al 1990, **Level II**). However, dose-related side effects are relatively common (nausea and vomiting 34–42%, pruritus 9%, and urinary retention 12.5%) (Krane et al 1989, **Level III-1**; de Beer & Thomas 2003). As clinically significant respiratory depression has been reported, particularly with higher doses and in younger patients (Krane et al 1989, **Level III-1;** Valley & Bailey 1991, **Level IV**; Bozkurt et al 1997, **Level IV**), clinical utility is limited (de Beer & Thomas 2003). Side effects are potentially less with lipid soluble opioids, but while fentanyl may prolong caudal analgesia (Constant et al 1998, **Level II**), other studies have shown no benefit (Jones et al 1990, **Level II;** Campbell et al 1992, **Level II**).

Addition of clonidine (1–2 microgram/kg) to caudal local anaesthetic prolongs analgesia (Ansermino et al 2003, **Level I**). Effects on analgesic efficacy could not be assessed by meta-analysis due to variablility in study design and outcome measures. Clinically important sedation occurs with higher doses (5 microgram/kg) (Ansermino et al 2003, **Level I**).

Preservative free ketamine 0.25–0.5mg/kg prolongs analgesia without increasing side effects, but higher doses (1mg/kg) increase behavioural side effects (Ansermino et al 2003, **Level I**).

Epidural analgesia

As the epidural space is relatively large with loosely packed fat in neonates, catheters can be threaded from the sacral hiatus to lumbar and thoracic levels (Bosenberg et al 1988, **Level IV**; Hogan 1996). In older infants, various techniques have been suggested to improve correct placement including ultrasound, nerve stimulation and ECG guidance (Tsui 2002, **Level IV**; Tsui et al 2004, **Level IV**). Insertion of epidural catheters at the segmental level required for surgery is more reliable in older children, and has been shown to be safe in experienced hands with appropriate size equipment (Dalens et al 1986, **Level IV;** Eccoffey 1986, **Level IV**).

Continuous infusion (Murrell 1993, **Level IV**) or intermittent boluses (Bosenberg 1998, **Level IV**) of local anaesthetic provide satisfactory analgesia. In children 7–12 years of age, patient-controlled epidural analgesia (PCEA) provided similar analgesia to continuous infusion. Total local anaesthetic dose was reduced with PCEA but was of limited clinical significance as no difference in side effects could be detected (Antok et al 2003, **Level III-1**).

The loss of resistance to air technique has been implicated in causing venous air embolism in children, with 2.5–3.0 mL of air being enough to cause cardiovascular collapse (Guinard & Borboen 1993, **Level IV**; Shwartz & Eisenkraft 1993, **Level IV**). Saline may be a safer alternative but if air is to be used, the volume should be limited to a maximum of 1.0mL (Sethna & Berde 1993, **Level IV**). Epidural blockade has minimal haemodynamic effect in children, consistent with reduced reliance on sympathetic tone (Murat et al 1987, **Level IV**).

Continuous epidural infusions of bupivacaine (0.4mg/kg/hr) are safe and effective in children (Howard 2003b) and can provide similar levels of analgesia as systemic opioids (Wolf et al 1993, **Level II**). Due to reduced clearance and the potential for accumulation of bupivacaine, the hourly dose should be reduced (0.2mg/kg/hr) and the duration of therapy limited to 24–48 hours in neonates (Larsson et al 1997). Ropivacaine (Cucchiaro et al 2003) and levobupivacaine (Lerman et al 2003) have also been utilised in paediatric epidural infusions.

Epidural opioids alone have a limited role. Epidural morphine provides prolonged analgesia but no improvement in the quality of analgesia compared with systemic opioids (Haberkern et al 1996, **Level II**; Bozkurt 2002, **Level II**). Epidural fentanyl alone was less effective than both levobupivacaine alone and a combination of local anaesthetic and fentanyl (Lerman et al 2003, **Level II**).

A combination of local anaesthetic and opioid is frequently used in epidural infusions, but there is little controlled data to assess the relative merits of different regimens. Both improvements in analgesia (Lovstad & Stoen 2001, **Level II**) and no change (Carr et al 1998, **Level II**; Lerman et al 2003, **Level II**) have been shown with addition of fentanyl to local anaesthetic infusions. Similar analgesia has been shown with epidural fentanyl or morphine added to local anaesthetic (Lejus et al 1994, **Level II**; Reinoso-Barbero et al 2002, **Level II**) and a reduction in side effects with fentanyl was shown in one study (Lejus et al 1994, **Level II**).

Addition of clonidine (0.08–0.12 microgram/kg/hr) to epidural local anaesthetic infusions improves analgesia (De Negri et al 2001, **Level II**) but a lower dose was less effective than the addition of 10 microgram/mL morphine (Cucchiaro et al 2003, **Level II**).

Outcomes

Perioperative epidural analgesia modifies the stress response to surgery in children (Murat et al 1988, **Level II**; Wolf et al 1993, **Level II**; Wolf et al 1998, **Level II**). Suppression of the stress response may necessitate a local anaesthetic block that is more intense or extensive than required for analgesia; the risks of increased side effects or toxicity must be balanced against any potential benefit (Wolf et al 1998, **Level II**).

Improvements in respiratory outcome with regional analgesia have not been established in controlled comparative trials. Reductions in respiratory rate and oxygen saturation were less marked during epidural analgesia compared with systemic opioids, but the degree of difference was of limited clinical significance (Wolf & Hughes 1993, **Level II**). Case series report improvements in respiratory function and/or a reduced need for mechanical ventilation with regional analgesia techniques (Murrell et al 1993, **Level IV**; McNeely et al 1997a, **Level IV**; Bosenberg & Ivani 1998, **Level IV**; Hodgson et al 2000, **Level IV**). A meta-analysis of spinal versus general anaesthesia for inguinal herniorrhaphy in premature infants reported a reduction in postoperative apnoea in the spinal group (when infants having preoperative sedation were excluded) and a reduced need for postoperative ventilation (of borderline statistical significance) (Craven et al 2003, **Level I**).

Complications

Accidental intravascular injection remains the most life-threatening complication of caudal and epidural analgesia. As the sacrum is largely cartilaginous during infancy and early childhood, there is an increased risk of injecting local anaesthetic into the highly vascular medullary space of the sacrum (Veyckemans et al 1992, **Level IV**). No method of detection or prevention is infallible in anaesthetised children. High concentrations of volatile agents, especially halothane, may mask the effects of a test dose containing adrenaline (epinephrine), however pretreatment with atropine 10 microgram/kg may increase the detection rate (Desparmet et al 1990, **Level II**). Sevoflurane attenuates cardiovascular responses to adrenaline (epinephrine) 0.5 microgram/kg less than halothane and may be a better agent to facilitate detection (Kozek-Langenbecker et al 2000, **Level II**). Incremental slow injection, while monitoring for signs of systemic toxicity (particularly electrocardiogram changes and an increase in T-wave amplitude) is recommended (Broadman 1996; Fisher et al 1997, **Level IV**). Continuous infusions of local anaesthetic or repeat boluses in infants can lead to local anaesthetic toxicity and seizures (McCloskey et al 1992, **Level IV**). As protein binding and clearance of local anaesthetics is reduced in neonates, lower doses are recommended to reduce the risk of accumulation (Meunier et al 2001, **Level III-3**). Irritability may be the only warning sign of toxicity in infants, and careful assessment is required to ensure that this is not incorrectly attributed to inadequate analgesia. Guidelines for safe infusion rates that achieve adequate analgesia have been established (Berde 1992, **Level IV**; Meunier et al 2001, **Level III-3**).

Neurological damage attributable to paediatric regional analgesia is rare, but reports of accidental spinal cord damage highlight the need for careful patient selection (Breschan et al 2001, **Level IV;** Kasai et al 2003, **Level IV**; Rose 2003, **Level IV**). Almost all regional blocks are performed under general anaesthesia in children, and there is no clear evidence that this is associated with increased complications (Bosenberg & Ivani 1998, **Level IV**; Krane et al 1998, **Level IV**). A retrospective review of 24,005 cases of regional block revealed five serious adverse outcomes, including three deaths, associated with difficult epidural insertions in young infants (Flandin-Blety & Barrier 1995, **Level IV**). A prospective study including 15,013 central blocks (predominantly caudal) reported 1.5 minor complications per 1,000 (Giaufre et al 1996, **Level IV**).

Bacterial colonisation of catheters is more commonly associated with caudal than lumbar catheters (McNeely et al 1997b, **Level IV;** Kost-Byerly 1998, **Level IV**), but epidural space infection is rare in the absence of prolonged or repeated insertion or immunodeficiency syndromes (Stafford 1995, **Level IV**).

Intrathecal morphine

The use of subarachnoid morphine 20 microgram/kg has been shown to decrease postoperative morphine requirements for paediatric patients undergoing cardiac surgery (Suominen et al 2004, **Level II**). Intrathecal morphine in this group did not lead to earlier extubation or earlier discharge from intensive care. There was effective analgesia for a 12-hour period postoperatively, with time for first IV morphine being 12.3 hours compared with 8.7 hours in the control group ($P<003$). Total IV morphine consumption was reduced from 378.1 microgram/kg to 260.1 microgram/kg in the intrathecal morphine group (P<0.03).

Key messages

1. Topical local anaesthetic does not adequately control pain associated with circumcision in awake neonates (**Level I** [Cochrane Review]).
2. Perioperative local anaesthetic infiltration does not improve analgesia after tonsillectomy (**Level I** [Cochrane Review]).
3. Clonidine prolongs analgesia when added to caudal local anaesthetic blocks (**Level I**)
4. Clonidine improves analgesia when added to epidural local anaesthetic infusions (**Level II**).
5. Wound infiltration, peripheral nerve blocks, and caudal local anaesthetic provide effective analgesia after day-case surgery (**Level II**).
6. Caudal local anaesthetic and dorsal penile nerve block provide perioperative analgesia for circumcision (**Level II**).
7. Epidural infusions of local anaesthetic provide similar levels of analgesia as systemic opioids (**Level II**).
8. Epidural opioids alone are less effective than local anaesthetic or combinations of local anaesthetic and opioid (**Level II**).

The following tick boxes ☑ represent conclusions based on clinical experience and expert opinion.

☑ Caudal local anaesthetic blocks provide effective analgesia for lower abdominal, perineal and lower limb surgery and have a low incidence of serious complications.

☑ Continuous epidural infusions provide effective postoperative analgesia in children of all ages and are safe if appropriate doses and equipment are used by experienced practitioners, with adequate monitoring and management of complications.

CHAPTER 10

10.1.8 Acute pain in children with cancer

Pain is a common symptom in children with cancer and is associated with significant fear and distress (Ljungman et al 1999, **Level IV**). The pattern and sources of acute pain differ significantly in children with cancer compared with adults.

Cancer-related pain

Pain due to tumour infiltration is present at diagnosis in 49–60% of children. Pain associated with haematological malignancies usually resolves with initial chemotherapy treatment. Solid tumours are less common than in adults, but are more likely to be associated with persistent cancer-related pain. Neuropathic pain and bone pain may be components of cancer-related pain and require specific treatment (Ljungman et al 1996, **Level IV**; Ljungman et al 1999, **Level IV**).

Procedure-related pain

Children, their parents, and physicians and nurses all rate pain due to procedural interventions and treatment as more significant than cancer-related pain (Ljungman et al 1996; Ljungman et al 1999). Multiple diagnostic and therapeutic interventions (eg lumbar punctures, bone marrow aspirations, blood samples) are required during the course of treatment and necessitate treatment matched to the severity of the procedure and needs of the child (see Section 10.1.3). EMLA® was evaluated as superior to placebo for pain relief during central venous port access in children with cancer (Miser et al 1994, **Level II**). Outcomes for second and subsequent procedures may be improved if adequate analgesia is provided for the first procedure (Weisman 1998, **Level III-2**).

Treatment-related pain

Pain related to side effects of chemotherapy and radiotherapy is a constant and dominating problem for children with cancer ((Ljungman et al 2000, **Level IV**). Mucositis is a common side effect of many chemotherapeutic regimens (Cella et al 2003) and is a frequent indication for IV opioid therapy (Drake et al 2004). Opioid requirements are often high and escalate with the severity of mucositis (Dunbar et al 1995; Coda et al 1997). In patients aged 12–18 years, morphine by PCA or continuous infusion provided similar analgesia, but morphine intake and opioid-related side effects were lower in the PCA group (Mackie et al 1991, **Level II**). A systematic review (which included mainly adult studies) found no difference in pain control between PCA and continuous infusion, but reduced hourly opioid requirement and shorter duration of pain with PCA (Worthington et al 2004, **Level I**). PCA morphine and hydromorphone have similar efficacy (Collins et al 1996, **Level II**) but sufentanil is less effective (Coda et al 1997, **Level II**). Prolonged administration is often required (6–74 days) (Dunbar 1995, **Level IV**). If excessive or dose-limiting side effects occur, rotation to another opioid (morphine to fentanyl or fentanyl to hydromorphone) can produce improvement in the majority of patients, without loss of pain control (Drake et al 2004, **Level IV**). Postoperative pain related to surgical procedures for diagnostic biopsies, insertion of long-term IV access devices and tumour resection is also a frequent source of treatment-related pain. In children with cancer requiring morphine infusions, the highest rate of breakthrough pain was found in postoperative cases, of which 92% had solid tumours (Flogegard & Ljungman 2003, **Level IV**).

For management of acute cancer pain in general see Section 9.7; for the management of acute mucositis pain see Section 9.6.7.

Key messages

1. PCA and continuous opioid infusions are equally effective in the treatment of pain in mucositis, but opioid consumption is less with PCA (**Level I** [Cochrane Review]).
2. PCA morphine and hydromorphone are equally effective for the control of pain associated with oral mucositis (**Level II**).

The following tick box ☑ represents conclusions based on clinical experience and expert opinion.

☑ Procedure and treatment related pain are significant problems for children with cancer.

10.2 THE PREGNANT PATIENT

10.2.1 Management of acute pain during pregnancy

Pregnant women with pain that is severe enough to warrant drug treatment (self-administered or prescribed by attendants) represent a difficult cohort in that drugs given to them almost always cross the placenta. While most drugs are safe there are particular times of concern, notably the period of organogenesis (weeks 4–10) and just before delivery. Where possible, non-pharmacological treatment options should be considered before analgesic medications are used and ongoing analgesic use requires close liaison between the obstetrician and the medical practitioner managing the pain (Roche & Goucke 2003).

Drugs used in pregnancy

Drugs that might be prescribed during pregnancy have been categorised according to fetal risk by the Australian Drug Evaluation Committee (ADEC). The categories used are listed in Table 10.4 and the classification of some of the drugs that might be used in pain management is summarised in Table 10.5.

Paracetamol

Paracetamol is regarded as the analgesic of choice although detailed studies are lacking (Niederhoff & Zahradnik 1983).

Non-steroidal anti-inflammatory drugs

NSAIDs are Category C drugs. While relatively safe in early and mid pregnancy, they can precipitate fetal cardiac and renal complications in late pregnancy, as well as interfere with fetal brain development and the production of amniotic fluid; they should be discontinued in the 32nd gestational week (Ostensen & Skomsvoll 2004). Use of NSAIDs during pregnancy is associated with increased risk of miscarriage (Nielsen et al 2001, **Level III-2**; Li et al 2003, **Level III-2**).

Fetal exposure to NSAIDs has been associated with persistent pulmonary hypertension in the neonate (Alano et al 2001, **Level III-2**).

Opioids

Most opioids are Category C drugs. Most of the experience that provides information about the effects on neonates of therapeutically administered opioids does not come from pain therapy, but opioid abuse; pregnant patients who abuse opioids or who are on maintenance programs represent an increasing group of parturients. Neonatal abstinence syndrome occurs in 30–90% of infants exposed to heroin or methadone in utero (Zelson et al 1973, **Level III-2**). The effect of maternal methadone dosage on severity of neonatal withdrawal is reported as closely associated (Dashe et al 2002, **Level IV**) or non-existent (Berghella et al 2003, **Level IV**). Prolonged antenatal opioid intake can necessitate weaning over weeks (Zelson 1975); first data suggest neonatal abstinence syndrome does not occur with buprenorphine use (Schindler et al 2003).

Overall, the use of opioids to treat pain in pregnancy appears safe (Wunsch et al 2003). However, a link between opioid use and low birth weight (Hulse et al 1997, **Level III-2**) as well as increased risk of strabismus in babies has been reported (Gill et al 2003, **Level IV**).

Specific pain syndromes

Meralgia paresthetica

This variable condition comprising some or all of the sensations of pain, tingling and numbness in the lateral thigh affects pregnant women in particular, with an increased odds ratio of 12 in comparison with a non-pregnant population (van Slobbe et al 2004, **Level III-2**). Therapies reported but not studied include ice packs, local infiltration with steroid and local anaesthetic, transcutaneous electrical nerve stimulation (TENS), drug therapy (tricyclic antidepressants, antiepileptics) and surgical intervention (van Diver & Camann 1995).

Symphysial diastasis

This occasionally disabling disorder (sometimes called osteitis pubis) involving separation of the symphysis pubis during pregnancy, and immediately after delivery in some, has a quoted incidence of 1:600 (Taylor & Sonson 1986, **Level IV**).

Key messages

1. Use of non-steroidal anti-inflammatory drugs during pregnancy is associated with increased risk of miscarriage (**Level III-2**).
2. Use of opioids in pregnancy does not cause fetal malformations, but may result in neonatal abstinence syndrome (**Level III-2**).

The following tick boxes ☑ represent conclusions based on clinical experience and expert opinion.

☑ For pain management in pregnancy non-pharmacological treatment options should be considered where possible before analgesic medications are used.

☑ Use of medications for pain in pregnancy should be guided by published recommendations; ongoing analgesic use requires close liaison between the obstetrician and the medical practitioner managing the pain.

☑ NSAIDs should be used with caution in the last trimester of pregnancy and should be avoided after the 32nd week.

Table 10.4 ADEC drug categorisation according to fetal risk

A	Drugs which have been taken by a large number of pregnant women and women of childbearing age without any proven increase in the frequency of malformations or other direct or indirect harmful effects on the fetus having been observed.
B1	Drugs which have been taken by only a limited number of pregnant women and women of childbearing age, without an increase in the frequency of malformation or other direct or indirect harmful effects on the human fetus having been observed. Studies in animals have not shown evidence of an increased occurrence of fetal damage.
B2	Drugs which have been taken by only a limited number of pregnant women and women of childbearing age, without an increase in the frequency of malformation or other direct or indirect harmful effects on the human fetus having been observed. Studies in animals are inadequate or may be lacking, but available data show no evidence of an increased occurrence of fetal damage.
B3	Drugs which have been taken by only a limited number of pregnant women and women of childbearing age, without an increase in the frequency of malformation or other direct or indirect harmful effects on the human fetus having been observed. Studies in animals have shown evidence of an increased occurrence of fetal damage, the significance of which is considered uncertain in humans.
C	Drugs which, owing to their pharmacological effects, have caused or may be suspected of causing, harmful effects on the human fetus or neonate without causing malformations. These effects may be reversible. Accompanying texts should be consulted for further details.
D	Drugs which have caused, are suspected to have caused or may be expected to cause, an increased incidence of human fetal malformations or irreversible damage. These drugs may also have adverse pharmacological effects. Accompanying texts should be consulted for further details.
X	Drugs which have such a high risk of causing permanent damage to the fetus that they should not be used in pregnancy or when there is a possibility of pregnancy.

Notes: For drugs in the B1, B2 and B3 categories, human data are lacking or inadequate and subcategorisation is therefore based on available animal data. The allocation of a B category does NOT imply greater safety than the C category. Drugs in category D are not absolutely contraindicated in pregnancy (eg anticonvulsants). Moreover, in some cases the 'D' category has been assigned on the basis of 'suspicion'.

Due to legal considerations in this country, sponsor companies have, in some cases, applied a more restrictive category than can be justified on the basis of the available data.

In some cases there may be discrepancies between the published Product Information and the information in this booklet due to the process of ongoing document revision.

Source: ADEC (1999). © Commonwealth of Australia. Reproduced with permission (see notes on verso page).

Table 10.5 Categorisation of drugs used in pain management

Drug	Cat	Comments
Opioids alfentanil, buprenorphine, dextromoramide, dextropropoxyphene, fentanyl, hydromorphone, methadone, morphine, oxycodone, papaveretum, pentazocine, pethidine, phenoperidine, remifentanil, tramadol	C	Opioid analgesics may cause respiratory depression in the newborn infant. Withdrawal symptoms in newborn infants have been reported with prolonged use of this class of drugs.
codeine, dihydrocodeine	A	Prolonged high-dose use of codeine prior to delivery may produce codeine withdrawal symptoms in the neonate
Paracetamol	A	
Aspirin	C	Aspirin inhibits prostaglandin synthesis. When given late in pregnancy, it may cause premature closure of the fetal ductus arteriosus, delay labour and birth. Aspirin increases the bleeding time both in the newborn infant and in the mother because of its antiplatelet effects. Products containing aspirin should be avoided in the last trimester. Low-dose aspirin (100mg/day) does not affect bleeding time.
Other NSAIDs diclofenac, diflunisal, ibuprofen, indomethacin (indometacin), ketoprofen, ketorolac, mefenamic acid, nabumetone, naproxen, phenylbutazone, piroxicam, sodium salicylate, sulindac, tenoxicam, tiaprofenic acid	C	These agents inhibit prostaglandin synthesis and, when given during the latter part of pregnancy, may cause closure of the fetal ductus arteriosus, fetal renal impairment, inhibition of platelet aggregation and delayed labour and birth. Continuous treatment with NSAIDs during the last trimester of pregnancy should only be given on sound indications. During the last few days before expected birth, agents with an inhibitory effect on prostaglandin synthesis should be avoided.
Local anaesthetics		
bupivacaine, cinchocaine, lignocaine (lidocaine), mepivacaine, prilocaine	A	
etidocaine, ropivacaine	B1	
procaine hydrochloride	B2	
Antidepressants		
SSRIs: citalopram, fluoxetine, fluvoxamine, paroxetine, sertraline	C	SSRIs have had limited use in pregnancy without a reported increase in birth defects. The use of SSRIs in the third trimester may result in a withdrawal state in the newborn infant.

CHAPTER 10

Drug	Cat	Comments
Tricyclic antidepressants:		
amitriptyline, clomipramine, desipramine, dothiepin (dosulepin), doxepin, imipramine, nortriptyline, protriptyline, trimipramin	C	Withdrawal symptoms in newborn infants have been reported with prolonged maternal use of this class of drugs.
Other antidepressants:		
mirtazapine, moclobemide, nefazodone	B3	
venlafaxine	B2	
Anticonvulsants		
carbamazepine	D	Spina bifida occurs in about 1% of pregnancies in which carbamazepine is used as monotherapy. Carbamazepine taken during pregnancy also has been associated with minor craniofacial defects, fingernail hypoplasia and developmental disability. Carbamazepine also can cause coagulation defects with consequent risk of haemorrhage in the fetus and the newborn infant which may be preventable by the prophylactic administration of vitamin K to the mother prior to delivery.
phenytoin sodium	D	This drug taken during pregnancy has been associated with craniofacial defects, fingernail hypoplasia, developmental disability, growth retardation and less frequently, oral clefts and cardiac anomalies. This clinical pattern is sometimes called the 'fetal hydantoin syndrome'. Phenytoin also can cause coagulation defects with consequent risk of haemorrhage in the fetus and the newborn infant which may be preventable by the prophylactic administration of vitamin K to the mother prior to delivery.
sodium valproate	D	If taken in the first trimester of pregnancy, sodium valproate (valproic acid) is associated with a 1–2% risk of neural tube defects (especially spina bifida) in the exposed fetus. Women taking sodium valproate (valproic acid) who become pregnant should be encouraged to consider detailed mid-trimester morphology ultrasound for prenatal diagnosis of such abnormalities.
clonazepam	C	Clonazepam is a benzodiazepine. These drugs may cause hypotonia, respiratory depression and hypothermia in the newborn infant if used in high doses during labour. Withdrawal symptoms in newborn infants have been reported with this class of drugs.
gabapentin	B1	
lamotrigine, tiagabine, topiramate	B3	

Drug	Cat	Comments
Antiemetics, antinauseants		
Phenothiazines:		
prochlorperazine, promethazine, thiethylperazine	C	When given in high doses during late pregnancy, phenothiazines have caused prolonged neurological disturbances in the infant.
Others:		
dimenhydrinate, diphenhydramine, metoclopramide	A	
dolasetron, granisetron, ondansetron	B1	
domperidone, hyoscine, hyoscine hydrobromide	B2	
tropisetron	B3	

Source: ADEC (1999). © Commonwealth of Australia. Reproduced with permission (see notes on verso page).

10.2.2 Management of pain during delivery

Pain during labour and delivery represents a complex interaction of multiple physiological and psychological factors involved in parturition. Women's desires for and expectations of pain relief during labour and delivery vary widely. High quality relief does not necessarily equate with a high level of satisfaction (Shapiro et al 1998, **Level IV**).

Appropriate pain relief in labour should not be denied (ACOG 2002). Women experiencing painful and traumatic labour without a feeling of control are more likely to suffer from post-traumatic stress disorder (Creedy et al 2000, **Level IV**) with sexual avoidance, fear of childbirth, or postnatal depression (Bailham & Joseph 2003).

Systemic analgesia in labour pain

Opioid analgesics used in labour result in significantly less pain relief than epidural and other regional analgesic techniques (Sharma et al 1997, **Level II**). Their use also decreases fetal heart rate variability and increases by 3–4-fold the number of infants requiring resuscitation at birth or needing naloxone compared with regional analgesia (Halpern et al 1999, **Level I**), as well as worsening fetal acid-base balance (Reynolds et al 2002, **Level I**). Intrapartum parenteral pethidine decreased neonatal rooting reflexes and successful first breast feed (Righard & Aldade 1990, **Level III-2**).

Women can become sedated but remain in pain despite repeated IV doses of pethidine or morphine (Olofsson et al 1996; Sharma et al 1997, **Level II**). There are insufficient data to evaluate the comparative efficacy and safety of any IM opioid (Elbourne & Wiseman 1998 **Level I**).

IV administration has greater efficacy than equivalent IM dosing (Isenor & Penny-MacGillivray 1993, **Level II**).

A quantitative assessment of the efficacy of nitrous oxide inhalational analgesia is currently not possible. However, although it is not a potent labour analgesic, it is safe (Rosen 2002, **Level I**). The maternal and fetal effects and impact on the progress of labour are benign (Westling et al 1992; Carstoniu et al 1994, **Level II**).

Epidural and combined spinal-epidural analgesia in labour pain

Epidural analgesia is more effective in reducing pain than non-regional methods of analgesia (Howell 1999, **Level I**; Liu & Sia 2004, **Level I**). Compared with non-epidural methods, epidural or spinal-epidural analgesia in nulliparous labour does not increase the caesarean section rate, but is associated with longer labour and a higher rate of instrumental delivery (Howell 1999 **Level I**; Liu & Sia 2004, **Level I**). By excluding trials that include induced labour, the increase in instrumental delivery rate is no longer significant (Liu & Sia 2004, **Level I**).

The requirement for pain relief in early labour is associated with an increased risk of caesarean delivery; this risk is independent of the method of analgesia, suggesting that epidural analgesia should not be withheld in early labour (Sharma et al 2003, **Level I**).

Combined spinal-epidural in comparison with epidural analgesia reduces time to effective analgesia and maternal satisfaction but increases the incidence of pruritus (Hughes et al 2004, **Level I**). Both techniques are associated with similar obstetric and neonatal outcomes (Hughes et al 2004, **Level I**) and a similar incidence of hypotension and of transient fetal heart rate changes (Patel et al 2003, **Level II**).

Low dose (0.1%) bupivacaine/opioid infusions in comparison with 0.25% bupivacaine bolus injection reduce motor block and instrumental vaginal delivery rate (Comet Study Group 2001, **Level II**). There is no significant difference in any outcome between use of bupivacaine and ropivacaine (Halpern & Walsh 2003, **Level I**). Patient-controlled epidural analgesia without background infusion reduces local anaesthetic use, motor block and need for anaesthetic intervention compared with continuous epidural infusion (van der Vyver 2002, **Level I**).

The addition of opioid to epidural local anaesthetic improves the quality and duration of pain relief and reduces local anaesthetic requirement, but increases pruritus compared with equieffective local anaesthetic alone (Lyons et al 1997, **Level II**); it also improves maternal satisfaction (Murphy et al 1991, **Level II**).

Pethidine (meperidine) is effective when administered epidurally by bolus dose, continuous infusion and by epidural patient-controlled analgesia; it is more lipid soluble than morphine (but less than fentanyl and its analogues), thus its onset and offset of epidural analgesic action is more rapid than morphine (Ngan Kee 1998, **Level IV**). Epidural pethidine has been used predominantly in the obstetric setting. After caesarean section epidural pethidine resulted in better pain relief and less sedation than IV pethidine (Paech 1994, **Level II**) but inferior analgesia compared with intrathecal morphine, albeit with less pruritus, nausea and drowsiness (Paech 2000, **Level II**).

Single-injection intrathecal opioids are as effective as epidural local anaesthetics for the management of pain in early labour; there is increased pruritus but no effect on nausea or mode of delivery (Bucklin et al 2002, **Level I**). Intrathecal opioids increase the risk of fetal bradycardia (NNH 28) and maternal pruritus (NNH 1.7) in comparison with non-intrathecal opioid analgesia (Mardirosoff et al 2002, **Level I**).

Epidural techniques do not increase the risk of long-term backache (Wight & Halpern 2003, **Level I**).

Compared with systemic opioid analgesia, epidural analgesia is associated with maternal fever (4-fold risk), probably due to the association of rising temperature with prolonged labour and nulliparity (Philip et al 1999, **Level II**).

There is no correlation between successful breast feeding at 6–8 weeks and epidural labour analgesia with opioids and local anaesthetics (Halpern et al 1999, **Level III-2**).

Other regional techniques in labour pain

Paracervical block is more effective than IM opioids (Jensen et al 1984, **Level II**) but requires supplementation more frequently than epidural analgesia (Manninen et al 2000, **Level II**). There is insufficient evidence to support its safety and serious fetal complications may occur (Asling et al 1970; Shnider et al 1970) although a role in hospitals without obstetric anaesthesia services has been suggested (Levy et al 1999, **Level III-2**).

Complementary and other methods of pain relief in labour pain

Childbirth training may have a limited effect on the pain of labour (Melzack et al 1981, **Level III-2**). Continuous or one-to-one support by a midwife or trained layperson during labour reduces analgesic use, operative delivery and dissatisfaction, especially if the support person is not a member of the hospital staff, is present from early labour, or if an epidural analgesia service is not available (Hodnett et al 2003, **Level I**).

Music, audio-analgesia and aromatherapy have no effect on use of medication for pain relief (Smith et al 2003, **Level I**). TENS does not reduce labour pain, but there is evidence for a weak analgesic sparing effect (NNT 14) (Carroll 1997, **Level I**). Hypnosis increases satisfaction with pain relief and acupuncture decreases the need for analgesics (Smith et al 2003, **Level I**). Hypnosis used in labour also leads to a decreased requirement for pharmacological analgesia, increased incidence of spontaneous vaginal delivery and decreased use of labour augmentation (Cyna et al 2004, **Level I**).

The injection of sterile water intradermally over the lumbosacral area is transiently very painful but reduces severe lower back pain during labour for at least 60 minutes. It is more effective than back massage, baths, mobilisation or TENS (Labrecque et al 1999, **Level II**; Martensson & Wallin 1999, **Level II**).

Key messages

1. Continuous or one-to-one support by a midwife or trained layperson during labour reduces analgesic use, operative delivery and dissatisfaction (**Level I**).
2. Epidural and combined spinal-epidural analgesia provide superior pain relief for labour and delivery compared with systemic analgesics (**Level I**).
3. Combined spinal-epidural in comparison with epidural analgesia reduces time to effective analgesia and improves maternal satisfaction but increases the incidence of pruritus (**Level I** [Cochrane Review]).
4. Epidural analgesia does not increase the incidence of caesarean section and long-term backache (**Level I**).
5. Epidural analgesia is associated with increased duration of labour and may increase rate of instrumental vaginal delivery (**Level I**).
6. There is no significant difference in any outcome between use of bupivacaine and ropivacaine for epidural labour analgesia (**Level I**).
7. Patient-controlled epidural analgesia without background infusion reduces local anaesthetic use and motor block compared with continuous epidural infusion (**Level I**).
8. Single-injection intrathecal opioids provide comparable early labour analgesia to epidural local anaesthetics with increased pruritus (**Level I**).
9. Systemic opioids in labour increase the need for neonatal resuscitation and worsen acid-base status compared with regional analgesia (**Level I**).
10. Nitrous oxide has some analgesic efficacy and is safe during labour (**Level I**).
11. Acupuncture reduces analgesic requirements in labour (**Level I** [Cochrane Review]).
12. Hypnosis used in labour reduces analgesic requirements and use of labour augmentation and increases the incidence of spontaneous vaginal delivery (**Level I**).
13. TENS does not reduce labour pain (**Level I**).
14. Systemic opioids are less effective than regional analgesia for pain in labour (**Level II**).
15. Paracervical block is more effective than intramuscular opioid analgesia but there is insufficient evidence to support its safety (**Level II**).
16. Lumbosacral intradermal injection of sterile water is painful, but reduces labour pain (**Level II**).

10.2.3 Pain management during lactation

A number of general principles apply when administering analgesic and antiemetic drugs for pain management during lactation:

- the choice of drugs should be based on knowledge of their potential impact on breast feeding and on the breast fed infant secondary to transfer in human milk; and
- the lowest possible effective maternal dose of analgesic is recommended, breast feeding is best avoided at times of peak drug concentration in milk, and the infant should be observed for effects of medication transferred in breast milk.

The effects of many analgesic and antiemetic drugs during lactation have not been adequately investigated, leaving clinical decisions to be made on evidence derived from pharmacokinetic or observational studies, case reports and anecdote. For most drugs, information on infant outcome is inadequate (based on single dose or short-term administration or on case reports) or absent, so maternal consent is advisable and caution is warranted.

The principles of passage of drugs in human milk (Ilett et al 1997) including drugs relevant to pain management (Rathmell et al 1997; Spigset & Hagg 2000; Bar-Oz et al 2003) have been reviewed. High lipid solubility, low molecular weight, low protein binding and the unionised state favour secretion into breast milk; low oral bioavailability limits neonatal exposure. The neonatal exposure is often 0.5–4% of the maternal dose, but infant drug metabolism may be impaired. Until about the third to fourth postpartum day only very small amounts of colostrum are secreted, so early breast feeding is unlikely to pose a hazard, even from drugs administered in the peripartum period.

Drugs that might be prescribed during lactation have been categorised according to their risk for the baby. Some of the drugs that might be used in pain management are listed with comments in Table 10.6.

Non-opioids

The weight-adjusted maternal dose of paracetamol transferred to the neonate is about 2% (Notarianni 1987). Although neonatal glucuronide conjugation may be deficient, the drug is considered safe given that there have been no reports of adverse effects and the fact that this represents a small fraction of the recommended single infant dose of 10mg/kg.

NSAIDs must be considered individually, but in general milk levels are low because they are weak acids and extensively plasma protein bound.

In particular, ibuprofen has very low transfer (< 1% weight-adjusted maternal dose), is short-acting, free of active metabolites and has the best documented safety. Diclofenac and ketorolac are minimally transported into breast milk and short-term or occasional use is compatible with breast feeding. The safety of naproxen is less clear but it is also considered compatible (Rathmell et al 1997).

Despite similar proportional transfer as paracetamol, salicylates are eliminated slowly by the neonate, cause platelet dysfunction and have been associated with Reye's syndrome; aspirin in analgesic doses cannot be recommended as safe (Bar-Oz et al 2003).

Indomethacin (indometacin) is found in low levels in breast milk (transfer < 1%) and a single report of neonatal seizures did not establish a causal association. However, it is less than ideal because of central maternal side effects, such as agitation and psychosis, in previously healthy postnatal women (Clunie et al 2003, **Level IV**). There are no data available on the COX-2-specific inhibitors such as parecoxib.

Opioids

With some provisos, the short-term use of opioids is generally considered safe during lactation (Ravin 1995). Most opioids are secreted into breast milk in low doses and with the possible exception of pethidine there is little evidence to suggest significant adverse neurobehavioural effects.

Good pain relief can improve milk production (Hirose et al 1996, **Level I**), but observational studies of maternal opioid use during labour suggest that sucking activity and duration is affected, potentially reducing infant weight gain (Kotelko et al 1995, **Level III-2**).

An association between opioid exposure in breast milk and episodes of apnoea and cyanosis in infants has been described (Naumburg & Meny 1988, **Level IV**), leading some to suggest that opioids should be avoided if the neonate experiences such events during the first week of life. Chronic exposure or repeated high doses of opioid may pose problems for the infant, although even neonatal concentrations within the analgesic range may not cause adverse effects or subsequent withdrawal symptoms (Robieux et al 1990, **Level IV**).

Repeated dosing of epidural, IV and IM morphine after caesarean section has been investigated both in the immediate and later postoperative periods (Ravin 1995). About 6% of the weight-adjusted maternal dose is transferred in breast milk (Feilberg et al 1989), but the oral bioavailability in the infant is low (about 25%) so only small amounts reach the infant. Although morphine-3 and 6-glucuronide transfer has not been adequately investigated, the absence of effects on the infant even following patient-controlled IV analgesia with morphine supports its safety. Pharmacokinetic studies suggest the more lipophilic opioids such as fentanyl and alfentanil are unlikely to cause problems. Following repeated fentanyl dosing during labour or a single dose after delivery, the weight-adjusted maternal dose received by the neonate is 3%, levels in colostrum become undetectable within several hours and the nursing infant appears unaffected (Steer et al 1992, **Level IV**).

A single dose of pethidine appears safe, peaking in breast milk after 2 hours, with transfer of less than 1% of the weight-adjusted maternal dose, and undetectable levels by 24 hours. However norpethidine accumulates in breast milk with repeated use and has very slow neonatal elimination. Infants exposed to patient-controlled IV pethidine are less alert and oriented on days 3 and 4 after caesarean section than those of mothers receiving morphine (Wittels et al1990, **Level III-2**), even if the systemic dose is reduced by preceding use of epidural morphine (Wittels et al 1997, **Level II**).

Codeine and oxycodone have milk to plasma ratios of more than 1 but infant ingestion is less than 2% of maternal dose and on the basis of no apparent adverse effects they are considered acceptable. Methadone and dextropropoxyphene are also considered compatible with breast feeding (Ravin 1995).

The distribution of tramadol into human breast milk has only been studied after a single dose and although transfer was acceptably low, there are insufficient data to support its safety.

Other medications related to pain relief

Local anaesthetics show acceptable milk to plasma ratios (Ortega et al 1999) and are considered safe, based on minimal measurable levels after epidural administration or antiarrhythmic IV lignocaine (lidocaine) infusion (Rathmell et al 1997).

Pain management is frequently associated with concurrent control of nausea and vomiting. There is very little information about antiemetics and in almost all cases the manufacturers do not recommend use during lactation (for recommendations see Table 10.6). Animal studies suggest possible central nervous system effects in the newborn, but human anecdotal experience is favourable.

Ondansetron is secreted in animal milk but no human data are available. It has been used during pregnancy without effect on the fetus.

Metoclopramide peaks in milk at 2–3 hours and the infant exposure is minimal compared with doses used therapeutically in infants (Kauppila et al 1983).

Table 10.6 The lactating patient and drugs used in pain management

Drug	Comments
Opioids	
buprenorphine, codeine, dextropropoxyphene, fentanyl, hydromorphone, methadone, morphine, oxycodone, pentazocine, tramadol	Safe to use
Paracetamol	Safe to use
Aspirin	Avoid due to theoretical risk of Reye's syndrome; ibuprofen is preferred
Other NSAIDs	
Non-selective NSAIDs,	Safe to use
COX-2 Selective NSAIDs	Limited data; appear safe
Local anaesthetics	
bupivacaine, cinchocaine, levobupivacaine lignocaine (lidocaine), mepivacaine, prilocaine, ropivacaine	Unlikely to cause problems

Drug	Comments
Antidepressants	
SSRIs: citalopram, fluvoxamine, paroxetine, sertraline	Use of SSRIs during lactation appears safe if indicated. Contact specialised information service
fluoxetine	Use an alternative SSRI because of fluoxetine's long half-life
Tricyclic antidepressants (TCAs): amitriptyline, clomipramine, dothiepin (dosulepin), doxepin, imipramine, nortriptyline, trimipramin	TCAs have been used to treat postnatal depression. Avoid doxepin if possible; a single case of neonatal respiratory depression has been reported
Other antidepressants: moclobemide	Appears to be safe; contact specialised information service
mirtazapine, nefazodone, venlafaxine	Contact specialised information service
Anticonvulsants	
carbamazepine	Safe to use; monitor infant for drowsiness and poor suckling
phenytoin sodium	May be used
sodium valproate	Safe to use at low dosage
clonazepam	Risk of sedation in infant; contact specialised information service
gabapentin, tiagabine	No data available
lamotrigine, topiramate	Excreted in breast milk; contact specialised information service
Antiemetics, antinauseants	
Phenothiazines: prochlorperazine	Safe to use
promethazine	Safe to use; however, may cause drowsiness or tiredness in mother
Others: dimenhydrinate	Safe to use occasional doses
metoclopramide	Used during first months of breast feeding to stimulate lactation
dolasetron, granisetron, ondansetron, tropisetron	Contact specialised information service; no data available, although 1 or 2 doses after delivery should not be a concern
domperidone	Used during first months of breast feeding to stimulate lactation; mother may be less drowsy than with metoclopramide
hyoscine hydrobromide	Safe to use occasional doses

Source: Adapted with permission from *Australian Medicines Handbook 2004*.

Key messages

The following tick boxes ☑ represent conclusions based on clinical experience and expert opinion.

☑ Prescribing medications during lactation requires consideration of possible transfer into breast milk, uptake by the baby and potential adverse effects for the baby; it should follow available prescribing guidelines.

☑ Local anaesthetics, paracetamol and several NSAIDs, in particular ibuprofen, are considered to be safe in the lactating patient.

☑ Morphine, fentanyl and oxycodone are also considered safe in the lactating patient and should be preferred over pethidine.

10.2.4 Pain in the puerperium

Pain during the puerperium is common and of multiple aetiologies, most often being perineal or uterine cramping pain initially and breast pain from the fourth postpartum day (Dewan et al 1993). This section of the report does not consider the management of other types of pain, including that after caesarean section, back pain, pubic symphysis diastasis pain, muscle and haemorrhoidal pain, headache or other neurological pain.

Women are often inadequately warned and remain ill informed of the best available treatments for postnatal pain. Pain after childbirth coincides with new emotional, physical and learning demands and may trigger postnatal depression. Compared with the management of intrapartum pain, pain during this period is often neglected and many aspects of the management of postnatal pain have not been subjected to scientific research. Therefore pain is frequently poorly managed, many women consider that they have not achieved good relief, and those with health problems indicate they would have liked more help or advice (Brown & Lumley 1998). Severe perineal and uterine pain limit mobility during maternal-infant bonding and unrelieved perineal pain is the most common reason for failure to resume sexual relations after birth. Breast, especially nipple, pain may result in abandonment of breast feeding.

Perineal pain

The majority of women in developed countries will suffer perineal trauma and a quarter still have perineal pain 10 days after delivery (Sleep et al 1984; Albers et al 1999). A number of obstetric and surgical factors are reputed to contribute to perineal trauma and episiotomy. The severity of pain may be increased by perineal haematomas, tears of the rectum or anal sphincter, inexperience of the surgeon performing perineal repairs (Albers et al 1999, **Level III-3**) and repair using non-absorbable or non-subcuticular skin sutures (Kettle & Johanson 1999, **Level I**). The restricted or liberal use of episiotomy does not influence the degree of perineal pain (Carroli & Belizan 1999, **Level I**).

Non-pharmacological treatments

The intermittent application of cold, as an icepack or cool gel pad, is probably the most commonly used form of localised treatment for perineal pain and oedema. Wound healing is not delayed, but ice should be covered to prevent direct skin

CHAPTER 10

contact and the risk of burns to adjacent areas (Steen & Cooper 1998). The localised application of purpose-designed cool gel pads is more effective in relieving moderate or severe pain at 48 hours postpartum than icepacks or anti-inflammatory steroid-based foam (Steen et al 2000, **Level II**). Cold and warm baths are also widely used to alleviate perineal pain (Sleep & Grant 1988) and appear equally effective (Hill 1989, **Level II**). There is no evidence to support the use of additives (eg salt or lavender oil) (Sleep & Grant 1998, **Level II**). Ultrasound and pulsed electromagnetic energy therapies have been inadequately evaluated and unless a part of current practice should not be instituted until further evidence of efficacy is available (Hay-Smith 1998, **Level I**).

Pharmacological treatments

Paracetamol is a moderately effective analgesic for perineal pain during the first 24 hours after birth. NSAIDs such as ibuprofen are as or more effective (Hedayati et al 2003, **Level I**) and preferable to paracetamol combined with codeine as the latter leads to more side effects (eg nausea, constipation) (Peter et al 2001, **Level II**). The topical application of lignocaine (lidocaine) ointment to the perineum during the second stage of labour reduces immediate perineal pain briefly but it is not an effective treatment of established perineal pain (Minassian et al 2002, **Level II**). Combinations of steroid and local anaesthetic are also not effective (Greer & Cameron 1984, **Level II**).

Breast pain

On the fourth postpartum day about 40% of women experience moderate to severe breast or nipple pain (Dewan et al 1993). Painful breasts are a common reason why women cease breast feeding (Snowden et al 2001). Management is firstly directed toward remedying the cause, whether this be infant-related (incorrect attachment, sucking, oral abnormalities); lactation-related (breast engorgement, blocked ducts or forceful milk ejection); nipple trauma; dermatological or infective problems (Candida or mastitis) or other causes (Amir 2003).

Nipple pain and cracking is usually resolved by temporarily discontinuing breast feeding, expressing milk and correcting the positioning and attachment of the baby. There is no evidence supporting various creams, gels or sprays (Inch & Renfew 1989, **Level I**).

Infective mastitis is most commonly from Staphylococcus aureus and can be treated with appropriate antibiotics (usually flucloxacillin) and analgesics, while breast milk is expressed and discarded. Non-infective mastitis is equally common and is managed by continuation of breast feeding, milk expression and analgesics (Inch & Renfew 1989, **Level III-3**).

The key to preventing breast engorgement is encouragement of unrestricted infant feeding (Moon & Humenick 1989, **Level III-3**). Binding of the breasts is ineffective in reducing the symptoms of engorgement (Brooten 1983, **Level II**). Symptomatic therapies have been inadequately investigated, but cabbage leaves and cabbage extract cream are no more effective than placebo (Snowden et al 2001, **Level I**). Similarly, ultrasound is not effective and observed benefit may be due to the effect of radiant heat or massage (Snowden et al 2001, **Level I**).

Oxytocin is ineffective (Ingelman-Sundberg 1953, **Level II**). Protease enzymes and homeopathic treatments with anti-inflammatory properties are effective but are not available in Australia (Snowden et al 2001, **Level I**). Hormonal treatments such as bromocriptine suppress lactation (Shapiro & Thomas 1984, **Level II**) but lead to a 'rebound' effect at cessation and side effects can be severe (hypertension, myocardial infarction and seizures).

Uterine pain

Uterine pain or 'after pains' often worsen with increasing parity, are experienced by most multiparous women and result from the release of oxytocin from the posterior pituitary gland, especially in response to breast feeding. Lower abdominal pain may be mild to severe, accompanied by back pain and is described as throbbing, cramping and aching.

Both paracetamol (Skovlund et al 1991a, **Level II**) and NSAIDs (Huang et al 2002, **Level II**) are modestly effective compared with placebo and are similar to each other (Skovlund et al 1991b, **Level II**).

Key messages

1. Routine episiotomy does not reduce perineal pain (**Level I**).
2. Paracetamol and NSAIDs are effective in treating perineal pain after childbirth (**Level I**).
3. The use of codeine for perineal pain after childbirth leads to more side effects than the use of NSAIDs (**Level II**).
4. Paracetamol and NSAIDs are equally, but only modestly effective in treating uterine pain (**Level II**).
5. The application of cooling, in particular with cooling gel pads, and the use of warm baths is effective in treatment of perineal pain after childbirth (**Level II**).
6. Bromocriptine should be avoided for the treatment of breast pain in the puerperium because of the potential for serious adverse effects (**Level II**).

The following tick boxes ☑ represent conclusions based on clinical experience and expert opinion.

☑ Pain after childbirth requires appropriate treatment as it coincides with new emotional, physical and learning demands and may trigger postnatal depression.

☑ Management of breast and nipple pain should target the cause.

10.3 THE ELDERLY PATIENT

Prevalence of persistent pain in older people increases with advancing age, but prevalence studies of acute pain are rare. In Australia, 5% of people aged 65 years or older have acute pain of less than 1 month's duration that interferes with activity (Kendig et al 1996). Conditions that are common in elderly people and that may lead to acute pain include acute exacerbations of arthritis, osteoporotic fractures of the spine, cancer and pain from other acute medical conditions including ischaemic heart disease, herpes zoster and peripheral vascular disease. Advances in anaesthetic and surgical techniques also mean that increasingly elderly patients are undergoing more major surgery (Richardson & Bresland 1998).

Factors that can combine to make effective control of acute pain in the elderly person more difficult than in younger patients include: a higher incidence of coexistent diseases and concurrent medications which increases the risk of drug-drug and disease-drug interactions; age-related changes in physiology, pharmacodynamics and pharmacokinetics; altered responses to pain; and difficulties with assessment of pain, including problems related to cognitive impairment (Macintyre et al 2003).

10.3.1 Pharmacokinetic and pharmacodynamic changes

The changes in pharmacokinetics and pharmacodynamics in elderly people and consequent alterations that might be required in some drug regimens are summarised in Table 10.8. These changes are generally attributable to ageing alone but may be compounded by the higher incidence of degenerative and other concurrent diseases in elderly people.

Assessment of the pharmacodynamic changes associated with ageing is difficult. When such studies have been done with opioids, most have used a surrogate measure of effect other than clinical pain relief. For example, by studying the effects of fentanyl and alfentanil on the EEG it was concluded that the pharmacokinetics were unaffected by age, but that the sensitivity of the brain to these opioids was increased by 50% in the elderly person (Scott & Stanski 1987). Whether this can be attributed to changes in the number or function of opioid receptors in the central nervous system or whether it is due to an increased free fraction of opioids in the central nervous system is unclear. In older rats there are fewer μ- and κ-opioid receptors (Vuyk 2003).

Table 10.7 Changes in drug administration regimens in elderly people

Physiological changes in elderly people		Likely pharmacokinetic result	Possible changes needed to drug regimens
Whole body			
Cardiac output	↓ 0–20%	↑ peak concentration after bolus dose	Smaller initial dose and slower rate of IV injection
Changes in fat/muscle/ total body water ratio		Changes in distribution volume; ↑ elimination half-life	Possible ↓ dose/kg
fat	↑ 10–50%		
muscle mass	↓ 20%		
total body water	↓ 10%		
Plasma albumin	↓ 20%	Altered free fraction of drug	Variable effect on bolus dose
alpha 1 glycoprotein	↑ 30–50%		
Drug binding	↑ (variable)	Little effect on clearance of high extraction drugs	Little effect on maintenance dose of high extraction drugs
Liver			
Liver blood flow	↓ 25–40%	↓ clearance of flow limited drugs	↓ maintenance dose
Hepatic enzymes			
phase I (eg oxidation)	↓ 25%		
phase II	Little change	↓ hepatic clearance of some enzyme limited drugs	
Kidney			
Nephron mass	↓ 30%	↓ clearance of renally excreted drugs	↓ maintenance dose of renally cleared drugs and drugs with renally cleared active metabolites
Renal blood flow	↓ 10% / decade	↓ clearance of some active metabolites	
Plasma flow at 80 years	↓ 50%		
Glomerular filtration rate	↓ 30–50%		
Creatinine clearance	↓ 50–70%		
CNS			
Cerebral blood flow and metabolism	↓ 20%	↓distribution to the CNS	Little net effect on dose
Cerebral volume	↓ 20%	↓ apparent volume in the brain	
Concentration response	↑ 50% for some opioids	↑ response to opioids	↓ bolus dose during titration

Source: Reproduced from Macintyre et al (2003). Reprinted by permission of Hodder Arnold.

CHAPTER 10

10.3.2 Physiology and perception of pain

Recent reviews by Gibson and Farrell (2004) and Gibson (2003) summarise the age-related changes that occur in pain perception and the neurophysiology of nociception.

In general, in the nervous system of the elderly person, there are extensive alterations in structure, neurochemistry and function of both peripheral and central nervous systems, including neurochemical deterioration of the opioid and serotonergic systems. Therefore there may be changes in nociceptive processing, including impairment of the pain inhibitory system.

There is a decrease in the density of both myelinated and unmyelinated peripheral nerve fibres, an increase in the number of sensory fibres with signs of damage or degeneration, a slowing of the conduction velocity and reductions in substance P, calcitonin gene-related peptide and somatostatin levels.

Similar structural and neurochemical changes have been noted in the central nervous system. In elderly humans there are sensory neuron degenerative changes and loss of myelin in the spinal cord; in the aged rat there are decreases in noradrenergic and serotonergic neurons in Lamina I and substance P and calcitonin gene-related peptide levels. Age-related loss of neurons and dendritic connections is seen in the human brain, particularly in the cerebral cortex including those areas involved in nociceptive processing; synthesis, axonal transport and receptor binding of neurotransmitters also change (Gibson 2003; Gibson & Farrell 2004). There is also reduced efficacy of endogenous analgesic systems with significantly smaller increases in pain threshold following prolonged noxious stimulation.

Variations in pain perception are best determined in controlled situations where severity of pathology is controlled and mood state is not an active variable. This can be done with experimental pain stimuli, or to a lesser extent, with standard medical procedures such as venipuncture and wound dressings.

Using experimental pain stimuli it can be shown that pain thresholds are generally increased in the elderly adult (Gibson 2003, **Level I**). Elderly people tend to have higher thresholds for thermal stimuli while results from mechanical stimulation are equivocal and there may be no change over the age groups with electrical stimuli. The significance of these observations in the clinical setting remains uncertain although they could indicate some deficit in the early warning function of pain. A decrease in pain threshold could narrow the gap between identification of the pain stimulus and recognition of a stimulus that might cause injury.

There are a number of clinical reports, summarised by Gibson (2003), suggesting that pain symptoms and presentation may change in the elderly patient. Reports of acute pain are commonly related to abdominal pain (eg associated with infection, peptic ulcer or intestinal obstruction), or chest pain (eg myocardial ischaemia or infarction) and are in general agreement with the experimental finding of increased pain thresholds in the elderly person. Compared with the younger adult with the same clinical condition, the elderly adult may report less pain, report it later or report no pain at all.

In patients with angina, controlled for disease severity and medication use and exercised to produce a 1mm ST depression, there was a longer time to onset of pain in elderly subjects (Miller et al 1990, **Level IV**, Ambepitiya et al 1993, **Level IV**). Elderly patients, matched for surgical procedure, also reported less pain in the postoperative period: pain intensity decreased by 10–20% each decade after 60 years of age (Thomas et al 1998, **Level IV**). Elderly men undergoing prostatectomy reported less pain on a present pain intensity scale and McGill Pain Questionnaire (but not a visual analogue scale [VAS]) in the immediate postoperative period and used less patient-controlled opioid analgesia than younger men undergoing the same procedure (Gagliese & Katz 2003, **Level III-2**). In a study of pain following placement of an IV cannula (a relatively standardised pain stimulus), elderly patients reported significantly less pain than younger patients (Li et al 2001, **Level IV**).

Studies looking at age-related changes in pain tolerance are limited but, in general and using a variety of experimental pain stimuli, there is a reduced ability in elderly people to endure or tolerate strong pain (Gibson 2003, **Level I**). This could mean that severe pain may have a greater impact on the elderly person.

10.3.3 Assessment of pain

Cognitive impairment

Undertreatment of acute pain is more likely to occur in cognitively impaired patients (Parmelee 1996; Bell 1997; Feldt et al 1998; Morrison & Siu 2000). The number of pain complaints and reported pain intensity decrease with increasing cognitive impairment (Parmelee et al 1993; Farrell et al 1996). Reasons for this could include a diminished memory, impairment of capacity to report, or it could be that less pain is experienced (Farrell et al 1996).

Delirium (confusion) is a common form of acute cognitive impairment in elderly people, especially during acute illnesses and in the postoperative setting (Bekker & Weeks 2003). Risk factors associated with the development of delirium include old age, infection, pre-existing dementia, pre-existing depression, hypoxaemia, anaemia, certain drugs (eg anticholinergic drugs, psychoactive drugs, benzodiazepines, opioids, some antiemetics), drug withdrawal (eg alcohol, benzodiazepines), fluid and electrolyte imbalance, and unrelieved pain (Bekker & Weeks 2003; Macintyre et al 2003).

Measurement of pain

Patient self-report measures of pain

Unidimensional measures of pain intensity (see Chapter 2) commonly used to quantify pain in the acute care setting include the VAS, verbal numerical rating scale (VNRS) and verbal descriptor scale (VDS), although visual and hearing impairments may cause occasional difficulties in elderly people (Workman et al 1989; Gagliese & Melzack 1997).

In a comparison of five pain scales in an experimental setting (the VAS, VNRS, numerical rating scale [NRS, a calibrated VAS], VDS and Faces Pain Scale), all the scales could effectively discriminate different levels of pain sensation in elderly people. However the

VDS was the most sensitive and reliable and considered to be the best choice in the elderly adult, including those with mild to moderate cognitive impairment, although it ranked second to the NRS for patient preference (Herr et al 2004, **Level III-2**). In the clinical setting, the VDS may also be a more reliable measure than the VAS or VNRS (Ferrell et al 1995; Gagliese & Melzack 1997, Gagliese & Katz 2003, **Level III-2**) but less reliable than the box scale (similar to the NRS) in both cognitively impaired and intact elderly patients (Chibnall & Tait 2001, **Level IV**).

Patients with mild to moderate cognitive impairment may need more time to understand and respond to questions regarding pain (Egbert 1996; Gagliese & Melzack 1997). Immediate reports of present pain may be reasonably accurate and as valid as those of cognitively intact patients (Parmelee et al 1993; Parmelee 1996) but recall of past pain is less likely to be as reliable (Parmelee et al 1993; Feldt et al 1998).

Other measures of pain

Assessment of pain in non-communicative patients is more difficult. Behaviours such as restlessness, frowning, and grimacing or sounds such as grunting or groaning have been used in attempts to assess pain severity (Bell 1997). In cognitively intact adults some of these behaviours have been shown to correlate reasonably well with patient self-report of pain (Bell 1997) but they may not always be valid indicators of pain in the non-verbal adult (Ferrell et al 1995; Farrell et al 1996). Clinician observations of facial expressions and sounds may be accurate measures of the presence of pain but not pain intensity in patients with advanced dementia (Manfredi at el 2003). Faces pain scales have also been used in cognitively impaired patients (Herr et al 2004).

10.3.4 Drugs used in the management of acute pain in elderly people

While sections 10.3.4 and 10.3.5 concentrate on the use of analgesic drugs and techniques in the elderly patient, as with other patients, physical and psychological strategies should also be employed.

CHAPTER 10

Non-steroidal anti-inflammatory drugs and paracetamol

Elderly patients are more likely to suffer adverse gastric and renal side effects following administration of NSAIDs and may also be more likely to develop cognitive dysfunction (Merry & Power 1995; Drage & Schug 1996; Phillips et al 1997; RCA 1998). Renal failure is of particular concern in elderly people, as they are more likely to have pre-existing renal impairment, cirrhosis, cardiac failure, or be using diuretic or antihypertensive medications (Drage & Schug 1996, RCA 1998). There is also greater potential for interactions with other drugs such as warfarin, low molecular weight heparin, oral hypoglycaemic agents, lithium, phenytoin, and drugs that are potentially nephrotoxic (eg aminoglycosides) (RCA 1998).

Selective COX-2 inhibitors have a significantly lower incidence of gastrointestinal complications and have no antiplatelet effects, which might be of some advantage in the elderly patient (Brooks & Day 2000). However, the incidence of other adverse effects including effects on renal function, are similar to non-selective NSAIDs (Brooks & Day 2000).

There is no consistent evidence on the effect of ageing on clearance of paracetamol but there is probably no need to reduce the dose given in elderly people (Divoll et al 1982; Miners et al 1988; Bannwarth et al 2001).

Opioids and tramadol

Dose-response in elderly people

Elderly patients require less opioid than younger patients, however, a large interpatient variability still exists and doses must be titrated to effect in all patients (Macintyre & Jarvis 1996, **Level IV**; Woodhouse & Mather 1997, **Level IV**; Vigano et al 1998, **Level IV**). The decrease is much greater than would be predicted by age-related alterations in physiology and seems to have a significant pharmacodynamic component (Macintyre et al 2003).

In the clinical setting there is evidence of an age-related 2–4-fold decrease in morphine and fentanyl requirements (Macintyre & Jarvis 1996, **Level IV**; Woodhouse & Mather 1997, **Level IV**; Gagliese et al 2000, **Level IV**). This is in agreement with the findings by Scott and Stanski (1987) that the sensitivity of the brain to fentanyl and alfentanil was increased by 50% in elderly people. The decrease in opioid requirement is not associated with reports of increased pain (Macintyre & Jarvis 1996, **Level IV**).

In patients over 75 years the elimination half-life of tramadol is slightly prolonged (Lee at al 1993), therefore lower daily doses may be required.

Opioid metabolites

Reduced renal function in the elderly patient could lead to a more rapid accumulation of active opioid metabolites (eg morphine-6-glucuronide, morphine-3-glucuronide, hydromorphone-3-glucuronide, nordextropropoxyphene, norpethidine, desmethyl-tramadol) (see Section 4.1).

Side effects of opioids

The fear of respiratory depression in elderly people, especially those with respiratory disease, often leads to inadequate doses of opioid being given for the treatment of their pain. However, as with other patients, significant respiratory depression can generally be avoided if appropriate monitoring (ie of sedation) is in place (see Section 4.1).

The incidence of nausea/vomiting and pruritus in the postoperative period lessens with increasing age (Quinn et al 1994). In elderly people, fentanyl may cause less depression of postoperative cognitive function than morphine and a trend towards less confusion (Herrick et al 1996, **Level II**). Some antiemetics, particularly those with anticholinergic properties, are more likely to cause side effects in elderly people (Egbert 1996).

Local anaesthetics

Age-related decreases in clearance and moderate increases in the terminal half-life of bupivacaine have been shown (Veering et al 1987; Veering et al 1991). Elderly patients are more sensitive to the effects of local anaesthetic agents because of a slowing of conduction velocity in peripheral nerves and a decrease in the number of neurons in the spinal cord (Saeden & Glass 2003).

Tricyclic antidepressants

Clearance of tricyclic antidepressant (TCA) drugs may decrease with increasing patient age and lower initial doses are recommended in elderly people (Bryson & Wilde 1996).

Elderly people may be particularly prone to the side effects of TCAs including sedation, confusion, orthostatic hypotension, dry mouth, constipation and urinary retention; adverse effects appear to be most common with amitriptyline (Bryson & Wilde 1996; Baron et al 1998). In addition, clinical conditions that may require TCAs to be administered with caution are more common in elderly people. These include prostatic hypertrophy, narrow angle glaucoma, cardiovascular disease and impaired liver function (Bryson & Wilde 1996). ECG abnormalities may be a contraindication to the use of TCAs in elderly people (Baron et al 1998).

Anticonvulsants

As liver and renal function decline with increasing age, elimination of anticonvulsants such as carbamazepine and gabapentin respectively may be reduced (Bernus et al 1997). As with TCAs, initial doses should be lower than for younger patients and any increases in dose should be titrated slowly (Drage & Schug 1996; Baron et al 1998).

Ketamine

There are no good data on the need or otherwise to alter ketamine doses in the elderly patient. In aged animals, however, there are changes in the composition of the NMDA receptor site and also a significant decrease in binding (Vuyk 2003). This suggests, apart from any pharmacokinetic changes, that ketamine doses may need to be lower in the elderly patient.

10.3.5 Patient-controlled analgesia

Many pharmacological and non-pharmacological treatments may be used in the management of acute pain in elderly people, either alone or in combination. However, differences between older and younger patients are more likely to be seen in treatments using analgesic drugs.

PCA is an effective method of pain relief in elderly people (Egbert et al 1990; Gagliese et al 2000; Mann et al 2000). To be used successfully, the patient needs to have reasonably normal cognitive function. Patients who have preoperative evidence of dementia or become confused postoperatively (more likely in the elderly patient) may not be suitable candidates for PCA.

Compared with IM morphine analgesia in elderly men, PCA resulted in better pain relief, less confusion and fewer severe pulmonary complications (Egbert et al 1990, **Level II**). In elderly patients PCA also resulted in significantly lower pain scores compared with intermittent subcutaneous (SC) morphine injections (Keita et al 2002, **Level II**).

10.3.6 Epidural analgesia

In the general patient population epidural analgesia can provide the most effective pain relief of all analgesic therapies used in the postoperative setting (see Section 7.2). Elderly patients given epidural PCA (using a mixture of bupivacaine and sufentanil) had lower pain scores at rest and movement, higher satisfaction scores and more rapid recovery of bowel function compared with those using IV PCA (Mann et al 2000, **Level II**).

Epidural opioid requirements decrease as patient age increases (Ready et al 1987). Closure of intervertebral foramina and increased epidural compliance in elderly patients also mean that there will be an increased spread of analgesia after administration of a fixed dose of local anaesthetic agent (Simon et al 2002; Vuyk 2003). Combinations of a local anaesthetic and opioid are commonly used for epidural analgesia so it would seem reasonable to use age-based doses or infusion rates when this combination is used.

Elderly patients may be more susceptible to some of the adverse effects of epidural analgesia, including hypotension (Crawford et al 1996; Simon et al 2002).

Key messages

1. Experimental pain thresholds to a variety of noxious stimuli are increased in elderly people but there is also a reduction in tolerance to pain (**Level I**).
2. PCA and epidural analgesia are more effective in elderly people than conventional opioid regimens (**Level II**).
3. Reported frequency and intensity of acute pain in clinical situations may be reduced in the elderly person (**Level III-2**).
4. Common unidimensional self-report measures of pain can be used in the elderly patient in the acute pain setting; in the clinical setting, the verbal descriptor scale may be more reliable than others (**Level III-2**).
5. There is an age-related decrease in opioid requirements; significant interpatient variability persists (**Level IV**).
6. The use of NSAIDs and COX-2 inhibitors in elderly people requires extreme caution; paracetamol is the preferred non-opioid analgesic (**Level IV**).

The following tick boxes ☑ represent conclusions based on clinical experience and expert opinion.

☑ The assessment of pain and evaluation of pain relief therapies in the elderly patient may present problems arising from differences in reporting, cognitive impairment and difficulties in measurement.

☑ Measures of present pain may be more reliable than past pain, especially in patients with some cognitive impairment.

☑ The physiological changes associated with ageing are progressive. While the rate of change can vary markedly between individuals, these changes may decrease the dose (maintenance and/or bolus) of drug required for pain relief and may lead to increased accumulation of active metabolites.

10.4 Aboriginal and Torres Strait Islander peoples

The appropriate assessment and treatment of pain in Aboriginal and Torres Strait Islander peoples needs to take into account a number of factors including cultural and language differences between the patient and health care worker. Unfortunately, there has been a lack of systematic study of pain in this group of Australians and so most information is anecdotal.

Despite having significant pain, some patients may present late depending on access to health care facilities and attitudes to Western biomedical models of health care. Honeyman and Jacob (1996, **Level IV**) studied back pain in a small Central Australian community and found that while prevalence was high in this non-urban community, it was uncommon for Aboriginal people to present with this complaint.

Stoic behaviour may lead to undertreatment of pain and cultural issues, including marked shyness with strangers (especially where there is a gender difference), gratuitous concurrence (saying 'yes' to be polite), different health belief systems and language differences, may complicate management (Howe et al 1998, **Level IV**). There could be a fear of hospitals due to past experiences with government services, cultural inappropriateness, institutional racism and a fear of dying in hospital.

Pain assessment by some conventional methods may not be appropriate. A verbal descriptor scale but not a numerical rating scale was a useful measure of pain (Sartain & Barry 1999, **Level III-3**). This is consistent with the fact that specific numbers and numerical scales are not part of many Aboriginal language systems. More descriptive terms are used for quantification. In a study of Aboriginal women after surgery, it was found that they had culturally appropriate ways of expressing and managing pain that were not well-understood by non-Aboriginal nurses (Fenwick & Stevens 2004).

Use of Aboriginal interpreters, health workers and liaison officers to assess pain is beneficial as in some cases English skills, although present, are limited and interpreters can help with non-verbal communication issues.

Aboriginal and Torres Strait Islander peoples can use PCA effectively if given adequate information about the technique. However, communication is often difficult and so techniques such as continuous opioid infusion techniques tend to be used more commonly in Aboriginal and Torres Strait Islander peoples than in other patient groups (Howe et al 1998, **Level IV**). In addition, consent for invasive procedures such as epidural analgesia may be difficult to obtain; there may be communication difficulties or the patient may need to discuss the proposed consent with other members of the family.

Medical comorbidities such as renal impairment are more common in Aboriginal and Torres Strait Islander peoples as well as New Zealand Maoris (Bramley et al 2004, **Level IV**; McDonald & Russ 2003, **Level IV**). This may affect the choice of analgesics (see Section 10.5).

Key messages

1. The verbal descriptor scale may be a better choice of pain measurement tool than verbal numerical rating scales (**Level III-3**).
2. Medical comorbidities such as renal impairment are more common in Aboriginal and Torres Strait Islander peoples and New Zealand Maoris, and may influence the choice of analgesic agent (**Level IV**).
3. Clinicians should be aware that pain may be under-reported by this group of patients (**Level IV**).

The following tick box ☑ represents conclusions based on clinical experience and expert opinion.

☑ Communication may be hindered by social, language and cultural factors.

10.5 OTHER ETHNIC GROUPS AND NON-ENGLISH SPEAKING PATIENTS

Australia is a culturally diverse nation with a relatively large immigrant population. In the 2001 Census 73% of people were born in Australia and English was the only language spoken at home by 80% of these. The three most common languages used at home other than English were Chinese languages (2.1%), Italian (1.9%) and Greek (1.4%).

There is a need to understand different cultures when considering pain assessment and management. This extends beyond the language spoken, because an individual's culture also influences their beliefs, expectations, methods of communication and norms of behaviour, as do the culture and attitudes of the health care provider (Green et al 2003; Davidhizar & Giger 2004).

It has been noted that communication problems may make it difficult to adequately help non-English speaking patients with interactive pain management (eg PCA use, requesting analgesia when needed), difficult to gain consent for invasive analgesic techniques (eg epidural or plexus catheters) and hard to assess their degree of pain (Howe et al 1998, **Level IV**).

It is important for clinicians to be aware of both verbal and non-verbal indicators of pain and be sensitive to both emotive and stoic behaviours in an individual's response.

Some cultural attitudes may limit pain-relief seeking behaviour. For example, it may be perceived by some patients as inappropriate to use a nurse's time to ask for analgesics or asking for pain relief may be seen as a weakness (Green et al 2003). When language is an obstacle, care should be used when enlisting non-professional interpreters to translate, because family members and friends of the patient may impose their own values when conveying the information to the clinician, and the patient may be reluctant to openly express themselves in front of people they know.

Strategies used to facilitate cross-cultural pain education and management include bilingual handouts describing varying methods of pain control and VAS scales with carefully chosen anchor terms or the use of faces scales (see Chapter 2); the numerical rating scale, for example has been translated and validated in many languages (Davidhizar & Giger 2004).

A series of pain scales in a number of different languages has been produced by the British Pain Society to assist in the assessment of people whose first language is not English. These are available at www.britishpainsociety.org/pain_scales.html.

One case series of 454 patients found that although prescription details of PCA varied with patient ethnicity, the actual self-administered doses of opioid were similar (Ng et al 1996, **Level IV**). Although limited, this series suggests that, provided patients are educated in use of PCA, it may help overcome some of the barriers to postoperative analgesia provision in a multicultural environment.

Key messages

1. Multilingual printed information and pain measurement scales are useful in managing patients from different cultural or ethnic backgrounds (**Level IV**).
2. With appropriate instruction, PCA may help overcome some of the barriers to postoperative analgesia provision in a multicultural environment (**Level IV**).

The following tick box ☑ represents conclusions based on clinical experience and expert opinion.

☑ Ethnic and cultural background can significantly affect the ability to assess and treat acute pain.

CHAPTER 10

10.6 The patient with obstructive sleep apnoea

Acute pain management in a patient with obstructive sleep apnoea (OSA) presents two main problems: choice of the most appropriate form of analgesia and the most suitable location in which to provide it. These difficulties arise primarily from the risk of exacerbating OSA by the administration of opioid analgesics.

Approximately 1 in 5 adults have at least mild OSA, 1 in 15 have moderate or worse OSA and 75–80% of those who could benefit from treatment remain undiagnosed (Young et al 2004). Therefore, many patients with undiagnosed OSA will have had treatment for acute pain without significant morbidity. This implies that the overall risk is quite low.

Evidence of the risks associated with analgesia and OSA is very limited. The use of opioid medications in patients with OSA appears to be a common factor in most cases where complications, including death, have been reported following intermittent IM, patient-controlled IV and epidural analgesia (Reeder et al 1991; VanDercar et al 1991; Etches 1994; Ostermeier et al 1997; Cullen 2001; Lofsky 2002; Parikh et al 2002). However, caution is required when interpreting these reports. Most of the cases involved what appear to be excessive opioid doses (eg excessive bolus dose or a background infusion with PCA) and/or inadequate monitoring (eg sedation levels were not checked and/or increasing sedation was not recognised as an early indicator of respiratory depression) and/or protocol failures and/or concurrent administration of sedatives.

A significantly higher incidence of serious postoperative complications and longer hospital stay after joint replacement surgery was reported in patients with OSA compared with matched controls (Gupta et al 2001, **Level III-3**). However, after outpatient surgery, a preoperative diagnosis of OSA was not associated with an increase in adverse events or unplanned hospital admission (Sabers et al 2003, **Level III-3**).

There has been no comparison of opioid and non-opioid analgesia for patients with OSA. Expert opinion, however, consistently suggests that non-opioid analgesics and regional techniques should be considered, either as an alternative to opioids or to help limit the amount of opioid required (Benumof 2001; Loadsman & Hillman 2001).

Morbid obesity is strongly associated with OSA (Young et al 2004) and the use of PCA with appropriate bolus doses and monitoring in morbidly obese patients has been reported to be no less safe than regional or other systemic opioid analgesic techniques, although the studies lacked power (Kyzer et al 1995, **Level II**; Choi et al 2000, **Level IV**; Charghi et al 2003, **Level IV**).

While oxygen therapy alone may not prevent the disruptions of sleep pattern or symptoms such as daytime somnolence and mental function that may occur in patients with OSA, it can reduce the likelihood of significant hypoxaemia (Phillips at el 1990; Landsberg et al 2001). As patients with OSA are more at risk of hypoxaemia after surgery or if given opioids, the use of supplemental oxygen would seem appropriate despite concerns about reducing respiratory drive during the apnoeic periods (Lofsky 2002).

The use of continuous positive airway pressure (CPAP) may help to reduce the postoperative risks and is recommended in patients with OSA (Benumof 2001; Loadsman & Hillman 2001). The effectiveness of CPAP (used appropriately) in the prevention of OSA in the postoperative setting is supported by case reports (Reeder et al 1991; Rennotte et al 1995; Mehta et al 2000). Concerns about the risk of CPAP causing gastric distension and anastomotic leaks after upper gastrointestinal surgery appear to be unfounded (Huerta et al 2002, **Level III-2**).

The effective use of CPAP in the setting of acute pain management may require a higher level of supervision than that available in the general surgical ward; most reports of the successful use of postoperative CPAP utilise extended periods of high-dependency nursing (Reeder et al 1991; Rennotte et al 1995; Mehta et al 2000). Advice on the most appropriate environment for the care of OSA patients requiring analgesia is based on expert opinion only and suggests that the severity of OSA, efficacy of any current therapy, relevant comorbidities (eg cardiac) and the analgesia required be taken into consideration (Benumof 2001; Loadsman & Hillman 2001).

Key messages

1. Patients with OSA may be at higher risk of complications after surgery and from opioid analgesia (**Level III-3**).
2. CPAP does not increase the risk of anastomotic leak after upper gastrointestinal surgery (**Level III-2**).

The following tick box ☑ represents conclusions based on clinical experience and expert opinion.

☑ Management strategies that may increase the efficacy and safety of pain relief in patients with OSA include the provision of appropriate multimodal opioid-sparing analgesia, CPAP, monitoring and supervision (in a high-dependency area if necessary) and supplemental oxygen.

10.7 THE PATIENT WITH CONCURRENT HEPATIC OR RENAL DISEASE

The clinical efficacy of most analgesic drugs is altered by impaired renal or hepatic function, not simply because of altered clearance of the parent drug, but also through accumulation of toxic or therapeutically active metabolites. Some analgesic agents can aggravate pre-existing renal and hepatic disease, causing direct damage and thus altering their metabolism.

A brief summary of the effects that renal or hepatic disease may have on some of the drugs used in pain management, as well as alterations that might be required in analgesic drug regimens, is given in Tables 10.9 and 10.10.

10.7.1 Patients with renal disease

The degree to which analgesic drug regimens require alteration in patients with renal impairment depends to a large extent on whether the drug has active metabolites that are dependent on the kidney for excretion or if the drug may further impair renal function. The available data indicates the following (see Table 10.9 for references).

- Analgesics that exhibit the safest pharmacological profile in patients with renal impairment are alfentanil, buprenorphine, fentanyl, ketamine, paracetamol (except with compound analgesics) and sufentanil. None of these drugs deliver a high active metabolite load or have a significantly prolonged clearance.
- Oxycodone can usually be used without any dose adjustment in patients with renal impairment as oxymorphone, one of its main metabolites, is only weakly active and contributes minimally to any clinical effect.

- Amitriptyline, bupivacaine, levobupivacaine, lignocaine (lidocaine), clonidine, gabapentin, codeine, hydromorphone, methadone, morphine and tramadol have been used in patients with renal disease, but, depending on the degree of impairment, may require a reduction in dose. Levobupivacaine, with similar clearance mechanisms, may be safer than bupivacaine because of a higher therapeutic ratio. Ropivacaine has not been studied in patients with significant renal disease.
- NSAIDs, dextropropoxyphene and pethidine should not be used in the presence of significant renal impairment.

10.7.2 Patients with hepatic disease

Not all patients with hepatic disease have impaired liver function. In patients with hepatic impairment, most analgesic drugs have reduced clearance and increased oral bioavailability, but the significance of these changes in the clinical setting has not been studied in depth. The available data indicates the following (see Table 10.10 for references).

- Sufentanil clearance is unlikely to be impaired with uncomplicated mild cirrhosis.
- Tramadol may need to be given at lower doses.
- Methadone is contraindicated in the presence of severe liver disease because of the potential for greatly prolonged clearance.
- The clearance of local anaesthetics may be significantly impaired; they should be administered cautiously and in decreased doses.
- Carbamazepine and valproate should be avoided as the risk of fulminant hepatic failure is higher in this population.
- Paracetamol may accumulate unpredictably and lead to hepatic necrosis. If it is used in the presence of mild cirrhosis there should be regular monitoring of hepatic function. The drug should be avoided in patients with greater degrees of hepatic impairment.

Key messages

The following tick box ☑ represents conclusions based on clinical experience and expert opinion.

☑ Consideration should be given to choice and dose regimen of analgesic agents in patients with hepatic and particularly renal impairment.

Table 10.8 Analgesic drugs in patients with renal impairment

Drug	Comments	Recommendations *NB doses must still be titrated to effect for each patient*	References
Opioids			
Alfentanil	No active metabolites 92% protein bound; increases in free fraction may result from alterations in protein binding	No dose adjustment required.	Davies et al 1996 Mercadante & Arcuri 2004
Buprenorphine	Inactive and weakly active (norbuprenorphine) metabolites; predominantly biliary excretion	No dose adjustment required	Davies et al 1996 Mercadante & Arcuri 2004
Codeine	Prolonged sedation and respiratory arrest have been reported in patients with renal impairment Neuro-excitation may occur at standard doses.	Dose adjustment recommended Recommend using an alternative agent where possible	Davies et al 1996 Mercadante & Arcuri 2004
Dextro-propoxyphene	Accumulation of active metabolite (nordextropropoxyphene) can lead to CNS and CVS toxicity	Dose adjustment recommended Use of alternative agent recommended	Mercadante & Arcuri 2004 AMH 2004
Dihydrocodeine	Metabolic pathway probably similar to codeine	Insufficient evidence: use not recommended	Davies et al 1996
Fentanyl	No active metabolites	No dose adjustment required	Mercadante & Arcuri 2004
Hydromorphone	Neurotoxicity from accumulation of H3G possible	Dose adjustment recommended Recommend alternative agent if high doses likely to be needed	Mercadante & Arcuri 2004 Babul et al 1995
Methadone	Predominantly inactive metabolites but 20% excreted unchanged via kidneys	Dose adjustment recommended in severe renal impairment	Davies et al 1996 Mercadante & Arcuri 2004

CHAPTER 10

Drug	Comments	Recommendations *NB doses must still be titrated to effect for each patient*	References
Morphine	Major metabolites M3G and M6G excreted via kidney. M6G is an opioid agonist; delayed sedation from M6G has been reported in renal failure Neurotoxicity from accumulation of M3G possible Oral administration results in proportionally higher metabolite load Morphine and its metabolites are cleared during haemodialysis but are not significantly affected by continuous ambulatory peritoneal dialysis (has similar clearance values to end stage renal failure)	Dose adjustment recommended Recommend alternative agent if high doses likely to be needed	Davies et a 1996 Mercadante & Arcuri 2004 D'Honneur et al 1994 Mercadante et al 1997 Angst et al 2000 Richtsmeier et al 1997 Hanna al 1993 Pauli-Magnus et al 1999
Oxycodone	Main metabolites are noroxycodone and oxymorphone; oxymorphone is weakly active but with minimal clinical effect	No dose adjustment required	AMH 2004
Pethidine	Accumulation of norpethidine can lead to neuroexcitation including seizures	Dose adjustment required Use of alternative agent recommended	Stone et al 1993 Davies et al 1996 Simopoulos et al 2002 Mercadante & Arcuri 2004
Sufentanil	Minimally active metabolite	No dose adjustment required	Davis et al 1988 AMH 2004
Tramadol	Increased tramadol-like effects from active metabolite O-desmethyltramadol (M1)	Dose adjustment recommended Use of alternative agent recommended with significant renal impairment	Mercadante & Arcuri 2004 MIMS 2004

Drug	Comments	Recommendations *NB doses must still be titrated to effect for each patient*	References
Other drugs			
Local anaesthetics	Increases in free fraction may result from alterations in protein binding No significant difference in plasma concentration of levobupivacaine (axillary block), bupivacaine (supraclavicular block), lignocaine (lidocaine) (interscalene block) in patients with chronic renal failure	Risk of toxicity may be affected by abnormalities in acid-base balance and/or potassium levels	Crews et al I 2002 Rice et al 1991 McEllistrem et al 1989
NSAIDs & COX-2 inhibitors	Can affect renal function	Use with caution in patients with mild renal impairment and avoid in patients with severe renal impairment	Royal College of Anaesthetists 1999
Clonidine	Half-life is increased in severe renal failure 50% metabolised by the liver; remained excreted unchanged by the kidney	Dose adjustment recommended	Lowenthakl et al 1993 Khan et al 1999
Tricyclic antidepressants	Amitriptyline is metabolised in the liver to nortriptyline, the active agent.	Limited data; metabolite accumulation may increased the risk of side effects	Liebermann et al 1985
Ketamine	Dehydronorketamine levels are increased but it has only 1% of potency of ketamine	Limited data; probable that no dose adjustment is required	Koppel et al 1990
Gabapentin	Impaired renal function results in higher plasma levels and longer elimination half-life	Dose adjustment recommended on basis of creatinine clearance	Blum et al 1994

Table 10.9 Analgesic drugs in patients with hepatic impairment

Drug	Comments	Recommendations *NB doses must still be titrated to effect for each patient*	References
Opioids			
Alfentanil	No significant difference in half-life found in children undergoing liver transplant	Limited data: no dose adjustment required	Davis et al 1989
Dextro-propoxyphene	Reduced oxidation leading to reduced clearance	Limited data: dose adjustment may be required	Tegeder et al 1999
Fentanyl	Disposition appears to be unaffected	Limited data: no dose adjustment required	Tegeder et al 1999
Morphine	Hepatic impairment does not appear to have a significant effect on morphine pharmacokinetics; even in patients with cirrhosis there is a large hepatic reserve for glucuronidation Increased oral bioavailability of morphine due to its normal high first pass metabolism when given via this route	In most patients no dose adjustment required	Mercadante & Arcuri 2004 Kaiko 1991
Pethidine	Reduced oxidation leading to reduced clearance	Limited data: dose adjustment may be required; use not recommended	Tegeder et al 1999
Sufentanil	No difference in clearance or elimination	No dose adjustment required	Chauvin et al 1989 Tegeder et al 1999
Tramadol	Reduced oxidation leading to reduced clearance	Limited data: dose adjustment may be required	Tegeder et al 1999

Drug	Comments	Recommendations *NB doses must still be titrated to effect for each patient*	References
Other drugs			
Local anaesthetics	Amide-type local anaesthetics undergo hepatic metabolism and clearance may be reduced in hepatic disease	Limited data: dose adjustment may be required with prolonged use	Bodenham & Park 1990
Paracetamol	Metabolised in the liver; small proportion metabolised to the potentially hepatotoxic metabolite *N*-acetyl-*p*-benzoquinonemine. This is normally inactivated by hepatic glutathione. Clearance is reduced.	Should be used with caution or in reduced doses with active liver disease, alcohol-related liver disease and glucose-6-phosphate dehydrogenase deficiency	al-Swayeh et al 2000 Moore&Marshall 2003 Romero-Sandoval et al 2003 Futter et al 2001 Zapater et al 2004
Carbemazepine	Hepatic enzymes are raised in about 6% of patients treated; has been reported to cause hepatic failure (rare). Primarily metabolised in the liver.	Dose adjustment may be required; use not recommended in severe hepatic impairment	Hadzic et al 1990 AMH 2004
Valproate	Abnormalities in liver function have been reported in up to 44% of patients; has been reported to cause hepatic failure (rare).	Dose adjustment may be required; use not recommended in severe hepatic impairment	Thompson et al 2000 Caparros-Lefebvre et al 1993

10.8 THE OPIOID-TOLERANT PATIENT

10.8.1 Definitions

Misunderstandings in the terminology related to substance abuse (see Section 10.9), tolerance, addiction and physical dependence may confuse health care providers and lead to inappropriate and/or suboptimal pain management. With this in mind, consensus statements with agreed definitions for addiction, tolerance and physical dependence have been developed by the American Pain Society, the American Academy of Pain Medicine and the American Society of Addiction Medicine (American Acad Pain Med et al 2004).

Table 10.10 Definitions for tolerance, physical dependence, addiction and substance abuse

Tolerance	A decrease in the effect of a drug over time so that a progressive increase in the amount of that drug is required to achieve the same effect. Tolerance develops to desired (eg analgesia) and undesired (eg euphoria, opioid-related sedation, nausea or constipation) effects at different rates.
Physical dependence	A physiological adaptation to a drug whereby abrupt discontinuation or reversal of that drug, or a sudden reduction in its dose, leads to a withdrawal (abstinence) syndrome. Withdrawal can be terminated by administration of the same or similar drug.
Addiction	A disease that is characterised by aberrant drug-seeking and drug-taking behaviours that may include cravings, compulsive drug use and loss of control over drug use, despite the risk of physical, social and psychological harm. While psychoactive drugs have an addiction liability, psychological, social and genetic factors may play a more important role in the development of addiction than exposure to the drug alone.
Pseudoaddiction	Behaviours that may seem inappropriately drug-seeking but are a result of undertreatment of pain and resolve when pain relief is adequate.
Substance abuse disorder	When the extent and pattern of substance use interferes with the psychological and sociocultural integrity of the person. For example, there may be recurring problems with social and personal interactions or with the legal system, recurrent failures to fulfil work or family obligations, or patients may find themselves in physically hazardous situations.

Source: Weissman & Haddox (1989), American Psychiatric Association (1994), Jage & Bey (2000a), American Academy of Pain Medicine et al (2004) and Mitra & Sinatra (2004).

10.8.2 Patient groups

Three main groups of opioid-tolerant patients are encountered in surgical and other acute pain settings:

- patients with chronic cancer or non-cancer pain being treated with opioids, some of whom (up to 19%) may exhibit features opioid addiction (Fishbain et al 1992);
- patients with a substance abuse disorder either using illicit opioids or on an opioid maintenance treatment program (see Section 10.9);
- patients who have developed acute opioid tolerance due to perioperative opioid administration, particularly opioids of high potency; and
- recognition of the presence of opioid tolerance may not be possible if the patient's history is not available or accurate. If a patient is requiring much larger than expected opioid doses and other factors that might be leading to the high requirements have been excluded, opioid tolerance should be considered.

CHAPTER 10

10.8.3 Managing acute pain in opioid-tolerant patients

Evidence for the most appropriate management of acute pain in opioid-tolerant patients is limited and advice is based primarily on comparative studies, case series, case reports and expert opinion. In all cases, close liaison with other treating clinicians is required.

Long-term use of opioids results in tolerance to the some of the effects of opioids including analgesia, nausea, sedation and respiratory depression but not to miosis or constipation (Mitra & Sinatra 2004, **Level IV**). Cross-tolerance with other opioids also occurs (Jage & Bey 2000a).

Opioid requirements are therefore usually significantly higher in opioid-tolerant patients. After a variety of surgical procedures, opioid-tolerant patients using PCA required approximately three times more opioid than their opioid-naive counterparts (de Leon-Casasola et al 1993, **Level III-2**; Rapp et al 1995, **Level III-2**).

Opioid-tolerant patients have been shown, in the experimental setting, to be relatively pain intolerant and show increased sensitivity with cold pressor and thermal testing (Doverty et al 2001, **Level III-2**).

Opioid-tolerant patients reported higher pain scores (both resting and dynamic) and remained under the care of acute pain services longer than other patients (Rapp et al 1995, **Level III-2**). Compared with opioid-tolerant patients with cancer pain, opioid-tolerant patients with non-cancer pain had higher rest and dynamic pain scores and required longer acute pain service input, but there was no difference in opioid requirements (Rapp et al 1995, **Level III-2**). In addition, staff relied more on functional measures of pain than on pain scores to assess pain intensity in these patients (Rapp et al 1994, **Level IV**).

The incidence of opioid-induced nausea and vomiting may be lower in opioid-tolerant patients although the risk of excessive sedation may be higher; in part this could be due to the greater use of sedatives in opioid-tolerant patients in this study (Rapp et al 1995, **Level III-2**).

Management of these patients should focus on (Jage & Bey 2000a):

- prevention of withdrawal;
- effective analgesia; and
- symptomatic treatment of affective disorders and behavioural disturbances.

Intravenous PCA is a useful modality for pain relief in opioid-tolerant patients, provided that pain intensity and opioid consumption are carefully monitored and background requirements are provided if the patient cannot take their usual opioid; larger bolus doses will often be needed (Macintyre & Ready 2001; Mitra & Sinatra 2004, **Level IV**). Opioid rotation (ie using an opioid that is different from their preadmission opioid) may be of use particularly with an agent of higher intrinsic opioid agonist activity (de Leon-Casasola & Lema 1994, **Level IV**).

Withdrawal from opioids should be prevented by maintenance of normal preadmission opioid regimens where possible, or appropriate substitutions with another opioid or the same opioid via another route (Mitra & Sinatra 2004). It may be of benefit to check preadmission opioid doses with the patient's doctor or pharmacist; the use of unauthorised additional opioids (licit or illicit) or of lower doses than prescribed, may affect both pain relief and the risk of adverse effects.

Neuraxial opioids have been used effectively in opioid-tolerant patients; although higher doses may be required and may not result in an increase in adverse effects (Wang 1979, **Level IV**). Effective analgesia using intrathecal or epidural opioids will not necessarily prevent symptoms of opioid withdrawal (de Leon-Casasola 1994, **Level IV**; Mitra & Sinatra 2004).

Ketamine may reduce opioid requirements in opioid-tolerant patients (Bell 1999, **Level IV**; Eilers et al 2001, **Level IV**; Sator-Katzenschlager et al 2001, **Level IV**).

While multimodal analgesic regimens (eg NSAIDs, paracetamol, ketamine, tramadol, regional analgesia) will be of benefit, opioid-tolerant patients are at risk of opioid withdrawal if a purely non-opioid analgesic regimen or tramadol is used (Thomas & Suresh 2000; Mitra & Sinatra 2004) (see also Section 10.9). For this reason opioid antagonists (naloxone, naltrexone) or mixed agonist-antagonists (eg buprenorphine, pentazocine) should be also avoided as their use may precipitate acute withdrawal reactions (Mitra & Sinatra 2004).

Discharge planning must take into account the potential for prescribed opioids to be abused or misused. Appropriate use of non-opioid analgesic where possible, communication with the primary physician and patient education and support must all be considered.

Key messages

1. Opioid-tolerant patients report higher pain scores and have a lower incidence of opioid-induced nausea and vomiting (**Level III-2**).
2. Ketamine may reduce opioid requirements in opioid-tolerant patients **(Level IV)**.

The following tick boxes ☑ represent conclusions based on clinical experience and expert opinion.

☑ Usual preadmission opioid regimens should be maintained where possible or appropriate substitutions made.

☑ Opioid-tolerant patients are at risk of opioid withdrawal if non-opioid analgesic regimens or tramadol alone are used.

☑ PCA settings may need to include a background infusion to replace the usual opioid dose and a higher bolus dose.

☑ Neuraxial opioids can be used effectively in opioid-tolerant patients although higher doses may be required and these doses may be inadequate to prevent withdrawal.

☑ Liaison with all clinicians involved in the treatment of the opioid-tolerant patient is important.

10.9 THE PATIENT WITH A SUBSTANCE ABUSE DISORDER

A substance abuse disorder (SAD) exists when the extent and pattern of substance use interferes with the psychological and sociocultural integrity of the person. For example, there may be recurring problems with social and personal interactions or with the legal system, recurrent failures to fulfil work or family obligations, or patients with SAD may find themselves in physically hazardous situations (eg driving a car while under the influence of the substance), also putting others at risk (American Psychiatric Association 1994).

Effective management of acute pain in patients with SAD may be complex due to (Jage & Bey 2000a):

- psychological and behavioural characteristics associated with a substance abuse disorder;
- presence of the drug (or drugs) of abuse;
- medications used to assist with drug withdrawal and/or rehabilitation;
- complications related to drug abuse including organ impairment and infectious diseases; and
- the presence of tolerance, physical dependence and the risk of withdrawal.

Evidence for the most appropriate management of acute pain in patients with SAD is limited and advice is based primarily on case series, case reports and expert opinion.

Effective analgesia may be difficult, may be required for longer periods than in other patients and often requires significant deviations from 'standard' treatment protocols (Jage & Bey 2000a). In addition, ethical dilemmas can arise as a result of the need to balance concerns of undermedication against anxieties about safety and possible abuse or diversion of the drugs (Mitra & Sinatra 2004). In all cases, close liaison with other treating clinicians and drug and alcohol services is required.

The first step in managing patients with SAD is identifying the problem, although obtaining an accurate history can sometimes be difficult. Polysubstance abuse is common and many of these patients will use drugs from different groups, the most common of which include central nervous system (CNS) depressant drugs such as alcohol, opioids and benzodiazepines, or CNS-stimulant drugs including cocaine, amphetamines (amfetamines) and amphetamine-like drugs, cannabis and other hallucinogens; the group from which the drugs come determines their withdrawal characteristics (if any) and their interaction with acute pain therapy (Jage & Bey 2000a; Mitra & Sinatra 2004).

Management of pain in patients with SAD should focus on (Jage & Bey 2000a):

- prevention of withdrawal;
- effective analgesia; and
- symptomatic treatment of affective disorders and behavioural alterations.

Pain management in patients with a SAD often presents significant challenges with respect to their fears, expectations and responses to interventions. Inappropriate behaviours can be prevented to a significant extent by the development of a respectful, honest and open approach to communication which includes an understanding that complete relief of pain may not be a realistic goal.

10.9.1 CNS depressant drugs

Although not inevitable, abuse of CNS-depressant drugs (eg opioids, alcohol) is associated with physical dependence and the development of tolerance (Jage & Bey 2000a) (see Section 10.8). Withdrawal from CNS-depressant drugs produces symptoms of CNS and autonomic hyperexcitability, the opposite of the effects of the CNS-depressant drugs themselves (Jage & Bey 2000a).

Opioids

Long-term use of opioids results in tolerance to some of the effects of opioids including analgesia, nausea, sedation and respiratory depression, but not to miosis or constipation (Mitra & Sinatra 2004). Cross-tolerance with other opioids occurs although the degree is inconsistent; there is no cross-tolerance with benzodiazepines or alcohol (Jage & Bey 2000a). See Section 10.8 for managing acute pain in opioid-tolerant patients.

Withdrawal from opioids is characterised by excitatory and autonomic symptoms including abdominal cramping, muscle aches and pain, insomnia, dysphoria, anxiety, restlessness, nausea and vomiting, diarrhoea, rhinorrhea and sneezing, trembling, yawning, runny eyes and piloerection or 'gooseflesh' (Jage & Bey 2000a). Unlike withdrawal from alcohol or benzodiazepines (see below), withdrawal from opioids alone does not result in seizures.

The time of onset of withdrawal symptoms after cessation of the drug will depend on the duration of action of the opioid.

Alcohol and benzodiazepines

There is no cross-tolerance between opioids and alcohol or benzodiazepines and there is therefore no pharmacological reason to use higher than 'standard' initial opioid doses in patients with an alcohol or benzodiazepine SAD (Jage & Bey 2000a). Benzodiazepines exhibit cross-tolerance with alcohol and are commonly used in managing alcohol withdrawal (Shand et al 2003).

Alcohol and/or benzodiazepine abuse is relatively common and prevention of withdrawal should be a clinical priority in all patients.

Alcohol

Alcohol withdrawal may occur as soon as 6–24 hours after alcohol intake is ceased; excitation and autonomic hyperactivity occurs leading to tremors, increases in heart and respiratory rates and blood pressure, nausea and vomiting, hyperthermia, sweating, anxiety, agitation, confusion and auditory, visual disturbances including hallucinations and seizures (Shand et al 2003).

Benzodiazepines

The pattern of withdrawal symptoms from benzodiazepines is similar to that of alcohol withdrawal; features of benzodiazepine withdrawal include myoclonic jerks and seizures. The time interval between cessation of the drug and the onset of withdrawal will vary according to the duration of action of the benzodiazepine (more likely following abrupt cessation of drugs with a short half life). Adequate benzodiazepine replacement should be provided to prevent withdrawal (Mitra & Sinatra 2004).

Cannabinoids

Cannabinoids, the active components in marijuana, have been shown to interact with opioid-mediated analgesia and may lead to increased sedation (Kumar et al 2001, **Level IV**; Pertwee 2001, **Level IV**). However, there is little support for reduced or increased opioid requirements in patients chronically exposed to cannabis (Kumar et al 2001). Significant withdrawal syndromes associated with abrupt cessation of cannabis use are infrequent (Jage & Bey 2000a).

10.9.2 CNS stimulant drugs

Abuse of CNS-stimulant drugs (eg cocaine, amphetamines [amfetamines], ecstasy) is associated with a psychological rather than physical dependence and only a low degree of tolerance; these drugs do not exhibit any cross-tolerance with opioids (with the possible exception of cannabinoids; see below) and while behavioural and autonomic effects are seen during acute exposure, withdrawal symptoms are predominantly affective rather than physical (Jage & Bey 2000b). There is no pharmacological reason for the use of higher than usual initial opioid doses (Jage & Bey 2000b).

10.9.3 Drugs used in the treatment of substance abuse disorders

Methadone

Methadone is a long-acting pure opioid agonist used in the management of patients with an opioid SAD. In the acute pain setting (where possible) methadone should be continued as usual at the same dose. If there is any doubt about the dose, it may be prudent to give half the reported dose and repeat in 6–8 hours if needed and if the patient is not sedated. If the patient is unable to take methadone by mouth, substitution with parenteral methadone or other opioids will be required in the short term (Jage & Bey 2000a; Mitra & Sinatra 2004).

Naltrexone

Naltrexone is used in the management of patients with an opioid or alcohol SAD. The usual maintenance dose is 25–50mg daily.

Naltrexone is an orally administered pure opioid antagonist that binds to opioid receptors for over 24 hours following a single dose, which can create difficulties in the acute pain setting. In humans, the half-time of brain opioid receptor blockade by naltrexone, measured by radioactive carfentanil binding, was between 72 and 108 hours (Lee et al 1988, **Level IV**).

There is experimental evidence of μ-opioid receptor upregulation following antagonist withdrawal (Millan et al 1988) and abrupt discontinuation of naltrexone may therefore lead to a period of increased opioid sensitivity.

It has been recommended that, where possible, naltrexone be stopped for at least 24 hours before surgery (Jage & Bey 2000a, Mitra & Sinatra 2004). In these patients and in patients requiring surgery within this 24-hour period, multimodal analgesic regimens (eg NSAIDs, paracetamol, ketamine, tramadol and regional analgesia) should also be employed. In patients having dental surgery and pretreated with either naltrexone or placebo, ibuprofen was, not surprisingly, more effective than codeine or placebo in those patients who had been given naltrexone (Hersh et al 1993, **Level II**).

As the effect of naltrexone diminishes after it has been ceased, the amount of opioid required to maintain analgesia may also need to be decreased in order to avoid signs of excessive opioid dose (in particular, respiratory depression).

Reintroduction of naltrexone should be done in consultation with the prescribing practitioner.

Buprenorphine

Buprenorphine is a partial opioid agonist used in the treatment of opioid addiction and is commonly prescribed in doses of 8–32mg (Roberts & Meyer-Witting, in press).

There are no good data on which to base the management of patients on buprenorphine maintenance programs requiring pain relief. In elective surgery, a decision needs be made whether or not to continue buprenorphine. If it is to be stopped, conversion to another opioid (eg methadone) would be required; this is a potentially complicated procedure (Roberts & Meyer-Witting, in press).

Continuation of buprenorphine has been suggested although it may be difficult to obtain good analgesia with full agonist opioids. Multimodal analgesic strategies, including opioid agonists (eg fentanyl, morphine) should be used (Mitra & Sinatra 2004; Roberts & Meyer-Witting, in press).

Close liaison with all treating clinicians and drug and alcohol services should occur. If buprenorphine has been ceased, its reintroduction should be managed in consultation with the prescribing practitioner.

10.9.4 Recovering patients

Patients in drug-free recovery may be concerned about the risk of relapse into the active SAD if they are given opioids for the management of their acute pain (Jage & Bey 2000b). Effective communication and planning, the use of multimodal analgesic strategies, reassurance that the risk of reversion to an active SAD is small, and information that ineffective analgesia can paradoxically lead to relapses in recovering patients, are important and help avoid under treatment (Jage & Bey 2000a, Mitra & Sinatra 2004).

Key messages

The following tick boxes ☑ represent conclusions based on clinical experience and expert opinion.

☑ Naltrexone should be stopped at least 24 hours prior to elective surgery.

☑ Patients who have completed naltrexone therapy should be regarded as opioid naïve; in the immediate post-treatment phase they may be opioid-sensitive.

☑ Maintenance methadone regimens should be continued where possible.

☑ Buprenorphine maintenance may be continued; if buprenorphine is ceased prior to surgery conversion to an alternative opioid is required.

☑ There is no cross-tolerance between CNS stimulants and opioids.

REFERENCES

ACOG (2002) Clinical management guidelines for obstetrician-gynecologists. Obstetric analgesia and anesthesia. *ACOG Practice Bulletin* 100: 177–91.

ADEC (1999) *Prescribing Medicines in Pregnancy*. 4th Edition. Canberra: Australian Drug Evaluation Committee. Copyright Commonwealth of Australia.

Alano MA, Ngougmna E, Ostrea EM at al (2001) Analysis of nonsteroidal antiinflammatory drugs in meconium and its relation to persistent pulmonary hypertension of the newborn *Pediatrics* 107: 519–23.

Albers L, Garcia J, Renfew M et al (1999) Distribution of genital tract trauma in childbirth and related postnatal pain. *Birth* 26: 11–15.

Allen DC, Jorgensen C, Sims C (1999) Effect of tropisetron on vomiting during patient-controlled analgesia in children. *Br J Anaesth* 83: 608–10.

Ambepitiya GB, Iyengar EN, Roberts ME (1993) Review: silent myocardial exertional myocardial ischaemia and perception of angina in elderly people. *Age Ageing* 22: 302–07.

Ambuel B, Hamlett KW, Marx CM et al (1992) Assessing distress in pediatric intensive care environments: the COMFORT scale. *J Pediatr Psychol* 17: 95–109.

American Academy of Pain Medicine, American Pain Society, American Society of Addiction Medicine (2004) *Definitions Related to the Use of Opioids for the Treatment of Pain 2001*. (www.ampainsoc.org/advocacy/opioids2.htm).

American Psychiatric Association (1994) *Diagnostic and Statistical Manual of Mental Disorders*. 4th edition, Washington DC: American Psychiatric Association.

AMH (2004) *Australian Medicines Handbook*. Adelaide: Australian Medicines Handbook Pty Ltd.

Amir LH (2003) Breast pain in lactating women-mastitis or something else? *Aus Fam Phys* 2: 141–45.

Anderson B, Kanagasundarum S, Woollard G (1996) Analgesic efficacy of paracetamol in children using tonsillectomy as a pain model. *Anaesth Int Care* 24: 669–73.

Anderson BJ, Holford NH, Woollard GA et al (1999) Perioperative pharmacodynamics of acetaminophen analgesia in children. *Anesthesiology* 90: 411–21.

Anderson BJ, van Lingen RA, Hansen TG et al (2002) Acetaminophen developmental pharmacokinetics in premature neonates and infants: a pooled population analysis. *Anesthesiology* 96: 1336–45.

Anderson BJ (2004) Comparing the efficacy of NSAIDs and paracetamol in children. *Paediatr Anaesth* 14: 201–17.

Angst MS, Bührer M, Lötsch J (2000) Insidious intoxication after morphine treatment in renal failure: delayed onset of morphine-6-glucuronide action. *Anesthesiology* 92: 1473–76.

Annequin D, Carbajal R, Chauvin P, Gall O et al (2000) Fixed 50% nitrous oxide oxygen mixture for painful procedures: a French survey. *Pediatrics* 105: E47.

Ansermino M, Basu R, Vandebeek C et al (2003) Nonopioid additives to local anaesthetics for caudal blockade in children: a systematic review. *Paediatr Anaesth* 13: 561–73.

Antok E, Bordet F, Duflo F et al (2003) Patient-controlled epidural analgesia versus continuous epidural infusion with ropivacaine for postoperative analgesia in children. *Anesth Analg* 97: 1608–11.

Arana A, Morton NS, Hansen TG (2001) Treatment with paracetamol in infants. *Acta Anaesth Scand* 45: 20–29.

Asling JH, Shnider SM, Margolis AJ et al (1970) Paracervical block anesthesia in obstetrics. II. Etiology of fetal bradycardia following paracervical block anesthesia. *Am J Obstet Gynecol* 107: 626–34.

Babul N, Darke AC, Hagen N (1995) Hydromorphone metabolite accumulation in renal failure. *J Pain Sympt Manage* 3: 184–86.

Bailham D & Joseph S (2003) Post-traumatic stress following childbirth: a review of the emerging literature and directions for research and practice. *Psych, Health & Med* 8: 159–68.

Bannwarth B, Pehourcq F, Lagrange F et al (2001) Single and multiple dose pharmacokinetics of acetaminophen (paracetamol) in polymedicated very old patients with rheumatic pain. *J Rheumatol* 28: 182-4.

Baron R, Wasner G, Lindner V (1998) Optimal treatment of phantom limb pain in the elderly. *Drugs Aging*12: 361–76.

Bar-Oz B, Bulkowstein M, Benyamini L et al (2003) Use of antibiotic and analgesic drugs during lactation. *Drug Saf* 26: 925–35.

Beasley SW & Tibballs J (1987) Efficacy and safety of continuous morphine infusion for postoperative analgesia in the paediatric surgical ward. *Aust N Z J Surg* 57: 233–37.

Bekker AY & Weeks EJ (2003) Cognitive function after anaesthesia in the elderly. *Best Pract Res Clin Anaesthesiol* 17: 259–72.

Bell ML (1997) Postoperative pain management for the cognitively impaired older adult. *Sem Periop Nurs* 6: 37–41.

Bell RF (1999) Low-dose subcutaneous ketamine infusion and morphine tolerance. *Pain* 83: 101–03.

Benumof JL (2001) Obstructive sleep apnea in the adult obese patient: implications for airway management. *J Clin Anesth* 13: 144–56.

Berde CB, Lehn, BM et al (1991) Patient-controlled analgesia in children and adolescents: a randomized, prospective comparison with intramuscular administration of morphine for postoperative analgesia. *J Pediatr* 118: 460–66.

Berde CB (1992) Convulsions associated with pediatric regional anesthesia. *Anesth Analg* 75: 164–66.

Berghella V, Lim PJ, Hill MK et al (2003) Maternal methadone dose and neonatal withdrawal. *Am J Obstet Gynecol* 189: 312–17.

Bernus B, Dickinson RG, Hooper WD et al (1997) Anticonvulsant therapy in aged patients. Clinical pharmacokinetic considerations. *Drugs Aging* 10: 278–89.

Birmingham PK, Tobin MJ, Henthorn TK et al (1997) Twenty-four hour pharmacokinetics of rectal acetominophen analgesia in children. *Anesthesiology* 1997; 87: 244–252.

Blum RA, Comstock TJ, Sica DA et al (1994) Pharmacokinetics of gabapentin in subjects with various degrees of renal function.*Clin Pharmacol Ther* 56: 154–59.

Bodenham A, Park GR (1990) Plasma Concentrations of bupivacaine after Intercostal Nerve Block in Patients after Orthotopic Liver Transplantation. *Br J Anaesth* 64: 436–41.

Borland ML, Jacobs I, Geelhoed G (2002) Intranasal fentanyl reduces acute pain in children in the emergency department: a safety and efficacy study. *Emerg Med (Fremantle)* 14: 275–80.

Bosenberg AT, Bland BA, Schulte-Steinberg O et al (1988) Thoracic epidural anesthesia via caudal route in infants. *Anesthesiology* 69: 265–69.

Bosenberg AT (1998) Epidural analgesia for major neonatal surgery. *Paed Anaesth* 8: 479–83.

CHAPTER 10

Bosenberg AT & Ivani G (1998) Regional anaesthesia – children are different. *Paed Anaesth* 8: 447–50.

Bouwmeester NJ, Anand KJ, van Dijk M et al (2001) Hormonal and metabolic stress responses after major surgery in children aged 0–3 years: a double-blind, randomized trial comparing the effects of continuous versus intermittent morphine. *Br J Anaesth* 87: 390–99.

Bouwmeester NJ, van den Anker JN, Hop WC et al (2003) Age- and therapy-related effects on morphine requirements and plasma concentrations of morphine and its metabolites in postoperative infants. *Br J Anaesth* 90: 642–52.

Bozkurt P, Kaya G, Yeker Y (1997) Single-injection lumbar epidural morphine for postoperative analgesia in children. *Regional Anesthesia* 22: 212–17.

Bozkurt P (2002) The analgesic efficacy and neuroendocrine response in paediatric patients treated with two analgesic techniques: using morphine epidural and patient controlled analgesia. *Paed Anaesth* 12: 248–54.

Brady-Fryer B, Wiebe N, Lander JA (2004) Pain relief for neonatal circumcision. *The Cochrane Database of Systematic Reviews*, Issue 3. Art. No.: CD004217. DOI: 10.1002/14651858.CD004217.pub2.

Bramley D, Herbert P, Jackson R et al (2004) Indigenous disparities in disease-specific mortality' a cross-country comparison: New Zealand, Australia, Canada and the United States. *NZ Med J* 117: U1215.

Bray RJ (1983) Postoperative analgesia provided by morphine infusion in children. *Anaesthesia* 38: 1075–78.

Bray RJ, Woodhams AM, Vallis CJ et al (1996a) Morphine consumption and respiratory depression in children receiving postoperative analgesia from continuous morphine infusion or patient-controlled analgesia. *Paediatr Anaesth* 6: 129–34.

Bray RJ, Woodhams AM, Vallis CJ et al (1996b) A double-blind comparison of morphine infusion and patient controlled analgesia in children. *Paediatr Anaesth* 6: 121–27.

Breau LM, McGrath PJ, Camfield CS (2002a) Psychometric properties of the non-communicating children's pain checklist-revised. *Pain* 99: 349–57.

Breau LM, Finley GA, McGrath PJ et al (2002b) Validation of the Non-communicating Children's Pain Checklist-Postoperative Version. *Anesthesiology*. 96: 528–35.

Breschan C, Krumpholz R, Jost R et al (2001) Intraspinal haematoma following epidural anaesthesia. *Paed Anaesth* 11: 105–08.

Broadman LM (1996) Complications of pediatric regional anesthesia. *Reg Anesth* 21: 64–70.

Brooks PM & Day RO (2000) COX-2 inhibitors. *Med J Aust* 173: 433–36.

Brooten D (1983) A comparison of four treatments to prevent and control pain engorgement in non-nursing mothers. *Nursing Res* 32: 225–29.

Brown S & Lumley J (1998) Maternal health after childbirth: results of an Australian population based survey. *Br J Obstet Gynaecol* 105: 156–61.

Brown TC, Eyres RL, McDougall RJ (1999) Local and regional anaesthesia in children. *Br J Anaesth* 83: 65–77.

Bryson HM & Wilde MI (1996) Amitriptyline. A review of its pharmacological properties and therapeutic use in chronic pain states. *Drugs Aging* 8: 459–76.

Bucklin BA, Chestnut DH, Hawkins JL (2002) Intrathecal opioids versus epidural local anesthetics for labor analgesia: A meta-analysis. *Reg Anesth Pain Med* 27: 23–30.

Buttner W & Finke W (2000) Analysis of behavioural and physiological parameters for the assessment of postoperative analgesic demand in newborns, infants and young children: a comprehensive report on seven consecutive studies. *Paediatr Anaesth* 10: 303–18.

Campbell A, Yentis SM, Fear DW et al (1992) Analgesic efficacy and safety of a caudal bupivacaine-fentanyl mixture. *Can J Anaesth* 39: 661–64.

Caparros-Lefebvre D, Lemonte-Houcke M, Prubot FR et al (1993) Unusual electronmicrosopic changes in valproate-associated liver failure. *Lancet* 341: 1604.

Carr AS, Fear DW, Sikich N et al (1998) Bupivacaine 0.125% produces motor block and weakness with fentanyl epidural analgesia in children. *Can J Anaesth* 45: 1054–60.

Carroli G, Belizan J (1999) Episiotomy for vaginal birth. *The Cochrane Database of Systematic Reviews* 1999, Issue 3. Art. No.: CD000081. DOI: 10.1002/14651858.CD000081.

Carroll D, Tramèr M, McQuay H et al (1997) Transcutaneous electrical nerve stimulation in labour pain: a systematic review. *Br J Obstet Gynaecol* 104: 169–75.

Carstoniu J, Levytam S, Norman P et al (1994) Nitrous oxide in early labor. Safety and analgesic efficacy assessed by a double-blind, placebo-controlled study. *Anesthesiology* 80: 30–35.

Casey WF, Rice LJ, Hannallah RS et al (1990) A comparison between bupivacaine instillation versus ilioinguinal/iliohypogastric nerve block for postoperative analgesia following inguinal herniorrhaphy in children. *Anesthesiology* 72: 637–39.

Cella D, Pulliam J, Fuchs H et al (2003) Evaluation of pain associated with oral mucositis during the acute period after administration of high-dose chemotherapy. *Cancer* 98: 406–12.

Champion GD, Goodenough B, von Baeyer CL et al (1998) Measurement of pain by self-report. In: Finley GA & McGrath PJ (Eds) *Measurement of Pain In Infants and Children. Progress in Pain Research and Management*, Volume 10. Seattle: IASP Press, pp123–60.

Charghi R, Backman S, Christou N et al (2003) Patient controlled IV analgesia is an acceptable management strategy in morbidly obese patients undergoing gastric bypass surgery. A retrospective comparison with epidural analgesia. *Can J Anaesth* 50: 672–78.

Chauvin M, Ferrier C, Haberer JP et al (1989) Sufentanil pharmacokinetics in patients with cirrhosis. *Anesth Analg* 68: 1–4.

Chen E, Joseph MH, Zeltzer LK (2000) Behavioral and cognitive interventions in the treatment of pain in children. *Pediatr Clin North Am* 47: 513–25.

Chibnall JT & Tait RC (2001) Pain assessment in cognitively impaired and unimpaired older adults: a comparison of four scales. *Pain* 92: 173–86.

Choi WY, Irwin MG, Hui TW et al (2003) EMLA cream versus dorsal penile nerve block for postcircumcision analgesia in children. *Anesth Analg* 96(2): 396–99.

Choi YK, Brolin RE, Bertil KJ et al (2000) Efficacy and safety of patient-controlled analgesia for morbidly obese patients following gastric bypass surgery. *Obes Surg* 10: 154–59.

Clunie M, Crone L-A, Klassen L et al (2003) Psychiatric side effects of indomethacin in parturients. *Can J Anaesth* 50: 586–88.

Coda BA, O'Sullivan B, Donaldson G et al (1997) Comparative efficacy of patient-controlled administration of morphine, hydromorphone, or sufentanil for the treatment of oral mucositis pain following bone marrow transplantation. *Pain* 72: 333–46.

Collins JJ, Geake J, Grier HE et al (1996) Patient-controlled analgesia for mucositis pain in children: a three-period crossover study comparing morphine and hydromorphone. *J Pediatr* 129: 722–28.

COMET Study Group (2001) Effects of low-dose mobile versus traditional epidural techniques on mode of delivery: a randomised controlled trial. Comparative Obstetric Mobile Epidural Trial. *Lancet* 358: 19–23.

Constant I, Gall O, Gouyet L et al (1998) Addition of clonidine or fentanyl to local anaesthetics prolongs the duration of surgical analgesia after single shot caudal block in children. *Br J Anaesth* 80: 294–98.

Cote CJ, Karl HW, Notterman DA et al (2000a) Adverse sedation events in pediatrics: analysis of medications used for sedation. *Pediatrics* 106: 633–44.

Cote CJ, Notterman DA, Karl HW et al (2000b) Adverse sedation events in pediatrics: a critical incident analysis of contributing factors. *Pediatrics* 105: 805–14.

Coulthard KP, Nielson HW, Schroder M et al (1998) Relative bioavailability and plasma paracetamol profiles of panadol suppositories in children. *J Paed Child Health* 34: 425–31.

Craig KD (1998) The facial display of pain. In: Finley GA & McGrath PJ (Eds) *Measurement of Pain In Infants and Children. Progress in Pain Research and Management*, Volume 10. Seattle: IASP Press, pp103–22.

Craven PD, Badawi N, Henderson-Smart DJ et al (2003) Regional (spinal, epidural, caudal) versus general anaesthesia in preterm infants undergoing inguinal herniorrhaphy in early infancy. *The Cochrane Database of Systematic Reviews* 2003, Issue 3. Art. No.: CD003669. DOI: 10.1002/14651858.CD003669.

Crawford ME, Møiniche S, Orbaek J et al (1996) Orthostatic hypotension during postoperative continuous thoracic epidural bupivacaine-morphine in patients undergoing abdominal surgery. *Anesth Analg* 83: 1028–32.

Creedy DK, Shochet IM, Horsfall J (2000) Childbirth and the development of acute trauma symptoms: Incidence contributing factors. *Birth Issues in Perinatal Care* 27: 104–11.

Crews JC, Weller RS, Moss J et al (2002) Levobupivacaine for axillary brachial plexus block: a pharmacokinetic and clinical comparison in patients with normal renal function or renal disease. *Anesth Analg* 95: 219–23.

Cross GD & Barrett RF (1987) Comparison of two regional techniques for postoperative analgesia in children following herniotomy and orchidopexy. *Anaesthesia* 42: 845–49.

Cucchiaro G, Dagher C, Baujard C et al (2003) Side-effects of postoperative epidural analgesia in children: a randomized study comparing morphine and clonidine. *Paediatr Anaesth* 13: 318–23.

Cullen DJ (2001) Obstructive sleep apnea and postoperative analgesia--a potentially dangerous combination. *J Clin Anesth* 13: 83–85.

Cummings EA, Reid GJ, Finley GA et al (1996) Prevalence and source of pain in pediatric inpatients. *Pain* 68: 25–31.

Cyna A, Parsons J, Jha S (2003) Caudal epidural block versus other methods of postoperative pain relief for circumcision in boys. *The Cochrane Database of Systematic Reviews* Issue 2. Art. No.: CD003005. DOI: 10.1002/14651858.CD003005.

Cyna AM, McAuliffe GL, Andrew M (2004) Hypnosis for pain relief in labour and childbirth: a systematic review. *Brit J Anaesth* 93: 505–11.

D'Honneur GD, Gilton A, Sandouk P et al (1994) Plasma and cerebrospinal fluid concentrations of morphine and morphine glucuronides after oral morphine the influence of renal failure. *Anesthesiology* 81: 87–93.

Dadure C, Pirat P, Raux O et al (2003) Perioperative continuous peripheral nerve blocks with disposable infusion pumps in children: a prospective descriptive study. *Anesth Analg* 97: 687–90.

Dalens B, Tanguy A, Haberer J-P (1986) Lumbar epidural anesthesia for operative and postoperative pain relief in infants and young children. *Anesth Analg* 65: 1069–73.

Dalens B & Hasnaoui A (1989) Caudal anesthesia in pediatric surgery. *Anesth Analg* 68: 83–89.

Dashe JS, Sheffield JS, Olscher DA et al (2002) Relationship between maternal methadone dosage and neonatal withdrawal. *Obstet Gynecol* 100: 1244–49.

Davidhizar R & Giger JN (2004) A review of the literature on care of clients in pain who are culturally diverse. *Int Nurs Rev* 51: 47–55.

Davies G, Kingswood C, Street M (1996) Pharmacokinetics of opioids in renal dysfunction. *Clin Pharmacokinetics* 31: 410–22.

Davis PJ, Stiller RL, Cook DR et al (1988) Pharmacokinetics of sufentanil in adolescent patients with chronic renal failure. *Anesth Analg* 67: 268–71.

Davis PJ, Stiller RL, Cook DR et al (1989) Effects of cholestatic hepatic disease and chronic renal failure on alfentanil pharmacokinetics in children. *Anesth Analg* 68: 579–83.

de Beer DA & Thomas ML (2003) Caudal additives in children--solutions or problems? *Br J Anaesth* 90: 487–98.

de Leon-Casasola OA, Myers DP, Donaparthi S et al (1993) A comparison of postoperative epidural analgesia between patients with chronic cancer taking high doses of oral opioids versus opioid-naïve patients. *Anesth Analg* 76: 302–07.

de Leon-Casasola OA & Lema MJ (1994) Epidural bupivacaine/sufentanil therapy for postoperative pain control in patients tolerant to opioid and unresponsive to epidural bupivacaine/morphine. *Anesthesiology* 80: 303–09.

De Negri P, Ivani G, Visconti C et al (2001) The dose-response relationship for clonidine added to a postoperative continuous epidural infusion of ropivacaine in children. *Anesth Analg* 93: 71–76.

DesparmetJ, Mateo J, Ecoffey C et al (1990) Efficiency of an epidural test dose in children anesthetised with halothane. *Anesthesiology* 72: 249–51.

Dewan G, Glazener C, Tunstall M (1993) Postnatal pain: a neglected area. *Br J Mid* 1: 63–66.

Divoll M, Abernathy DR, Ameer B et al (1982) Acetaminophen kinetics in the elderly. *Clin Pharmacol Ther* 32: 151–56.

Doverty M, Somogyi AA, White JM et al (2001) Methadone-maintenance patients are cross-tolerant to the antinociceptive effects of morphine. *Pain* 93: 155–63.

Doyle E, Robinson D, Morton NS et al (1993a) Comparison of patient-controlled analgesia with and without a background infusion after lower abdominal surgery in children. *Br J Anaesth* 71: 670–73.

Doyle E, Harper I, Morton NS et al (1993b) Patient-controlled analgesia with low dose background infusions after lower abdominal surgery in children. *Br J Anaesth* 71: 818–22.

Doyle E, Morton NS, McNicol LR (1994a) Comparison of patient-controlled analgesia in children by i.v. and s.c. routes of administration. *Br J Anaesth* 72: 533–36.

Doyle E, Mottart KJ, Marshall C et al (1994b) Comparison of different bolus doses of morphine for patient-controlled analgesia in children. *Br J Anaesth* 72: 160–63.

Doyle E, Byers G, McNicol LR et al (1994c) Prevention of postoperative nausea and vomiting with transdermal hyoscine in children using patient-controlled analgesia. *Br J Anaesth* 72: 72–76.

Drage MP & Schug SA (1996) Analgesia in the elderly. Practical treatment recommendations. *Drugs Aging* 9: 311–18.

Drake R, Longworth J, Collins JJ (2004) Opioid rotation in children with cancer. *J Palliat Med* 7: 419–22.

Dsida RM, Wheeler M, Birmingham PK et al (2002) Age stratified pharmacokinetics of ketorolac tromethamine in pediatric surgical patients. *Anesth Analg* 94: 266–70.

Dunbar PJ, Buckley P, Gavrin JR et al (1995) Use of patient-controlled analgesia for pain control for children receiving bone marrow transplant. *J Pain Symptom Manage* 10: 604–11.

Ecoffey C, Dubousset AM, Samii K (1986) Lumbar and thoracic epidural anesthesia for urologic and upper abdominal surgery in infants and children. *Anesthesiology* 65: 87–90.

Egbert AM, Parks LH, Short LM et al (1990) Randomised trial of postoperative patient-controlled analgesia v. intramuscular opioids in frail elderly men. *Arch Int Med* 150: 1897–1903.

Egbert AM (1996) Postoperative pain management in the frail elderly. *Clinics Geriatr Med* 12: 583–99.

Eilers H, Philip LA, Bickler PE et al (2001) The reversal of fentanyl-induced tolerance by administration of 'small-dose' ketamine. *Anesth Analg* 93: 213–14.

Elbourne D, Wiseman RA (1998)Types of intra-muscular opioids for maternal pain relief in labour. *The Cochrane Database of Systematic Reviews*.Issue 4. Art. No.: CD001237. DOI: 10.1002/14651858.CD001237.

Engelhardt T, Steel E, Johnston G et al (2003) Tramadol for pain relief in children undergoing tonsillectomy: a comparison with morphine. *Paediatr Anaesth* 13: 249–52.

Esmail Z, Montgomery C, Courtrn C et al (1999) Efficacy and complications of morphine infusions in postoperative paediatric patients. *Paediatr Anaesth* 9: 321–27.

Etches R (1994) Respiratory depression associated with patient-controlled analgesia: a review of eight cases. *Can J Anaesth* 41: 125–32.

Evans JK, Buckley SL, Alexander AH et al (1995) Analgesia for the reduction of fractures in children: A comparison of nitrous oxide with intramuscular sedation. *J Pediatr Orthop* 15: 73–77.

Farrell MJ, Katz B, Helme RD (1996) The impact of dementia on the pain experience. *Pain* 67: 7–15.

Feilberg VL, Rosenborg D, Christensen CM et al (1989) Excretion of morphine in human breast milk. *Acta Anaesthesiol Scand* 33: 426–28.

Feldt KN, Ryden MB, Miles S (1998) Treatment of pain in cognitively impaired compared with cognitively intact older patients with hip-fracture. *J Am Geriatr Soc* 46: 1079–85.

Fell D, Derrington MC, Taylor E et al (1988) Paediatric postoperative analgesia. A comparison between caudal block and wound infiltration of local anaesthetic. *Anaesthesai* 43: 107–10.

Fenwick C, Stevens J (2004) Postoperative pain experiences of central Australian aboriginal women: what do we understand? *Aust J Rural Health* 12: 22.

Ferrell BA (1995) Pain evaluation and management in the nursing home. *Ann Int Med* 123: 681–87.

Ferrell BA, Ferrell BR, Rivera L (1995) Pain in cognitively impaired nursing home patients. *J Pain Sympt Manage* 10: 591–98.

Findlow D, Aldridge LM, Doyle E (1997) Comparison of caudal block using bupivacaine and ketamine with ilioinguinal nerve block for orchidopexy in children. *Anaesthesia* 52: 1110–13.

Finkel JC, Rose JB, Schmitz ML et al (2002) An evaluation of the efficacy and tolerability of oral tramadol hydrochloride tablets for the treatment of postsurgical pain in children. *Anesth Analg* 94: 1469–73.

Finley G, McGrath PJ (Eds) (1998) *Measurement of Pain In Infants and Children. Progress in Pain Research and Management,* Volume 10. Seattle: IASP Press, pp103–122.

Fishbain DA, Rosomoff HL, Rosomoff RS (1992) Drug abuse, dependence, and addiction in chronic pain patients. *Clin J Pain* 8: 77–85.

Fisher QA, McComiskey CM, Hill JL et al (1993) Postoperative voiding interval and duration of analgesia following peripheral or caudal nerve blocks in children. *Anesth Analg* 76: 173–77.

Fisher QA, Shaffner DH, Yaster M (1997) Detection of intravascular injection of regional anaesthetics in children. *Can J Anaesth* 44: 592–98.

Fisher WJ, Bingham RM, Hall R (1999) Axillary brachial plexus block for perioperative analgesia in 250 children. *Paediatr Anaesth* 9: 435–38.

Fitzgerald M & Howard RF (2002) The neurobiologic basis of paediatric pain. In: Schecter NL, Berde CB, Yaster M (Eds) *Pain in Infants, Children and Adolescents.* Baltimore: Lippincott Williams and Wilkins, pp19–42.

Fitzgerald M & Walker S (2003) The role of activity in developing pain pathways. *Proceedings of the 10th World Congress on Pain. Progress in Pain Research and Management*, Vol. 24. Dostrovsky JO, Carr DB, Koltzenburg, M (Eds) IASP Press, Seattle, pp185–196; 2003.

Flandin-Blety C & Barrier G (1995) Accidents following extradural analgesia in children. The results of a retrospective study. Paediatric *Anaesthesia* 5: 41–46.

Flogegard H & Ljungman G (2003) Characteristics and adequacy of intravenous morphine infusions in children in a paediatric oncology setting. *Med Pediatr Oncol* 40: 233–38.

Franck LS, Greenberg CS, Stevens B (2000) Pain assessment in infants and children. *Pediatr Clin North Am* 47: 487–512.

Gaffney A, McGrath PJ, Dick B (2003) Measuring pain in children: developmental and instrument issues. In: Schecter NL, Berde CB, Yaster M (Eds) *Pain in Infants, Children and Adolescents.* Baltimore: Lippincott Williams and Wilkins, pp 128–141.

Gagliese L & Melzack R (1997) Chronic pain in elderly people. *Pain* 70: 3–14.

Gagliese L, Jackson M, Ritvo P et al (2000) Age is not an impediment to effective use of patient-controlled analgesia by surgical patients. *Anesthesiology* 93: 601–10.

Gagliese L & Katz J (2003) Age differences in postoperative pain are scale dependent: a comparison of measures of pain intensity and quality in younger and older surgical patients. *Pain* 103: 11–20.

Gall O, Annequin D, Benoit G et al (2001) Adverse events of pre-mixed nitrous oxide and oxygen for procedural sedation in children. *Lancet* 358: 1514–15.

Gaukroger PB, Tomkins DP, van der Walt JH (1989) Patient-controlled analgesia in children. *Anaesth Int Care* 17: 264–68.

Gaukroger PB, Chapman MJ, Davey RB (1991) Pain control in paediatric burns — the use of patient-controlled analgesia. *Burns* 17: 396–99.

Gauntlett I (2003) A comparison between local anaesthetic dorsal nerve block and caudal bupivacaine with ketamine for paediatric circumcision. *Paed Anaesth* 13: 38–42.

Giaufre E, Dalens B, Gombert A (1996) Epidemiology and morbidity of regional anesthesia in children: A one-year prospective survey of the French Language Society of Pediatric Anesthesiologists. *Anesth Analg* 83: 904–12.

Gibson SJ (2003) Pain and aging: the pain experience over the adult life span. In: Dostrovsky JO, Carr DB, Koltzenburg M (Eds) *Proceedings of the 10th World Congress on Pain*. Seattle: IASP Press, pp767–90.

Gibson SJ & Farrell M (2004) A review of age differences in the neurophysiology of nociception and the perceptual experience of pain. *Clin J Pain* 20: 227–39.

Gill AC, Oei J, Lewis NL et al (2003) Strabismus in infants of opiate-dependent mothers. *Acta Paediatr* 92: 379–85.

Green CR, Anderson KO, Baker TA et al (2003) The unequal burden of pain: confronting racial and ethnic disparities in pain. *Pain Med* 4: 277–94.

Green SM, Hummel CB, Wittlake WA et al (1999) What is the optimal dose of intramuscular ketamine for pediatric sedation? *Acad Emerg Med* 6: 21–26.

Greer IA & Cameron AD (1984) Topical pramoxine and hydrocortisone foam versus placebo in relief of postpartum episiotomy symptoms and wound healing. *Scott Med J* 29: 104–06.

Gregory PR & Sullivan JA (1996) Nitrous oxide compared with intravenous regional anesthesia in pediatric forearm fracture manipulation. *J Pediatr Orthop* 16: 187–91.

Grunau RV & Craig KD (1987) Pain expression in neonates: facial action and cry. *Pain* 28: 395–410.

Grunau RE (2000) Long-term consequences of pain in human neonates. In: Anand KJS, Stevens BJ, McGrath PJ (Eds) *Pain Research and Clinical Management* Volume 10. Amsterdam: Elsevier, pp 55–76.

Guinard J-P & Borboen M (1993) Probable venous air embolism during caudal anesthesia in a child. *Anesth Analg* 76: 1134–35.

Gupta RM, Parvizi J, Hanssen AD et al (2001) Postoperative complications in patients with obstructive sleep apnea syndrome undergoing hip or knee replacement: a case-control study. *Mayo Clinic Proc* 76: 897–905.

Haberkbern CM, Lynn AM, Geiduschek JM et al (1996) Epidural and intravenous bolus morphine for postoperative analgesia in infants. *Can J Anaesth* 43: 1203–10.

Habre W, Wilson D, Johnson CM (1999) Extrapyramidal side-effects from droperidol mixed with morphine for patient-controlled analgesia in two children. *Paediatr Anaesth* 9: 362–64.

Hadzic N, Portmann B, Davies ET et al (1990) Acute liver failure induced by carbemazepine. *Arch Dis Child* 65: 315–17.

Halpern SH, Levine T, Wilson DB et al (1999) Effect of labor analgesia on breastfeeding success. *Birth* 26: 83–88.

Halpern SH & Walsh V (2003) Epidural ropivacaine versus bupivacaine for labor: A meta-analysis. *Anesth Analg* 96: 1473–79.

Hanna MH, D'Costa F, Peat SJ et al (1993) Morphine-6-glucuronide disposition in renal impairment. *Br J Anaesth* 70: 511–14.

Hansen TG, Henneberg SW, Hole P (1996) Age-related postoperative morphine requirements in children following major surgery- an assessment using patient-controlled analgesia (PCA). *Eur J Pediatr Surg* 6: 29–31.

Hansen TG, O'Brien K, Morton NS et al (1999) Plasma paracetamol concentrations and pharmacokinetics following rectal administration in neonates and young infants. *Acta Anaesth Scand* 43: 855–59.

Hay-Smith EJC (1998) Therapeutic ultrasound for postpartum perineal pain and dyspareunia. *The Cochrane Database of Systematic Reviews* Issue 3. Art. No.: CD000495. DOI: 10.1002/14651858.CD000495.

Hedayati H, Parsons J, Crowther CA (2003) Rectal analgesia for pain from perineal trauma following childbirth. *The Cochrane Database of Systematic Reviews* Issue 2. Art. No.: CD003931. DOI: 10.1002/14651858.CD003931.

Hee HI, Goy RWL, Ng ASB (2003) Effective reduction of anxiety and pain during venous cannulation in children: a comparison of analgesic efficacy conferred by nitrous oxide, EMLA and combination. *Paediatr Anaesth* 3: 210–16.

Hendrickson M, Myre L, Johnson DG et al (1990) Postoperative analgesia in children: a prospective study in intermittent intramuscular injection versus continuous intravenous infusion of morphine. *J Pediatr Surg* 25: 185–90.

Herr KA, Spratt K, Mobily PR et al (2004) Pain intensity in older adults. *Clin J Pain* 20: 207–19.

Herrick IA, Ganapathy S, Komar W et al (1996) Postoperative cognitive impairment in the elderly. Choice of patient-controlled analgesia opioid. *Anaesthesia* 51: 356–60.

Hersh, EV, Ochs H, Quinn P et al (1993) Narcotic receptor blockade and its effect on the analgesic response to placebo and ibuprofen after oral surgery. *Oral Surg Oral Med Oral Pathol* 75: 539–46.

Hester NK (1979) The preoperational child's reaction to immunization. *Nurs Res* 28: 250–55.

Hicks CL, von Baeyer CL, Spafford PA et al (2001) The Faces Pain Scale-Revised: toward a common metric in pediatric pain measurement. *Pain* 93: 173–83.

Hill PD (1989) Effects of heat and cold on the perineum after episiotomy/laceration. *J Obstet Gynaecol Neo Nurs* 18: 124–29.

Hirose M, Hosokawa T, Tanaka Y (1997) Extradural buprenorphine suppresses breast feeding after Caesarean section. *Br J Anaesth* 9: 120–21.

Hodgson RE, Bosenberg AT, Hadley LG (2000) Congenital diaphragmatic hernia repair- impact of delayed surgery and epidural analgesia. *S Afr J Surg* 38: 31–34.

Hodnett ED, Gates S, Hofmeyr G J et al (2003)Continuous support for women during childbirth. *The Cochrane Database of Systematic Reviews* Issue 3. Art. No.: CD003766. DOI: 10.1002/14651858.CD003766.

Hoffman GM, Nowakowski R, Troshynski TJ et al (2002) Risk reduction in pediatric procedural sedation by application of an American Academy of Pediatrics/American Society of Anesthesiologists process model. *Pediatr* 109: 236–43.

Hogan QH (1996) Epidural anatomy examined by cryomicrotome section. Influence of age, vertebral level and disease. *Reg Anesth* 21: 395–406.

Holder KJ, Peutrell JM, Weir PM (1997) Regional anaesthesia for circumcision. Subcutaneous ring block of the penis and subpubic penile block compared. *Eur J Anaesthesiol* 14: 495–98.

Hollis LJ, Burton MJ, Millar JM (1999) Perioperative local anaesthesia for reducing pain following tonsillectomy. *The Cochrane Database of Systematic Reviews* Issue 3. Art. No.: CD001874. DOI: 10.1002/14651858.CD001874.

Honeyman PT & Jacobs EA (1996) Effects of culture on back pain in Australian Aboriginals. *Spine* 21: 841–43.

Hopkins CS, Underhill S, Booker PD (1990) Pharmacokinetics of paracetamol after cardiac surgery. *Arch Dis Child* 65: 971–76.

Howard RF, Hatch DJ, Cole TJ (2001) Inflammatory pain and hypersensitivity are selectively reversed by epidural bupivacaine and are developmentally regulated. *Anesthesiology* 95: 421–27.

Howard RF (2003a) Current status of pain management in children. *JAMA* 290: 2464–69.

Howard RF (2003b) Acute pain management in children. In: Rowbotham DJ & Macintyre PE (Eds) Clinical Pain Management. Acute Pain. London: Arnold, pp437–62.

Howe PW, Condon JR, Goodchild CS (1998) Anaesthesia for Aboriginal Australians. *Anaesth Int Care* 26: 86–91.

Howell CJ (1999) Epidural versus non-epidural analgesia for pain relief in labour. *The Cochrane Database of Systematic Reviews*. Issue 3. Art. No.: CD000331. DOI: 10.1002/14651858.CD000331.

Howell TK & Patel D (2003) Plasma paracetamol concentrations after different doses of rectal paracetamol in older children: a comparison of 1gm vs 40mg/kg. *Anaesthesia* 58: 69–73.

Huang YC, Tsai SK, Huang CH et al (2002) Intravenous tenoxicam reduces uterine cramps after caesarean delivery. *Can J Anesth* 49: 384–87.

Huerta S, DeShields S, Shpiner R et al (2002) Safety and efficacy of postoperative continuous positive airway pressure to prevent pulmonary complications after Roux-en-Y gastric bypass. *J Gastroint Surg* 6: 354–58.

Hughes D, Simmons SW, Brown J et al (2003) Combined spinal-epidural versus epidural analgesia in labour. *The Cochrane Database of Systematic Reviews*. Issue 4. Art. No.: CD003401. DOI: 10.1002/14651858.CD003401.

Hulse GK, Milne E, English DR et al (1997) The relationship between maternal use of heroin and methadone and infant birth weight. *Addiction* 92: 1571–79.

Ilett KF, Kristensen JH, Wojnar-Horton RE et al (1997) Drug distribution in human milk. *Aus Prescriber* 20: 35–40.

Inch S & Renfrew MJ (1989) Common breastfeeding problems. In: Chalmers I, Enkin M, Keirs M (Eds) *Effective Care in Pregnancy and Childbirth*. Oxford: Oxford University Press, pp1375–89.

Ingelman-Sundberg A (1953) Early puerperial breast engorgement. *Acta Paediatr Scand* 32: 399–402.

Irwin MG & Cheng W (1996) Comparison of subcutaneous ring block of the penis with caudal epidural block for post-circumcision analgesia in children. *Anaesth Int Care* 24: 365–67.

Isenor I & Penny-MacGillivray T (1993) Intravenous meperidine infusion for obstetric analgesia. *J Obstet Gynecol Neo Nurs* 22: 349–56.

Jage J & Bey T (2000a) Postoperative analgesia in patients with substance use disorders: Part I. *Acute Pain* 3: 141–56.

Jage J & Bey T (2000b) Postoperative analgesia in patients with substance use disorders: Part II. *Acute Pain* 3: 1–9.

Jensen F, Qvist I, Brocks V et al (1984) Submucous paracervical blockade compared with intramuscular meperidine as analgesia during labor: a double-blind study. *Obstet Gynecol* 64: 724–27.

Young G, Jewell D (2002) Interventions for preventing and treating pelvic and back pain in pregnancy. *The Cochrane Database of Systematic Reviews*, Issue 1. Art. No.: CD001139. DOI: 10.1002/14651858.CD001139.

Johnson CM (1994) Continuous femoral nerve blockade for analgesia in children with femoral fractures. *Anaesth Int Care* 22: 281–83.

Johnston CC, Stevens BJ, Craig KD et al (1993) Developmental changes in pain expression in premature, full-term, two- and four-month-old infants. *Pain* 52: 201-8.

Johnston, CC (1998) Psychometric issues in the measurement of pain. In: Finley GA & McGrath PJ (Eds) *Measurement of Pain In Infants and Children. Progress in Pain Research and Management*, Volume 10. Seattle: IASP Press, pp5–20.

Johnston CC, Stevens BJ, Boyer K et al (2003) Development of psychologic responses to pain and assessment of pain in infants and toddlers. In: Schecter NL, Berde CB, Yaster M (Eds) *Pain in Infants, Children and Adolescents.* Baltimore: Lippincott Williams and Wilkins, pp85–104.

Jones RDM, Gunawardene WMS, Yeung CK (1990) A comparison of lignocaine 2% with adrenaline 1: 200,000 and lignocaine 2% with adrenaline 1: 200,000 plus fentanyl as agents for caudal anaesthesia in children undergoing circumcision. *Anaesthesia Int Care* 18: 194–99.

Kaiko RF (1991) Relationships between opioid disposition and their pharmacological effects- an overview. *Postgrad Med J* 67 (Suppl 2): S44–S49.

Kaplowitz N (200)4 Acetaminophen hepatotoxicity: what do we know, what don't we know and what do we do next? *Hepatology* 40:23-26.

Kart T, Christrup LL, Rasmussen M (1997a) Recommended use of morphine in neonates, infants and children based on a literature review: Part 1--Pharmacokinetics. *Paediatr Anaesth* 7: 5–11.

Kart T, Christrup LL, Rasmussen M et al (1997b) Recommended use of morphine in neonates, infants and children based on a literature review. Part 2- Clinical use. *Paediatr Anaesth* 7: 93–101.

Kasai T, Yaegashi K, Hirose M et al (2003) Spinal cord injury in a child caused by an accidental dural puncture with a single-shot thoracic epidural needle. *Anesth Analg* 96: 65–67.

Kauppila A, Arvela P, Koivisto M et al (1983) Metoclopramide and breast feeding: transfer into milk and the newborn. *Eur J Clin Pharmacol* 25: 819–23.

Kazak AE, Penati B, Brophy P et al (1998) Pharmacologic and psychologic interventions for procedural pain. *Pediatr* 102: 59–66.

Keita H, Geachan N, Dahmani S et al (2002) Comparison between patient-controlled analgesia and subcutaneous morphine in elderly patients after total hip replacement. *Br J Anaesth* 90: 53–57.

Kendig H, Helme R, Teshuva K et al (1996) *Health Status of Older People Project: Preliminary Findings from a Survey of the Health and Lifestyles of Older Australians*. Melbourne: Victorian Health Promotion Foundation.

Kennedy RM, Porter FL, Miller PJ et al (1998) Comparison of fentanyl/midazolam with ketamine/midazolam for pediatric orthopedic emergencies. *Pediatr* 102: 956–63.

Kennedy RM, Luhmann JD, Luhmann SJ (2004) Emergency department management of pain and anxiety related to orthopedic fracture care: a guide to analgesic techniques and procedural sedation in children. *Paediatr Drugs* 6: 11–31.

Kettle C, Johanson RB (1999) Absorbable synthetic versus catgut suture material for perineal repair. *The Cochrane Database of Systematic Reviews* Issue 3. Art. No.: CD000006. DOI: 10.1002/14651858.CD000006.

Khan ZP, Ferguson CN, Jones RM (1999) Alpha-2 and imidazoline receptor agonists, their pharmacology and therapeutic role. *Anaesthesia* 54: 146–65.

Koh JL, Fanurik D, Harrison RD 92004) Analgesia following surgery in children with and without cognitive impairment. *Pain* 111: 239-44.

Kokinsky E, Thornberg E, Nilsson K et al (1999) Postoperative nausea and vomiting in children using patient-controlled analgesia: the effect of prophylactic intravenous dixyrazine. *Acta Anaesthesiol Scand* 43: 191–95.

Kokki H (2003) Nonsteroidal anti-inflammatory drugs for postoperative pain. A focus on children. *Pediatr Drugs* 5: 103–23.

Koppel C, Arndt I, Ibe K (1990) Effects of enzyme induction, renal and cardiac function on ketamine plasma kinetics in patients with ketamine long-term analgesosedation. *Eur J Drug Metab Pharmacokinetics* 15: 259–63.

Korpela R, Korvenoja P, Meretoja OA (1999) Morphine-sparing effect of acetaminophen in pediatric day-case surgery. *Anesthesiology* 91: 442–47.

Kost-Byerly S, Tobin JR, Greenberg RS et al (1998) Bacterial colonization and infection rates of continuous epidural catheters in children. *Anesth Analg* 86: 712–16.

Kotelko DM, Faulk DL, Rottman RL et al (1995) A controlled comparison of maternal analgesia: effects on neonatal nutritional sucking behaviour. *Anesthesiology* 83: A928.

Kozek-Langenecker S, Marhofer P, Jonas K et al (2000) Cardiovascular criteria for epidural test dosing in sevoflurane-and halothane-anesthetised children. *Anesth Analg* 90: 579–83.

Krane EJ, Tyler DC, Jacobson LE (1989) The dose response of caudal morphine in children. *Anesthesiology* 71: 48–52.

Krane EJ, Dalens BJ, Murat I et al (1998) The safety of epidurals placed during general anesthesia. *Reg Anesth Pain* Med 23: 433–38.

Krechel SW & Bildner J (1995) CRIES: a new neonatal postoperative pain measurement score. Initial testing of validity and reliability. *Paediatr Anaesth* 5: 53–61.

Krishna S, Hughes LF, Lin SY (2003) Postoperative hemorrhage with nonsteroidal anti-inflammatory drug use after tonsillectomy. A meta-analysis. *Arch Otolaryngol Head Neck Surg* 129: 1086–89.

Kumar RN, Chambers WA, Pertwee RG (2001) Pharmacological actions and therapeutic uses of cannabis and cannabinoids. *Anaesthesia* 56: 1059–68.

Kuppenheimer W & Brown R (2002) Painful procedures in pediatric cancer. A comparison of interventions. *Clin Psychol Rev* 22: 753–86.

Kussman BD & Sethna NF (1998) Pethidine-associated seizure in a healthy adolescent receiving pethidine for postoperative pain control. *Paediatr Anaesth* 8: 349–52.

Kyzer S, Ramadan E, Gersh M, Chaimoff C (1995) Patient-controlled analgesia following vertical gastroplasty: a comparison with intramuscular narcotics. *Obesity Surgery* 5: 18–21.

Labrecque M, Nouwen A, Bergeron M et al (1999) A randomized controlled trial of nonpharmacological approaches for relief of low back pain during labour. *J Fam Prac* 48: 259–63.

LaMontagne LL, Johnson BD, Hepworth JT (1991) Children's ratings of postoperative pain compared to ratings by nurses and physicians. *Issues in Comprehensive Pediatric Nursing.* 14: 241-7.

Landsberg R, Freidman M, Ascher-Landsberg J (2001) Treatment of hypoxemia in obstructive sleep apnea. *Am J Rhinol* 15: 311–13.

Larsson BA, Lonnqvist PA, Olsson GL (1997) Plasma concentrations of bupivacaine in neonates after continuous epidural infusion. *Anesth Analg* 84: 501–05.

Lawrence J, Alcock D, McGrath P et al (1993) The development of a tool to assess neonatal pain. *Neonatal Netw* 12: 59–66.

Lee CR, McTavish D, Sorkin EM (1993) Tramadol - a preliminary review of its pharmacokinetic and pharmacodynamic properties, and therapeutic potential in acute and chronic pain states. *Drugs* 46: 313–40.

Lee MC, Wagner HN Jr, Tanada S et al (1988) Duration of occupancy of opiate receptors by naltrexone. *J Nucl Med* 29: 1207–11.

Lejus C, Roussiere G, Testa S et al (1994) Postoperative extradural analgesia in children: comparison of morphine with fentanyl. *Br J Anaesth* 72: 156–59.

Lerman J, Nolan J, Eyres R et al (2003) Efficacy, safety, and pharmacokinetics of levobupivacaine with and without fentanyl after continuous epidural infusion in children. *Anesthesiology* 99: 1166–74.

Lesko SM & Mitchell AA (1995) An assessment of the safety of pediatric ibuprofen *JAMA* 273: 929–33.

Lesko SM & Mitchell AA (1999) The safety of acetaminophen and ibuprofen among children younger than two years old. *Pediatr* 104: e39.

Lesko SM, Louik C, Vezina RM et al (2002) Asthma morbidity after the short-term use of ibuprofen in children. *Pediatr* 109: E20.

Levy BT, Bergus GR, Hartz A et al (1999) Is paracervical block safe and effective? A prospective study of its association with neonatal umbilical artery pH values. *J Fam Pract* 48: 778–84.

Li DK, Liu L, Odouli R (2003) Exposure to non-steroidal anti-inflammatory drugs during pregnancy and risk of miscarriage: Population based cohort study. *BMJ* 327: 368.

Li SF, Greenwald PW, Gennis P et al (2001) Effect of age on acute pain perception of a standardized stimulus in the emergency department. *Ann Emerg Med* 38: 644–47.

Liebermann JA, Cooper TB, Suckow RF et al (1985) Tricyclic antidepressant and metabolite levels in chronic renal failure. *Clin Pharmacol Ther* 37: 301–07.

Litalien C & Jacqz-Aigrain E (2001) Risks and benefits of nonsteroidal anti-inflammatory drugs in children: a comparison with paracetamol. *Paediatr Drugs* 3: 817–58.

Litman RS, Berkowitz RJ, Ward DS. (1996) Levels of consciousness and ventilatory parameters in young children during sedation with oral midazolam and nitrous oxide. *Arch Pediatr Adolesc Med* 150: 671–75.

Litman RS, Kottra JA, Berkowitz RJ et al (1998) Upper airway obstruction during midazolam / nitrous oxide sedation in children with enlarged tonsils. *Pediatr Dent* 20: 318–20.

Litman RS (1999) Concious sedation with remifentanil and midazolam during brief painful procedures in children. *Arch Pediatr Adolesc Med* 153: 1085–88.

Liu EH & Sia AT (2004) Rates of caesarean section and instrumental vaginal delivery in nulliparous women after low concentration epidural infusions or opioid analgesia: Systematic review. *BMJ* 328: 1410.

Ljungman G, Kreugar A, Gordh T et al (1996) Treatment of pain in pediatric oncology: a Swedish nationwide survey. *Pain* 68: 385–94.

Ljungman G, Gordh T, Sorensen S et al (1999) Pain in paediatric oncology: interviews with children, adolescents and their parents. *Acta Paediatr* 88: 623–30.

Ljungman G, Gordh T, Sorensen S et al (2000) Pain variations during cancer treatment in children: a descriptive survey. *Pediatr Hematol Onco* 17: 211–21.

Lloyd-Thomas AR, Howard RF (1994) A pain service for children. *Paediatr Anaesth* 4: 3–15.

Loadsman JA & Hillman DR (2001) Anaesthesia and sleep apnoea. *Br J Anaesth* 86: 254–66.

Lofsky A (2002) Sleep apnea and narcotic postoperative pain medication: morbidity and mortality risk. *Anesthesia Patient Safety Foundation Newsletter* 17: 24.

Lovstad RZ & Stoen R (2001) Postoperative epidural analgesia in children after major orthopaedic surgery. A randomised study of the effect on PONV of two anaesthetic techniques: low and high dose i.v. fentanyl and epidural infusions with and without fentanyl. *Acta Anaesth Scand* 5: 482–88.

Lowenthal DT, Saris SD, Paran E et al (1993) The use of transdermal clonidine in the hypertensive patient with chronic renal failure. *Clin Nephrol* 39: 37–42.

Lynn AM, Nespeca MK, Opheim KE et al (1993) Respiratory effects of intravenous morphine infusions in neonates, infants, and children after cardiac surgery. *Anesth Analg* 77: 695–70.

Lynn A, Nespeca MK, Bratton SL et al (1998) Clearance of morphine in postoperative infants during intravenous infusion: the influence of age and surgery. *Anesth Analg* 86: 958–63.

Lynn AM, Nespeca MK, Bratton SL et al (2000) Intravenous morphine in postoperative infants: intermittent bolus dosing versus targeted continuous infusions. *Pain* 88: 89–95.

Lyons G, Columb M, Hawthorne L et al (1997) Extradural pain relief in labour: bupivacaine sparing by extradural fentanyl is dose dependent. *Br J Anaesth* 78: 493–97.

Machotta A, Risse A, Bercker S et al (2003) Comparison between instillation of bupivacaine versus caudal analgesia for postoperative analgesia following inguinal herniotomy in children. *Paediatr Anaesth* 13: 397–402.

Macintyre PE & Jarvis DA (1996) Age is the best predictor of postoperative morphine requirement. *Pain* 64: 357–64.

Macintyre PE & Ready LB (2001) *Acute Pain Management: A Practical Guide*. 2nd Edition. London: WB Saunders.

Macintyre PE, Upton R, Ludbrook GL (2003) Pain in the elderly. In: Rowbotham DJ & Macintyre PE (Eds) *Clinical Pain Management: Acute Pain*. London: Arnold.

Mackie AM, Coda BC, Hill HF (1991) Adolescents use patient-controlled analgesia effectively for relief from prolonged oropharyngeal mucositis pain. *Pain* 46: 265–69.

Madirosoff C, Dumont L, Boulvain M et al (2002) Fetal bradycardia due to intrathecal opioids for labour analgesia: a systematic review. *Br J Obstet Gynaecol* 109: 274–81.

Malviya S, Voepel-Lewis T, Tait AR et al (2001) Pain management in children with and without cognitive impairment following spine fusion surgery. *Paediatr Anaesth* 11: 453–58.

Manfredi PL, Breuer B, Meier DE et al (2003) Pain assessment in elderly patients with severe dementia. *J Pain Sympt Manage* 25: 48–52.

Mann C, Pouzeratte Y, Boccara G et al (2000) Comparison of intravenous or epidural patient-controlled analgesia in the elderly after major abdominal surgery. *Anesthesiology* 92: 433–41.

Manninen T, Aantaa R, Salonen M et al (2000) A comparison of the hemodynamic effects of paracervical block and epidural analgesia for labor analgesia. *Acta Anaesthesiol Scand* 44: 441–45.

Marret E, Flahault A, Samama CM et al (2003) Effects of postoperative, nonsteroidal, antiinflammatory drugs on bleeding risk after tonsillectomy: meta-analysis of randomized, controlled trials. *Anesthesiology*. 98,1497–502.

Marsh D, Dickenson A, Hatch D et al (1999) Epidural opioid analgesia in infant rats II: responses to carrageenan and capsaicin. *Pain* 82: 33–38.

Martensson L & Wallin G (1999) Labour pain treated with cutaneous injections of sterile water: a randomised controlled trial. *Br J Obstet Gynaecol* 106: 633–37.

Marx C, Stein STM, Nieder M et al (1997) Ketamine-midazolam versus meperidine-midazolam for pain procedures in pediatric oncology patients. *J Clin Oncol* 15: 94–102.

McCloskey JJ, Haun SE, Deshpande JK (1992) Bupivacaine toxicity secondary to continuous caudal epidural infusions in children. *Anesth Analg* 75: 287–90.

McDonald SP & Russ GR (2003) Current incidence, treatment patterns and outcomes of endstage renal disease among indigenous groups in Australia and New Zealand. *Nephrology* (Carlton) 8: 42–48.

McEllistrem RF, Schell J, O'Malley K et al (1989) Interscalene brachial plexus blockade with lidocaine in chronic renal failure--a pharmacokinetic study. *Can J Anaesth* 36: 59–63.

McEwan A, Sigston PE, Andrews KA et al (2000) A comparison of rectal and intramuscular codeine phosphate in children following neurosurgery. *Paediatr Anaesth* 10: 189–93.

McGrath PA, Seifert CE, Speechley KN et al (1996) A new analogue scale for assessing children's pain: an initial validation study. *Pain* 64: 435–43.

McGrath PJ, Johnson G, Goodman JT (1985) CHEOPS: a behavioural scale for rating postoperative pain in children. In: Fields HL, Dubner R, Cervero F (Eds) *Advances in Pain Research and and Therapy*, Volume 9. New York: Raven Press, pp395–402.

McGrath PJ (1998) Behavioural measures of pain. In: Finley GA & McGrath PJ (Eds) *Measurement of Pain In Infants and Children. Progress in Pain Research and Management*, Volume 10. Seattle: IASP Press, pp83–102.

McNeely JK & Trentadue NC (1997) Comparison of patient-controlled analgesia with and without nighttime morphine infusion following lower extremity surgery in children. *J Pain Symptom Manage* 13: 268–73.

McNeely JK, Farber NE, Rusy LM et al (1997a) Epidural analgesia improves outcome following pediatric fundoplication. *Reg Anesth* 22: 16–23.

McNeely JK, Trentadue NC, Rusy LM, Farber NE (1997b) Culture of bacteria from lumbar and caudal epidural catheters used for postoperative analgesia in children. *Reg Anesth* 22: 428–31.

McNicol R (1993) Postoperative analgesia in children using continuous s.c. morphine. *Br J Anaesth* 71: 752–56.

Mehta Y, Manikappa S, Juneja R et al (2000) Obstructive sleep apnea syndrome: anesthetic implications in the cardiac surgical patient. *J Cardiothor Vasc Anesth* 14: 449–53.

Melzack R, Taenzer P, Feldman P et al (1981) Labour is still painful after prepared childbirth training. *CMAJ* 125: 357–63.

Mercadante S, Caligara M, Sapio M et al (1997) Subcutaneous fentanyl infusion in a patient with bowel obstruction and renal failure. *J Pain Sympt Manage* 13: 241–44.

Mercadante S & Arcuri E (2004) Opioids and renal function. *J Pain* 5: 2–19.

Merkel SI, Voepel-Lewis T, Shayevitz JR et al (1997) The FLACC: a behavioral scale for scoring postoperative pain in young children. *Pediatr Nurs* 23: 293–97.

Merry A & Power I (1995) Perioperative NSAIDs: towards greater safety. *Pain Rev* 2: 268–91.

Meunier J-F, Goujard E, Dubousset A-M et al (2001) Pharmacokinetics of bupivacaine after continuous epidural infusion in infants with and without biliary atresia. *Anesthesiology* 95: 87–95.

Millan MJ, Morris BJ, Herz A (1988) Antagonist-induced opioid receptor up-regulation. I. Characterization of supersensitivity to selective mu and kappa agonists. *J Pharmacol Exp Ther* 247: 721–28.

Miller PF, Sheps DS, Bragdon EE et al (1990) Aging and pain perception in ischemic heart disease. *Am Heart J* 120: 22–30.

MIMS (2004) *MIMS Annual 2004*. MediMedia Australia Pty Ltd. (www.mims.com.au)

Minassian VA, Jazayeri A, Prien SD et al (2002) Randomised trial of lidocaine ointment versus placebo for the treatment of postpartum perineal pain. *Obstet Gynecol* 100: 1239–43.

Miners JO, Penhall R, Robson RA et al (1988) Comparison of paracetamol metabolism in young adult and elderly males. *Eur J Clin Pharmacol* 35: 156–60.

Miser AW, Goh TS, Dose AM et al (1994) Trial of a topically administered local anesthetic (EMLA cream) for pain relief during central venous port accesses in children with cancer. *J Pain Symptom Manage* 9: 259–64.

Mitra S & Sinatra RS (2004) Perioperative management of acute pain in the opioid-dependent patient. *Anesthesiology* 101: 212–27.

Møiniche S, Rømsing J, Dahl J et al (2003) Nonsteroidal antiinflammatory drugs and the risk of operative site bleeding after tonsillectomy: a quantitative systematic review. *Anesth Analg* 96: 68–77.

Moir MS, Bair E, Shinnick P et al (2000) Acetaminophen versus acetaminophen with codeine after pediatric tonsillectomy. *Laryngoscope* 110: 1824–27.

Monitto CL, Greenberg RS, Kost-Byerly S et al (2000) The safety and efficacy of parent-/nurse-controlled analgesia in patients less than six years of age. *Anesth Analg* 91: 573–79.

Moon JL & Humenick S (1989) Breast engorgement: contributing variables and variables amenable to nursing intervention. *J Obstet Gynaecol Neo Nurs* 18: 309–15.

Morris JL, Rosen DA, Rosen KR (2003) Nonsteroidal anti-inflammatory agents in neonates. *Paediatr Drugs* 5: 385–405.

Morrison RS & Siu AL (2000) A comparison of pain and its treatment in advanced dementia and cognitively intact patients with hip fracture. *J Pain Sympt Manage* 19: 240–48.

Morton NS (1993) Development of a monitoring protocol for safe use of opioids in children. *Paediatr Anaesth* 3: 179–84.

Morton NS & O'Brien K (1999) Analgesic efficacy of paracetamol and diclofenac in children receiving PCA morphine. *Br J Anaesth* 82: 715–17.

Munro FJ, Fisher S, Dickson U et al (2002) The addition of antiemetics to the morphine solution in patient-controlled analgesia syringes used by children after an appendicectomy does not reduce the incidence of postoperative nausea and vomiting. *Paediatr Anaesth* 12: 600–03.

Murat I, Delleur MM, Esteve C et al (1987) Continuous extradural anaesthesia in children. *Br J Anaesth* 69: 1441–50.

Murat I, Walker J, Esteve C et al (1988) Effect of lumbar epidural anaesthesia on plasma cortisol levels in children. *Can J Anaesth* 35: 20–24.

Murat I, Gall O, Tourniaire B (2003) Procedural pain in children: evidence-based best practice and guidelines. *Reg Anesth Pain Med* 28: 561–72.

Murphy JD, Henderson K, Bowden MI et al (1991) Bupivacaine versus bupivacaine plus fentanyl for epidural analgesia: effect on maternal satisfaction. *Br Med J* 302: 564–67.

Murrell D, Gibson PR, Cohen RC (1993) Continuous epidural analgesia in newborn infants undergoing major surgery. *J Paed Surgery* 28: 548–53.

Ngan Kee WD (1998) Epidural pethidine: pharmacology and clinical experience. *Anaesth Intensive Care* 26: 247-55.

Naumburg EG & Meny RG (1988) Breast milk opioids and neonatal apnea (letter). *AJDC* 142: 11–12.

Ng B, Dimsdale JE, Rollnik JD et al (1996) The effect of ethnicity on prescriptions for patient-controlled analgesia for post-operative pain. *Pain* 66: 9–12.

Niederhoff H & Zahradnik HP (1983) Analgesics during pregnancy. *Am J Med* 75: 117–120.

Nielsen GL, Sorensen HT, Larsen H et al (2001) Risk of adverse birth outcome and miscarriage in pregnant users of non-steroidal anti-inflammatory drugs: population based observational study and case-control study. *BMJ* 322: 266–70.

Notarianni LJ, Oldham HG, Bennett PN (1987) Passage of paracetamol into breast milk and its subsequent metabolism by the neonate. *Br J Clin Pharmacol* 24: 63–67.

Olkkola KT & Hamunen K (2000) Pharmacokinetics and pharmacodynamics of analgesic drugs. In: Anand KJS, Stevens BJ, McGrath PJ (Eds) *Pain Research and Clinical Management,* Volume 10. Amsterdam: Elsevier, pp135–58.

Olofsson C, Ekblom A, Ekman-Ordeberg G et al (1996) Lack of analgesic effect of systemically administered morphine or pethidine on labour pain. *Br J Obstet Gynaecol* 103: 968–72.

Ortega D, Viviand X, Lorec AM et al (1999) Excretion of lidocaine and bupivacaine in breast milk following epidural anesthesia for cesarean delivery. *Acta Anaesthesiol Scand* 43: 394–97.

Ostensen ME & Skomsvoll JF (2004) Anti-inflammatory pharmacotherapy during pregnancy. *Expert Opin Pharmacother* 5: 571–80.

Ostermeier AM, Roizen MF, Hautkappe M et al (1997) Three sudden postoperative respiratory arrests associated with epidural opioids in patients with sleep apnea. *Anesth Analg* 85: 452–60.

Ozer Z, Gorur K, Altunkan AA et al (2003) Efficacy of tramadol versus meperidine for pain relief and safe recovery after adenotonsillectomy. *Eur J Anaesthesiol* 20: 920–24.

Paech MJ, Moore JS, Evans SF (1994 Meperidine for patient-controlled analgesia after cesarean section. Intravenous versus epidural administration. *Anesthesiology*. 80: 1268-76.

Paech MJ, Pavy TJ, Orlikowski CE et al (2000) Postoperative intraspinal opioid analgesia after caesarean section; a randomised comparison of subarachnoid morphine and epidural pethidine. *Int J Obstet Anesth* 9: 238-45.

Pappas AL, Fluder EM, Creech S et al (2003) Postoperative analgesia in children undergoing myringotomy and placement equalization tubes in ambulatory surgery. *Anesth Analg* 96: 1621–24.

Parikh SN, Stuchin SA, Maca C et al (2002) Sleep apnea syndrome in patients undergoing total joint arthroplasty. *J Arthroplast* 17: 635–42.

Parker RI, Mahan RA, Giugliano D et al (1997) Efficacy and safety of intravenous midazolam and ketamine as sedation for therapeutic and diagnostic procedures in children. *Pediatrics* 99: 427–31.

Parmelee PA, Smith B, Katz IR (1993) Pain complaints and cognitive status among elderly institution residents. *J Am Geriatr Soc* 41: 517–22.

Parmelee PA (1996) Pain in cognitively impaired older persons. *Clin Geriatr Med* 12: 473–87.

Patel N, Fernando R, Robson S et al (2003) Fetal effects of combined spinal-epidural (CSE) vs. epidural labour analgesia: a prospective, randomised study. *Int J Obstet Anesth* 12(Supp 1): O01.

Pauli-Magnus C, Hofmann U, Mikus G et al (1999) Pharmacokinetics of morphine and its glucuronides following intravenous administration of morphine in patients undergoing continuous ambulatory peritoneal dialysis. *Nephrol Dialysis Transplant* 14: 903–09.

Paut O, Sallabery M, Schreiber-Deturmeny E et al (2001) Continuous fascia iliaca compartment block in children: a prospective evaluation of plasma bupivacaine concentrations, pain scores, and side effects. *Anesth Analg* 92: 1159–63.

Pendeville PE, Von Montigny S, Dort JP et al (2000) Double-blind randomized study of tramadol vs. paracetamol in analgesia after day-case tonsillectomy in children. *Eur J Anaesthesiol* 17: 576–82.

Pertwee RG (2001) Cannabinoid receptors and pain. *Prog Neurobiol* 63: 569–611.

Peter EA, Janssen PA, Grange CS et al (2001) Ibuprofen versus acetaminophen with codeine for relief of perineal pain after childbirth: a randomized controlled trial. *CMAJ* 165: 1203–09.

Peters, JW, Bandell Hoekstra, IE et al (1999) Patient-controlled analgesia in children and adolescents: a randomized controlled trial. *Paediatr Anaesth* 9: 235–41.

Peters JW, Koot HM, de Boer JB et al (2003a) Major surgery within the first 3 months of life and subsequent biobehavioral pain responses to immunization at later age: a case comparison study. *Pediatr* 111: 129–35.

Peters JW, Koot HM, Grynau RE et al (2003) Neonatal facial coding system for assessing postoperative pain in infants: item reduction is valid and feasible. *Clin J Pain* 19: 353-63.

Philip J, Alexander JM, Sharma SK et al (1999) Epidural analgesia during labor and maternal fever. *Anesthesiology* 90: 1271–75.

Phillips AC, Polisson RP, Simon LS (1997) NSAIDs and the elderly. Toxicity and economic implications. *Drugs Aging* 10: 119–30.

Phillips BA, Schmitt FA, Berry DT et al (1990) Treatment of obstructive sleep apnea. A preliminary report comparing nasal CPAP to nasal oxygen in patients with mild OSA. *Chest* 8: 325–30.

Pickering AE, Bridge HS, Nolan J (2002) Double-blind, placebo-controlled analgesic study of ibuprofen or rofecoxib on combination with paracetamol for tonsillectomy in children. *Br J Anaesthesia* 88: 72–77.

Powers SW (1999) Empirically supported treatments in pediatric psychology: procedure-related pain. *J Pediatr Psychol* 24: 131-45.

Quinn AC, Brown JH, Wallace PG et al (1994) Studies in postoperative sequelae: nausea and vomiting still a problem. *Anaesthesia* 49: 62–65.

RACP (2002) *Policy Statement on Circumcision.* Royal Australasian College of Physicians. (www.racp.edu.au/hpu/paed/circumcision/index.htm)

Ragg P & Davidson A (1997) Comparison of the efficacy of paracetamol versus paracetamol, codeine and promethazine (Painstop) for premedication and analgesia for myringotomy in children. *Anaesth Int Care* 25: 29–32.

Rapp SE, Wild LM, Egan KJ et al (1994) Acute pain management of the chronic pain patient on opiates: a survey of caregivers at University of Washington Medical Center. *Clin J Pain* 10: 133–38.

Rapp SE, Ready BL, Nessly ML (1995) Acute pain management in patients with prior opioid consumption: a case-controlled retrospective review. *Pain* 61: 195–201.

Rathmell JP, Viscomi CM, Ashburn MA (1997) Management of nonobstetric pain during pregnancy and lactation. *Anesth Analg* 85: 1074–87.

Ravin DS (1995) Narcotic analgesics and breastfeeding. *J Hum Lact* 11: 47–50.

RCA (1998) *Guidelines for the Use of Non-steroidal Anti-inflammatory Drugs in the Perioperative Period.* London: Royal College of Anaesthetists.

Ready LB, Chadwick HS, Ross B (1987) Age predicts effective epidural morphine dose after abdominal hysterectomy. *Anesth Analg* 66: 1215–18.

Reeder MK, Goldman MD, Loh L, et al (1991) Postoperative obstructive sleep apnoea. Haemodynamic effects of treatment with nasal CPAP. *Anaesthesia* 46: 849–53.

Reid MF, Harris R, Phillips PD et al (1987) Day-case herniotomy in children. A comparison of ilio-inguinal nerve block and wound infiltration for postoperative analgesia. *Anaesthesia* 42(6): 658–61.

Reinoso-Barbero F, Saavedra B, Hervilla S et al (2002) Lidocaine with fentanyl, compared to morphine, marginally improves postoperative epidural analgesia in children. *Can J Anaesth* 49: 67–67.

Rennotte MT, Baele P, Aubert G et al (1995) Nasal continuous positive airway pressure in the perioperative management of patients with obstructive sleep apnea submitted to surgery. *Chest* 107: 367–74.

Reynolds F, Sharma SK, Seed PT (2002) Analgesia in labour and fetal acid-base balance: A meta-analysis comparing epidural with systemic opioid analgesia. *BJOG* 109: 1344–53.

Rice AS, Pither CE, Tucker GT (1991) Plasma concentrations of bupivacaine after supraclavicular brachial plexus blockade in patients with chronic renal failure *Anaesthesia* 46: 354–57.

Richardson J & Bresland K (1998) The management of postsurgical pain in the elderly population. *Drugs Aging* 13: 17–31.

Richtsmeier AJ, Barnes SD, Barkin RL (1997) Ventilatory arrest with morphine patient-controlled analgesia in a child with renal failure. *Am J Ther* 4: 255–57.

Righard L & Aldade MO (1990) Effect of delivery room routines on success of first breast-feed. *Lancet* 336: 1105–07.

Roberts DM & Meyer-Witting M (2005) Buprenorphine: perioperative precautions and management strategies. *Anaesth Int Care* 33: 17–25.

Robieux I, Koren G, Vandenbergh H et al (1990) Morphine excretion in breast milk and resultant exposure of a nursing infant. *Clin Toxicol* 28: 365–70.

Roche SI & Goucke CR (2003) Management of acutely painful medical conditions. In: Rowbotham DJ & Macintyre PE (Eds) *Clinical Pain Management. Acute Pain.* London: Arnold

RømsingJ, Moller-sonnergaard J, Hertel S et al (1996) Postoperative pain in children: comparison between ratings of children and nurses. *J Pain Symptom manage* 11: 42–46.

Rømsing J, Ostergaard D, Drozdziewicz D et al (2000) Diclofenac or acetaminophen for analgesia in paediatric tonsillectomy outpatients. *Acta Anaesth Scand* 44: 291–95.

Rose JB (2003) Editorial: Spinal cord injury in a child after single-shot epidural anesthesia. *Anesth Analg* 96: 3–6.

Rosen MA (2002) Nitrous oxide for relief of labor pain: a systematic review. *Am J Obstet Gynecol* 186: S110–26.

Sabers C, Plevak DJ, Schroeder DR et al (2003) The diagnosis of obstructive sleep apnea as a risk factor for unanticipated admissions in outpatient surgery. *Anesth Analg* 96: 1328–35.

Sadean MR &Glass PSA (2003) Pharmacokinetics in the elderly. *Best Pract Res Clin Anaesthesiol* 17: 191–205.

Sartain JB & Barry JJ (1999) The impact of an acute pain service on postoperative pain management. *Anaesth Int Care* 27: 375–80.

Sator-Katzenschlager S, Deusch E, Maier P et al (2001) The long-term antinociceptive effect of intrathecal S(+)-ketamine in a patient with established morphine tolerance. *Anesth Analg* 93: 1032–34.

Schindler SD, Eder H, Ortner R et al (2003) Neonatal outcome following buprenorphine maintenance during conception and throughout pregnancy. *Addiction* 98: 103–10.

Sciard D, Matuszczak M, Gebhard R et al (2001) Continuous posterior lumbar plexus block for acute postoperative pain control in young children. *Anesthesiology* 95: 1521–23.

Scott JC & Stanski DR (1987) Decreased fentanyl and alfentanil requirements with age. A simultaneous pharmacokinetic and pharmacodynamic evaluation. *J Pharmacol Exp Ther* 240: 159–66.

Semple D, Russell S, Doyle E et al (1999) Comparison of morphine sulphate and codeine phosphate in children undergoing adenotonsillectomy. *Paediatr Anaesth* 9: 135–38.

Semsroth M, Plattner O, Horcher E (1996) Effective pain relief with continuous intrapleural bupivacaine after thoracotomy in infants and children. *Paediatr Anaesth* 6: 303–10.

Sethna NF & Berde CB (1993) Venous air embolism during identification of the epidural space in children. *Anesth Analg* 76: 925–27.

Shanahan EC, Marshall AG, Garrett CP (1983) Adverse reactions to intravenous codeine phosphate in children. A report of three cases. *Anaesthesia* 38: 40–43.

Shand F, Gates J, Faucett J et al (2003) *The Treatment of Alcohol Problems. A Review of the Evidence.* Sydney: National Drug and Alcohol Research Centre (NDARC)

Shapiro AG & Thomas L (1984) Efficacy of bromocriptine versus breast binders as inhibitors of postpartum lactation. *South Med J* 77: 719–21.

Shapiro A, Fredman B, Zohar E et al (1998) Delivery room analgesia: An analysis of maternal satisfaction. *Int J Obstet Anesth* 7: 226–30.

Sharma SK, Sidawi JE, Ramin SM et al (1997) Cesarean delivery: a randomized trial of epidural versus patient-controlled meperidine analgesia during labor. *Anesthesiology* 87: 487–94.

Sharma SK, Alexander JM, Wiley J et al (2003) Abstracts of the Society for Obstetric Anesthesia and Perinatology. *Anesthesiology* 98 (Suppl 1 SOAP): A69.

Shnider SM, Asling JH, Holl JW et al (1970) Paracervical block anesthesia in obstetrics. I. Fetal complications and neonatal morbidity. *Am J Obstet Gynecol* 107: 619–25.

Short JA, Barr CA, Palmer CD et al (2000) Use of diclofenac in children with asthma. *Anaesthesia* 55: 334–37.

Shwartz N & Eisenkraft JB (1993) Probable venous air embolism during epidural placement in an infant. *Anesth Analg* 76: 1136–38.

Simon MJC, Veering B, Stienstra R et al (2002) The effects of age on neural blockade and hemodynamic changes after epidural analgesia with ropivacaine. *Anesth Analg* 94: 1325–30.

Simopoulos TT, Smith HS, Peeters-Asdourian C et al (2002) Use of meperidine in patient-controlled analgesia and the development of a normeperidine toxic reaction. *Arch Surg* 137: 84–88.

Skovlund E, Fyllingen G, Landre H et al (1991a) Comparison of postpartum pain treatment using a sequential trial design. I Paracetamol versus placebo. *Eur J Clin Pharmacol* 40: 343–47.

Skovlund E, Fyllingen G, Landre H et al (1991b) Comparison of postpartum pain treatment using a sequential trial design: II Naproxen versus paracetamol. *Eur J Clin Pharmacol* 40: 539–42.

Sleep J, Grant A, Garcia J et al (1984) West Berkshire perineal management trial. *Br Med J* 289: 587–90.

Sleep J & Grant A (1988) Relief of perineal pain following childbirth: A survey of midwifery practice. *Midwifery* 4: 118–22.

Sleep J (1995) Postnatal perineal care revisited. In: Alexander J, Levy V, Roch S (Eds) *Aspects of Midwifery Care: a Research Based Approach.* London: Macmillan Press, pp132–53.

Sleep J & Grant A (1998) Effects of salt and Savlon bath concentrate postpartum. *Nurs Times* 84: 55–57.

Smith CA, Collins CT, Cyna AM et al(2003)Complementary and alternative therapies for pain management in labour. *The Cochrane Database of Systematic Reviews*, Issue 2. Art. No.: CD003521. DOI: 10.1002/14651858.CD003521

Snowden HM, Renfrew MJ, Woolridge MW (2001) Treatments for breast engorgement during lactation. *The Cochrane Database of Systematic Reviews* Issue 2. Art. No.: CD000046. DOI: 10.1002/14651858.CD000046.

Spigset O & Hagg S (2000) Analgesics and breast-feeding: Safety considerations. *Paediatr Drugs* 2: 223–38.

Splinter WM, Bass J, Komocar L (1995) Regional anaesthesia for hernia repair in children: local vs caudal anaesthesia. *Can J Anaesth* 42: 197–200.

Steen MP & Cooper KJ (1998) Cold therapy and perineal wounds: too cool or not too cool? *Br J Mid* 6: 572–79.

Steen M, Cooper K, Marchant P et al (2000) A randomised controlled trial to compare the effectiveness of ice packs and Epifoam with cooling maternity gel pads at alleviating postnatal perineal trauma. *Midwifery* 16: 48–55.

Steer PL, Biddle CJ, Marley WS et al (1992) Concentration of fentanyl in colostrum after an analgesic dose. *Can J Anaesth* 39: 231–35.

Stevens B, Johnston C, Petryshen P et al (1996) Premature Infant Pain Profile: development and initial validation. *Clin J Pain* 12: 13–22.

Stevens B (1998) Composite measures of pain. In: Finley GA & McGrath PJ (Eds) *Measurement of Pain In Infants and Children. Progress in Pain Research and Management*, Volume 10. Seattle: IASP Press, pp161–78.

Stevens B, Johnston C, Gibbins S (2000) In: Anand KJS, Stevens BJ, McGrath PJ (Eds) *Pain In Neonates. Pain Research and Clinical* Management, Volume 10. Amsterdam: Elsevier, pp101–34.

Stevens B, McGrath P, Gibbins S et al (2003) Procedural pain in newborns at risk for neurologic impairment. *Pain* 105: 27–35.

Stevens B, Yamada J, Ohlsson A (2004) Sucrose for analgesia in newborn infants undergoing painful procedures. The Cochrane Database of Systematic Reviews Issue 3. Art. No.: CD001069. DOI: 10.1002/14651858.CD001069.pub2

Steward DL, Welge JA, Myer CM (2002) Steroids for improving recovery following tonsillectomy in children. *The Cochrane Database of Systematic Reviews* 2002, Issue 3. Art. No.: CD003997. DOI: 10.1002/14651858.CD003997.

Stone PA, Macintyre PE, Jarvis DA (1993) Norpethidine toxicity and patient controlled analgesia. *Br J Anaesth* 71: 738–40.

Strafford MA, Wilder RT, Berde CB (1995) The risk of infection from epidural analgesia in children: a review of 1620 cases. *Anesth Analg* 80: 234–38.

Suominen PK, Ragg PG, McKinley DF et al (2004) Intrathecal morphine provides effective and safe analgesia in children after cardiac surgery. *Acta Anaesthesiol Scand* 48: 875–82.

Sweet SA & McGrath PJ (1998) Physiological measures of pain. In: Finley GA & McGrath PJ (Eds) *Measurement of Pain In Infants and Children. Progress in Pain Research and Management*, Volume 10. Seattle: IASP Press, pp59–82.

Taddio A, Goldbach M, Ipp M et al (1997) Effect of neonatal circumcision on pain responses during vaccination in boys. *Lancet* 345: 291–92.

Taddio A, Ohlsson A, Einarson TR et al (1998) A systematic review of lidocaine-prilocaine cream (EMLA) in the treatment of acute pain in neonates. *Pediatrics* 101: e1.

Tay CL & Tan S (2002) Diclofenac or paracetamol for analgesia in paediatric myringotomy outpatients. *Anaesth Int Care* 30: 55–59.

Taylor RN & Sonson RD (1986) Separation of the pubic symphysis. An underrecognized peripartum complication. *J Reprod Med* 31: 203–06.

Tegeder I, Lotsch J, Geisslinger G (1999) Pharmacokinetics of opioids in liver disease. *Clin Pharmacokinet* 37: 17–40.

Thomas AN & Suresh M (2000) Opiate withdrawal after tramadol and patient-controlled analgesia *Anaesthesia* 55: 826–27.

Thomas T, Robinson C, Champion D et al (1998) Prediction and assessment of the severity of post-operative pain and of satisfaction with management. *Pain* 75: 177–85.

Thomson MA, Lynch S, Strong R et al (2000) Orthotopic Liver Transplantation With Poor Neurologic Outcome in Valproate-Associated Liver Failure: A need for Critical Risk-Benefit Appraisal in the use of Valproate. *Transplant Proc* 32: 200–03.

Tobias JD & Baker DK (1992) Patient-controlled analgesia with fentanyl in children. *Clin Pediatr (Phila)* 31: 177–79.

Tobias JD, Lowe S, Hersey S et al (1995) Analgesia after bilateral myringotomy and placement of pressure equalization tubes in children: acetaminophen versus acetaminophen with codeine. *Anesth Analg* 81: 496–500.

Tobias JD (2001) Brachial plexus anaesthesia in children. *Paediatr Anaesth* 11: 265–75.

Treadwell MJ, Franck LS, Vichinsky E (2002) Using quality improvement strategies to enhance pediatric pain assessment. *Int J Qual Health Care* 14: 39–47.

Tsui BCH, Seal R, Koller J (2002) Thoracic epidural catheter placement via the caudal approach in infants by using electrocardiographic guidance. *Anesth Analg* 95: 326–30.

Tsui BCH, Wagner A, Cave D et al (2004) Thoracic and lumbar epidural analgesia via the caudal approach using electrical stimulation guidance in pediatric patients. A Review of 289 patients. *Anesthesiology* 100: 683.

Tyler DC, Pomietto M, Womack W (1996) Variation in opioid use during PCA in adolescents. *Paediatr Anaesth* 6: 33–38.

Valley RD & Bailey AG (1991) Caudal morphine for postoperative analgesia in infants and children: a report of 138 cases. *Anesth Analg* 72: 120–24.

van der Marel CD, Anderson BJ, van Lingen RA et al (2003) Paracetamol and metabolite pharmacokinetics in infants. *Eur J Clin Pharmacol* 59: 243–51.

van der Marel CD, Anderson BJ, Rømsing J et al (2004) Diclofenac and metabolite pharmacokinetics in children. *Paediatr Anaesth* 14: 443–51.

Van der Vyver M, Halpern S, Joseph G (2002) Patient-controlled epidural analgesia versus continuous infusion for labour analgesia: a meta-analysis. *Br J Anaesth* 89: 459–65.

van Dijk M, de Boer JB, Koot HM et al (2000) The reliability and validity of the COMFORT scale as a postoperative pain instrument in 0 to 3-year-old infants. *Pain* 84: 367–77.

van Dijk M, Bouwmeester NJ, Duivenvoorden HJ et al (2002) Efficacy of continuous versus intermittent morphine administration after major surgery in 0–3-year-old infants; a double-blind randomized controlled trial. *Pain* 98: 305–13.

Van Diver T & Camman W (1995) Meralgia paresthetica in the parturient. *Int J Obstet Anesth* 4: 109–12.

van Lingen RA, Deinum HT, Quak CM et al (1999) Multiple-dose pharmacokinetics of rectally administered acetaminophen in term infants. *Clin Pharmacol Ther* 66 : 509–15.

van Slobbe AM, Bohnen AM, Bernsen RM et al (2004) Incidence rates and determinants in meralgia paresthetica in general practice. *J Neurol* 251: 294–97.

VanDercar DH, Martinez AP, De Lisser EA (1991) Sleep apnea syndromes: a potential contraindication for patient-controlled analgesia. *Anesthesiology* 74: 623–4.

Veering BT, Burm AGL, van Kleef JW et al (1987) Epidural anaesthesia with bupivacaine: effects of age on neural blockade and pharmacokinetics. *Anesth Analg* 66: 589–93.

Veering BT, Burm AGL, Vletter AA et al (1991) The effect of age on the systemic absorption and systemic disposition of bupivacaine after subarachnoid administration. *Anesthesiology* 74: 250–57.

Veyckemans F, Van Obbergh LJ, Gouverneur JM (1992) Lessons from 1100 pediatric caudal blocks in a teaching hospital. *Reg Anesth* 17: 119–25.

Vigano A, Bruera E, Suarez-Almazor ME (1998) Age, pain intensity, and opioid dose in patients with advanced cancer. *Cancer* 83: 1244–50.

Viitanen H & Annila P (2001) Analgesic efficacy of tramadol 2 mg kg(-1) for paediatric day-case adenoidectomy. *Br J Anaesth* 86: 572–75.

Viitanen H, Tuominen N, Vaaraniemi H et al (2003) Analgesic efficacy of rectal acetaminophen and ibuprofen alone or in combination for paediatric day-case adenoidectomy. *Br J Anaesth* 91: 363–67.

Voepel-Lewis T, Merkel S, Tait AR (2002) The reliability and validity of the Face, Legs, Activity, Cry, Consolability observational tool as a measure of pain in children with cognitive impairment. *Anesth Analg* 95: 1224–29.

Vuyk J (2003) Pharmacokinetics in the elderly. *Best Practice and Research Clinical Anaesthesiology* 17: 207–18.

Walker SM, Meredith-Middleton J, Cooke-Yarborough C et al (2003) Neonatal inflammation and primary afferent terminal plasticity in the rat dorsal horn. *Pain* 105: 185–95.

Wang et al (1979) Pain relief by intrathecally applied morphine in man. *Anesthesiology* 50: 149–51.

Wathen JE, Roback MG, Mackenzie T et al (2000) Does midazolam alter the clinical effects of intravenous ketamine sedation in children? A double-blind, randomized, controlled, emergency department trial. *Ann Emerg Med* 36: 579–88.

Weisman SJ, Bernstein B, Schecter NL (1998) Consequences of inadequate analgesia during painful procedures in children. *Arch Pediatr Adolesc Med* 152: 147–49.

Weissman DE & Haddox JD (1989) Opioid pseudoaddiction – an iatrogenic syndrome. *Pain* 36: 363–66.

Weldon BC, Connor M, White PF (1993) Pediatric PCA: the role of concurrent opioid infusions and nurse-controlled analgesia. *Clin J Pain* 9: 26–33.

Westling F, Milsom I, Zetterstrom H et al (1992) Effects of nitrous oxide inhalation on the maternal circulation during vaginal delivery. *Acta Anaesthesiol Scand* 36: 175–81.

Wight WJ & Halpern SH (2003) Back pain and epidural analgesia for labor and delivery- a systematic review. *Anesthesiology* 98 (Suppl 1 SOAP): A131.

Williams DG, Patel A, Howard RF (2002) Pharmacogenetics of codeine metabolism in an urban population of children and its implications for analgesic reliability. *Br J Anaesth* 89: 839–45.

Williams DG &Howard RF (2003) Epidural analgesia in children. A survey of current opinions and practices amongst UK paediatric anaesthetists. *Paed Anaesth* 13: 769–76.

Wittels B, Scott DT, Sinatra RS (1990) Exogenous opioids in human breast milk and acute neonatal neurobehaviour: a preliminary study. *Anesthesiology* 73: 864–69.

Wittels B, Glosten B, Faure EAM et al (1997) Postcesarean analgesia with both epidural morphine and intravenous patient-controlled analgesia: neurobehavioural outcomes among nursing neonates. *Anesth Analg* 85: 600–06.

Wolf AR, Hughes D, Wade A et al (1990) Postoperative analgesia after paediatric orchidopexy: evaluation of a bupivacaine-morphine mixture. *Br J Anaesth* 64: 430–35.

Wolf AR, Hughes D, Hobbs AJ et al (1991) Combined morphine-bupivacaine caudals for reconstructive penile surgery in children: systemic absorption of morphine and postoperative analgesia. *Anaesth Int Care* 19: 17–21.

Wolf AR & Hughes D (1993) Pain relief for infants undergoing abdominal surgery: comparison of infusions of IV morphine and extradural bupivacaine. *Br J Anaesth* 70: 10–16.

Wolf AR, Eyres RL, Laussen PC et al (1993) Effect of extradural analgesia on stress responses to abdominal surgery in infants. *Br J Anaesth* 70: 654–60.

Wolf AR, Doyle E, Thomas E (1998) Modifying infant stress responses to major surgery: spinal vs extradural vs opioid analgesia. *Paed Anaesth* 8: 305–11.

Wong D & Baker C (1988) Pain in children: comparison of assessment scales. *Pediatric Nursing* 14: 9–17.

Woodhouse A & Mather LE (1997) The influence of age upon opioid use in the patient-controlled analgesia (PCA) environment. *Anaesthesia* 52: 949–55.

Workman BS, Ciccone V, Christophidis N (1989) Pain management for the elderly. *Aust Fam Phys* 18: 1515–27.

Worthington HV, Clarkson JE, Eden OB (2004) Interventions for treating oral mucositis for patients with cancer receiving treatment. *The Cochrane Database of Systematic Reviews* Issue 2. Art. No.: CD001973. DOI: 10.1002/14651858.CD001973.pub2.

Wunsch MJ, Stanard V, Schnoll SH (2003) Treatment of pain in pregnancy. *Clin J Pain* 19: 148–55.

Yeoman PM, Cooke R, Hain WR (1983) Penile block for circumcision? A comparison with caudal blockade. *Anaesthesia* 38: 862–66.

Young T, Skatrud J, Peppard PE (2004) Risk factors for obstructive sleep apnoea in adults. *JAMA* 291: 2013–16.

Zapater P, Lasso de la Vega MC, Horga JF et al (2004) Pharmacokinetic variations of acetaminophen according to liver dysfunction and portal hypertension status. *Aliment Pharmacol Ther* 20: 29–36.

Zelson C, Lee SJ, Casalino M (1973) Neonatal narcotic addiction. Comparative effects of maternal intake of heroin and methadone. *N Engl J Med* 289: 1216–20.

Zelson C (1975) Acute management of neonatal addiction. *Addict Dis* 2: 159–68.

Zwaveling J, Bubbers S, Van Meurs AH et al (2004) Pharmacokinetics of rectal tramadol in postoperative paediatric patients. *Br J Anaesth* 93: 224–27.

Appendix A

THE WORKING PARTY, CONTRIBUTORS AND REPRESENTATIVES ON THE MULTIDISCIPLINARY CONSULTATIVE COMMITTEE

Working party

Dr Pam Macintyre (Chair)
Director, Acute Pain Service
Department of Anaesthesia,
Hyperbaric and Pain Medicine
Royal Adelaide Hospital, Adelaide

Professor Ian Power
Professor of Anaesthesia, Critical
Care and Pain Medicine
The University of Edinburgh
Royal Infirmary, Edinburgh

Professor Stephan Schug
Professor of Anesthesia and Director
of Pain Medicine
Department of Anaesthesia and Pain
Medicine
Royal Perth Hospital and University of
Western Australia, Perth

Assoc Prof. David Scott
Deputy Director of Anaesthesia
Department of Anaesthesia
St. Vincent's Hospital, Melbourne

Dr Eric Visser
Consultant
Department of Anaesthesia and Pain
Medicine
Royal Perth Hospital, Perth

Dr Suellen Walker
Senior Lecturer in Paediatric
Anaesthesia and Pain Management
Great Ormond Street Hospital and
The Institute of Child Health
University College, London

Royal College of Anaesthetists Consultant to the Working Party

Dr Douglas Justins
Pain Management Centre
St Thomas' Hospital
London

Guideline Assessment Register Consultants

Professor Karen Grimmer
Director, Allied Health Evidence
University of South Australia

Assoc. Prof. Caroline Smith
Deputy Director, Allied Health
Evidence
University of South Australia

Editors

Elizabeth Hall
Ampersand Editorial & Design

Jenny Zangger
Ampersand Editorial & Design

Contributors

Dr Kirsten Auret
School of Medicine and Pharmacology
University of Western Australia, Perth

Dr David Barker
Department of Paediatric Anaesthesia
Womens and Childrens Hospital, Adelaide

Dr Steve Barrett
Department of Anaesthesia and Pain Management
Royal North Shore Hospital, Sydney

Dr Michael Barrington
Department of Anaesthesia
St. Vincent's Hospital, Melbourne

Dr Emma-Jane Bennett
Department of Anaesthesia and Pain Medicine
King Edward Memorial Hospital for Women, Perth

Dr Duncan Blake
Department of Anaesthesia and Pain Management
Royal Melbourne Hospital, Melbourne

Dr Penny Briscoe
Pain Management Unit
Royal Adelaide Hospital, Adelaide

Dr Gary Brown
Emergency Department
The Children's Hospital at Westmead, Sydney

Dr Richard Burstal
Department of Anaesthesia, Intensive Care and Pain Management
John Hunter Hospital, Newcastle

Dr Robyn Campbell
Pain Management Unit
Royal Adelaide Hospital, Adelaide

Dr George Chalkiadis
Department of Anaesthesia and Pain Management
Royal Children's Hospital, Melbourne

Dr John Collins
Pain and Palliative Care Service
The Children's Hospital at Westmead, Sydney

Dr Michael Cooper
Pain & Palliative Care Service
The Childrens Hospital at Westmead, Sydney

Prof Michael Cousins
President, ANZCA
Department of Anaesthesia and Pain Management
Royal North Shore Hospital, Sydney

Dr Meredith Craigie
Department of Anaesthesia
Flinders Medical Centre, Adelaide

DrJonathon de Lima
Department of Anaesthesia
The Children's Hospital at Westmead, Sydney

Dr Greg Emery
Department of Anaesthesia
St. Vincent's Hospital, Melbourne

Dr Daniel Fatovich
Department of Emergency Medicine
Royal Perth Hospital, Perth

Dr Julia Fleming
Peter MacCallum Cancer Centre, Melbourne

Dr Paul Glare
Central Sydney Palliative Care Service
Royal Prince Alfred Hospital, Sydney

Dr Roger Goucke
Department of Pain Management
Sir Charles Gairdner Hospital, Perth

Prof Robert Helme
National Ageing Research Institute
Melbourne

Dr Malcolm Hogg
Department of Pain Management
Prince of Wales Hospital, Sydney

Dr David Jarvis
Department of Anaesthesia,
Hyperbaric and Pain Medicine
Royal Adelaide Hospital, Adelaide

Professor Peter Kam
Department of Anaesthetics
St George Hospital, Sydney

Prof Anne-Maree Kelly
Department of Emergency Medicine
Western Hospital, Melbourne

Dr John Loadsman
Department of Anaesthetics
Royal Prince Alfred Hospital, Sydney

Dr Susie Lord
Division of Anaesthesia, Intensive
Care & Pain Management
John Hunter Hospital, Newcastle

Dr Pam Macintyre
Acute Pain Service
Department of Anaesthesia,
Hyperbaric and Pain Medicine
Royal Adelaide Hospital, Adelaide

Dr Ross MacPherson
Department of Anaesthesia and Pain
Management
Royal North Shore Hospital, Sydney

Dr Neil Maycock
Department of Anaesthesia,
Hyperbaric and Pain Medicine
Royal Adelaide Hospital, Adelaide

Dr Jennifer Morgan
Department of Anaesthesia and Pain
Medicine
Royal Perth Hospital, Perth

Dr David Murrell
Department of Anaesthesia
The Children's Hospital at Westmead,
Sydney

Dr Ted Murphy
Department of Anaesthesia,
Hyperbaric and Pain Medicine
Royal Adelaide Hospital, Adelaide

Assoc Prof Michael Nicholas
University of Sydney Pain
Management and Research Centre
Royal North Shore Hospital, Sydney

Dr Greg O'Sullivan
Department of Anaesthetics
St Vincent's Hospital, Sydney

A/Prof Michael Paech
School of Medicine and
Pharmacology
University of Western Australia, Perth

Dr Greta Palmer
Department of Anaesthesia and Pain
Management
Royal Childrens Hospital, Melbourne

Dr Tim Pavy
Department of Anaesthesia
King Edward Memorial Hospital, Perth

Tiina Piira
Pain Research Unit
Sydney Children's Hospital, Randwick

Professor Ian Power
Anaesthesia, Critical Care and Pain
Medicine
The University of Edinburgh
Royal Infirmary, Edinburgh

Dr John Reeves
Intensive Care Unit
Epworth Hospital, Melbourne

Dr Lindy Roberts
Departments of Anaesthesia and Pain Management
Sir Charles Gairdner Hospital, Perth

Dr Sharon Roche
Ocean Reef, Western Australia

Dr Glenda Rudkin
Specialist Anaesthetic Services, Adelaide

Dr James Sartain
Department of Anaesthesia and Intensive Care
Cairns Base Hospital, Cairns

Professor Stephan Schug
Departments of Anaesthesia and Pain Medicine
Royal Perth Hospital and University of Western Australia, Perth

Assoc Prof David Scott
Department of Anaesthesia
St. Vincent's Hospita, Melbournel

Dr Philip Siddall
University of Sydney Pain Management & Research Centre
Royal North Shore Hospital, Sydney

A/Prof Kevin Singer
Director, Centre for Musculoskeletal Studies
Department of Surgery
Royal Perth Hospital, Perth

Dr Brian Spain
Dept of Anaesthesia
Royal Darwin Hospital, Darwin

Dr Philip Stephens
Mater Health Services, Brisbane

Dr Jane Trinca
Barbara Walker Centre for Pain Management,
St Vincents Hospital, Melbourne

Dr Grant Turner
Department of Anaesthesia and Pain Medicine
Royal Perth Hospital, Perth

Dr Russell Vickers
University of Sydney Pain Management and Research Centre
Royal North Shore Hospital, Sydney

Dr Suellen Walker
Department of Anaesthesia
Great Ormond Street Hospital for Children
WellChild Pain Research Centre
Institute of Child Health
University College London, London

Dr Annie Woodhouse
Department of Anaesthesia and Pain Management
Royal North Shore Hospital, Sydney

Dr Paul Wrigley
Pain Management and Research Institute
Royal North Shore Hospital, Sydney

Representatives on the Multidisciplinary Consultative Committee

Aboriginal Health

Ms Josie Owens
Project Officer, SA Review of Aboriginal Palliative Care Resource Kit Project Department of Health and Aboriginal Health Nurse CNC
Royal Adelaide Hospital, Adelaide

Australian Medicines Handbook

Dr Ruth Hanley
Australian Medicines Handbook, Adelaide

Basic Sciences

Dr Richard Upton
Principle Medical Scientist/Senior Lecturer
Department of Anaesthesia, Hyperbaric and Pain Medicine
Royal Adelaide Hospital and University of Adelaide, Adelaide

Chiropractic

Dr Philip Bolton
School of Biomedical Science, Faculty of Health
University of Newcastle, Newcastle

Dr Keith Charlton
Forest Lake Chiropractic Centre, Forest Lake

Clinical Pharmacology

A/Prof Anne Tonkin
Dept of Clinical and Experimental Pharmacology
Medical School, University of Adelaide, Adelaide

Clinical Psychology

Assoc Prof Michael Nicholas
University of Sydney Pain Management and Research Centre
Royal North Shore Hospital, Sydney

Drug and Alcohol and Addiction Medicine

Dr Matt Gaughwin
Director, Drug and Alcohol Resource Unit
Drug and Alcohol Services Council
Royal Adelaide Hospital, Adelaide

Emergency Medicine

Prof Chris Baggoley
Director, Emergency Medicine
Royal Adelaide Hospital, Adelaide

Dr Garry Brown
Head, The Emergency Department
The Children's Hospital at Westmead, Sydney

Dr Daniel Fatovich
Department of Emergency Medicine
Royal Perth Hospital, Perth

Prof Anne-Maree Kelly
Director, Emergency Medicine
Western Hospital, Melbourne

General Practice

Prof Justin Beilby
Professor, University Department of General Practice
University of Adelaide and Royal Adelaide Hospital, Adelaide

General Surgery

Mr James Moore
Head, Colorectal Unit
Royal Adelaide Hospital, Adelaide

Intensive Care Medicine

Dr John Reeves
Director, Intensive Care Unit
Epworth Hospital, Melbourne

Neurosurgery

Prof Nigel Jones
University Department of Neurosurgery
Royal Adelaide Hospital, Adelaide

A/Prof Leigh Atkinson
Brisbane

New Zealand

Dr David Jones
Department of Anaesthesia
Dunedin Hospital, Dunedin

Nursing

Ms Fran Bermingham
CNC, Acute Pain Service
Flinders Medical Centre, Adelaide

Ms Lynne Haley
CNC, Pain Management Unit
Royal Adelaide Hospital, Adelaide

Obstetrics

A/Prof Jan Dickinson
School of Women's and Infants health
The University of Western Australia
King Edward Memorial Hospital, Perth

Oncology

Prof Ian Olver
Clinical Director
Cancer Centre
Royal Adelaide Hospital, Adelaide

Oral Surgery

Dr Russell Vickers
University of Sydney Pain Management and Research Centre
Royal North Shore Hospital, Sydney

Orthopaedic Surgery

Prof Peter Choong
Professor of Orthopaedics, University of Melbourne and Director of Orthopaedics, St Vincent's Hospital, Melbourne

Osteopathy

Dr Nick Penny
Australian Osteopathic Association

Palliative Care

Dr Kirsten Auret
Senior Lecturer in Palliative Care
University of Western Australia, Perth

Dr Paul Glare
Director, Central Sydney Palliative Care Service
Royal Prince Alfred Hospital, Sydney

Paediatrics

Dr John Collins
Head, Pain and Palliative Care Service
The Children's Hospital at Westmead, Sydney

Pharmacy

Stephanie Wiltshire
Project Pharmacist, Drug Committee
Royal Adelaide Hospital, Adelaide

Physicians

A/Prof Milton Cohen – rheumatologist
Arthritis and Pain Research Clinic
St Vincent's Medical Centre, Sydney

Dr Ray Garrick – neurologist
St Vincent's Clinic, Sydney

Prof Robert Helme
National Ageing Research Institute, Melbourne

Physiotherapy

Ms Lois Tonkin
Associate Clinical Lecturer, Physiotherapist-in-charge,
University of Sydney Pain Management and Research Centre,
Royal North Shore Hospital, Sydney

Psychiatry

Dr Faiz Noore
Nepean Hospital, Penrith

Rehabilitation Medicine

Dr Carolyn Arnold
Caulfield Pain Management & Research Centre, Melbourne

Rural and Remote Medicine

Dr John Hadok

Australian College of Rural and Remote

Medicine, Mackay

Thoracic Surgery

Mr Craig Jurisevic
Department of Cardiothoracic Surgery
Royal Adelaide Hospital, Adelaide

Consumer representative

Mr Duncan Love, Adelaide

APPENDIX A

Appendix B

Process report

This is the second edition of the report *Acute Pain Management: Scientific Evidence*. The first edition was written by a multidisciplinary committee headed by Professor Michael Cousins and published by the National Health and Medical Research Council (NHMRC) in 1999. In accordance with NHMRC requirements that guidelines be revised as further evidence accumulates, and with the move towards development of guidelines by external bodies, the Australian and New Zealand College of Anaesthetists (ANZCA) undertook responsibility for the revision of the document.

Since the first edition was published in 1999, a sizeable amount of new evidence relating to the management of acute pain has been published. The aim of this document is to summarise the available evidence to assist clinicians from a range of disciplines. The document is a compilation of current evidence relating to acute pain management in a wide range of patients and acute pain settings using a variety of treatment modalities. It aims to assist those involved in the management of acute pain, including the consumer, with the best current (up to January 2005) evidence-based information.

This report provides examples of the decision-making processes that were put in place to deal with the plethora of available evidence under consideration.

Development process

A working party was convened to coordinate and oversee the development process. The working party comprised Dr Pam Macintyre (Chair), Prof Ian Power, Prof Stephan Schug, Dr David Scott, Dr Eric Visser, Dr Suellen Walker and Dr Douglas Justins (Royal College of Anaesthetists, UK). A large panel of contributors was appointed to draft sections of the document and a multidisciplinary consultative committee was chosen to review the early drafts of the document and contribute more broadly as required. A list of members is attached at Appendix A, together with a list of contributing authors and working party members. Through the NHMRC Guidelines Assessment Register (GAR), the working party was provided with expert advice on the use of evidence-based findings and the application of NHMRC criteria by Professor Karen Grimmer from the University of South Australia.

Structures and processes for the revised edition were developed, and within these frameworks contributors were invited to review the evidence and submit content for specific sections according to their area of expertise. All contributors were given instructions about the process of the literature search, a copy of the NHMRC document *How to use the evidence: assessment and application of scientific evidence* (2000), and directed to the NHMRC website for copies of the first edition of the document as well as other publications that assist in the development of guidelines.

Two members of the working party were responsible for the initial editing of each section, the evaluation of the literature submitted with the contributions and checking for further relevant references. In a series of meetings the working party compiled and edited an initial draft with the assistance of editors experienced in NHMRC requirements and processes. Once the draft of the document had been prepared, it was sent to all contributors for comment as well as members of the multidisciplinary panel, before being redrafted for public consultation. To ensure general applicability, there was a very wide range of experts on the contributor and multidisciplinary committee, including medical, nursing, allied health and complementary medicine clinicians and consumers.

The second edition of *Acute Pain Management: Scientific Evidence* is based on the NHMRC's recommendations for guideline development. That is, these guidelines focus on improving patient outcomes, are based on the best evidence available, include statements concerning the strength of levels of evidence underpinning recommendations, and use a multidisciplinary approach involving all stakeholders (including consumers).

Consideration is being given to the preparation of specially formatted documents for the general practitioner and consumer.

Review of the evidence

This document is a revision of the initial guidelines published in 1999. Therefore most of the evidence included in the second review has been published from 1998 onwards, unless no more recent papers on a particular topic have been published since the 1999 review. Recent evidence-based guidelines have been published in the areas of acute musculoskeletal pain and of cancer pain, and recommendations relevant to the management of acute pain were drawn directly from these.

Search strategies

Searches of the electronic databases Medline or PubMed, Embase, Cochrane and DARE were conducted for each of the main topics included in the review. Searches were limited to articles concerning humans published in English, and literature published since 1998 was highlighted. The initial searches were inevitably broad, given the very wide scope of the topic. 'Pain', 'acute pain, 'postoperative pain' or 'analgesia' was searched with the key headings of the various sections and subsections of the document such as 'neuropathic', 'patient-controlled', 'epidural', 'paracetamol' and so on. For drugs and techniques a search was also made for 'efficacy' and 'complications'. Hand searches were also conducted of a large range of relevant journals from 1998 onwards and bibliographies of relevant papers were checked.

Preferred evidence

A review of acute pain management requires a broad focus on a range of topics (eg postoperative pain, musculoskeletal pain, migraine, pain associated with spinal cord injury etc). This broad focus inevitably produces a very large number of research publications. In order to provide the best information and to inform best practice, it was important to concentrate on the highest ranked, highest quality evidence available.

Secondary evidence: High quality systematic reviews of randomised-controlled trials (NHMRC Level I) were the preferred evidence source. This approach was efficient as many high quality systematic reviews of specific aspects of acute pain management have already been undertaken by the Cochrane Collaboration and other reputable evidence-synthesis groups (such as members of the Oxford Pain Group). Systematic reviews that included non-randomised controlled studies were assigned the level of evidence of their component studies, as outlined in the NHMRC designation of evidence levels (1999) (see below).

Primary evidence: Where Level I reviews were not available, the next preferred level of evidence was single randomised controlled trials (NHMRC Level II). Where these were not available, other experimental evidence or case studies were accepted as the best available evidence by the guideline developers (reflecting NHMRC Levels II and IV). According to NHMRC guidelines (1999), Level IV evidence is obtained from case series, either post-test or pre-test and post-test; the levels refer to evidence about interventions. Publications describing results of audits or papers that were comprehensive clinical reviews, for example, were also included as Level IV evidence.

Expert opinion: In the few instances where no relevant published evidence was available, expert opinion was included as the best available information.

Other evidence types: Not all evidence relating to the management of acute pain is intervention-based. In a number of instances, best practice has been derived from record audit, quality processes or single case reports.

Examples of evidence level decision-making: For examples of the decisions that were made about assigning levels to low quality evidence where there was limited evidence available, see the table below.

Quality scoring

Where Cochrane reviews or reviews from other reputable sources were available, no additional methodological quality evaluation was undertaken, and what was available in the review was accepted as the quality scoring for these guidelines. For the remaining systematic reviews containing controlled trials (Level I), methodological quality was evaluated using Oxman and Gyatt (1991). For the primary RCT evidence, methodological quality was evaluated using the Oxford Scale (Jadad et al 1996). No quality evaluation was undertaken for lower ranked evidence (Level III & IV).

The main area where the non-Cochrane reviews (Level I) generally lacked quality was the inclusion of published research only (thus potentially biasing their interpretation of available research evidence). All Level I literature was included in this document.

The areas where Level II studies often lacked methodological rigour were low patient numbers and the lack of capacity to truly double-blind. Where there was a range of available primary research evidence, studies with these methodological flaws were excluded and the highest available methodological quality studies were identified to support the document. Thus this document is underpinned by the highest level, highest methodological quality evidence available.

Conflicting evidence

If evidence was consistent, the most recent, highest level and highest quality references were used. If it was conflicting, the same approach was taken (identifying highest level, highest quality evidence) however examples were given of differences within the literature so that readers could appreciate the ongoing debate. In some instances, particularly in acute pain management in various patient populations, evidence was limited to case reports only, which was made clear in the document as the best available evidence in this instance.

Key messages

Key messages were based on the highest levels of evidence available. Key messages referring to information extracted from Cochrane meta-analyses were marked"Level I [Cochrane Review]".

Cost analyses

The area of acute pain management is remarkably deficient in research on costs and cost-benefit. Where this information was available it was reported. One obvious example is the costs associated with the adverse effects of treatment. Information to assist clinicians to better manage both pain and some of the adverse effects of treatment, as well as better individualise treatment for each patient, may assist in minimising such costs. This is noted as an area warranting further research.

Examples of decisions made assigning levels to evidence of lower quality	
Systematic reviews of articles designated Level IV were also cited as Level IV	A systematic review of case-series looking at effectiveness of pain relief before and after the introduction of an acute pain service (Werner et al 2002)
Evidence from audits or case series that directly affects patient safety cited as Level IV	The amount of morphine a patient requires is better predicted by their age rather than weight (adds to safety of prescribing) (Macintyre & Jarvis 1996) The routine use of a continuous infusion with patient-controlled analgesia (PCA) markedly increases the risk of respiratory depression (Schug & Torrie 1993) Sedation is a better early indicator of opioid-induced respiratory depression than a decrease in respiratory rate (Ready et al 1998) Delays in the diagnosis and treatment of an epidural abscess in a patient with neurological signs greatly increases the risk of an incomplete recovery (Davies et al 2004)
Evidence from a single case report or letter that directly affects patient safety cited as Level IV	Electrical corruption of PCA pumps resulting in uncontrolled delivery of syringe contents (Notcutt et al 1992) The need for antisyphon valves when using PCA in order to prevent inadvertent delivery of an excessive dose of opioid (Kwan 1995)

Public consultation

Following acceptance of the draft by the contributors and the multidisciplinary committee, its availability was advertised in national newspapers for public consultation on 6th and 13th of November 2004. The draft was also made available on the ANZCA website, and Colleges of many of the contributors and multidisciplinary consultative committee members were notified of the availability of the draft and asked to disseminate this information to their members.

The public was invited to provide comments on the draft and 13 submissions were received from the following individuals and organisations.

Dr Graeme Thomson
Director of Emergency Medicine, Angliss Hospital Vic

Prof Anne-Maree Kelly
Director of Emergency Medicine, Western Hospital, Footscray Vic

Dr James Sartain
Supervisor Acute Pain Service, Cairns Base Hospital Qld

Dr Daniel Fatovich
Specialist in Emergency Medicine, Royal Perth Hospital WA

Jacqui Beavis
Principal Pharmacist Family Health, Middlemore Hospital, Auckland NZ

Dr Greg Treston
Consultant-Emergency Medicine, Redcliffe Hospital Qld

Assoc Prof David Crankshaw
Depts of Pharmacology and Civil and Biomedical Engineering, University of Melbourne Vic

Prof Colin Torrance
Acute Care Nursing, Victoria University, Melbourne Vic

Dr Allan Cyna
Dept Womens Anaesthesia, Women's and Children's Hospital, Adelaide SA

Tiina Piira
Clinical psychologist/researcher, Pain Research Unit, Sydney Children's Hospital, Randwick NSW

Grazyna Jastrzab
CNC Pain Management, Prince of Wales Hospital, Sydney NSW

June Gorringe
CNC Pain Service, Royal Perth Hospital WA

Dr Alan Gijsbers
Drug and Alcohol Service, Royal Melbourne Hospital, Vic

The main areas of comment raised in these submissions included:

- emergency medicine;
- acute cardiac pain;
- migraine;
- paediatric pain;
- inhalation analgesia and methoxyflurane;
- use of hypnosis and acupuncture in acute pain management;

- patient-controlled analgesia use in patients with alcohol withdrawal; and
- management of acute pain in opioid-resistant patients.

The working party met to consider these submissions and the draft was revised accordingly.

Implementation, dissemination and revision

The Australian and New Zealand College of Anaesthetists (ANZCA) will be responsible for the dissemination, implementation, evaluation and updating of this document. The document will be available on the internet (formatted to allow for downloading and printing) as well as in hard copy. ANZCA will distribute hard copies to all its members and trainees, to state and territory health authorities, professional associations and professional journals. ANZCA will also notify the Colleges of all contributors and multidisciplinary consultative committee members of the availability of the document and ask them to disseminate the information to their members. In addition, the document has been endorsed by the Royal College of Anaesthetists in the United Kingdom, the *International Association for the Study of Pain* and the *Australian Pain Society*. This is further expected to heighten awareness of its availability. The document will also be promoted at relevant professional meetings and conferences and by editorials in professional journals.

The ANZCA working party responsible for this document will continue to monitor the literature relevant to acute pain management. As new evidence becomes available, further revision will be required. Unless earlier revision is indicated, it is anticipated that the document will be revised again in 2010.

Areas identified as requiring further research

The Working Party identified a number of areas that warrant urgent further research using appropriate research approaches. These relate primarily to:

1. The management (including pain assessment and education) of acute pain in specific patient groups including:
   - Elderly patients
   - Children
   - Patients who are cognitively impaired
   - Non-English speaking patients
   - Aboriginal and Torres Straight Islander peoples
   - Patients with obstructive sleep apnoea
   - Patients who are opioid-tolerant
   - Patients with a substance abuse disorder
   - Patients with or at risk of persistent postoperative pain
2. Issues of cost and cost-effectiveness.

It is the intention of the Working Party to bring these issues to the attention of NHMRC in order to support an agenda for research into currently under-researched areas of acute pain management, and to ensure that subsequent guideline developers can draw on better quality, higher level evidence in these areas. Strategies to assist in ongoing identification of areas of neglect or rapid change in pain management will be proposed when this document is submitted to NHMRC.

References

Davies DP, Wold RM, Patel RJ et al (2004) The clinical presentation and impact of diagnostic delays on emergency department patients with spinal epidural abscess. *J Emerg Med* 26: 285–91.

Jada AR et al (1996) Assessing the quality of reports of randomised trials: is blinding necessary. *Controlled Clinical Trials* 17: 1–12.

Kwan A (1995) Overdose of morphine during PCA. *Anaesthesia* 50: 919.

Macintyre PE &Jarvis DA (1996) Age is the best predictor of postoperative morphine requirements. *Pain* 64: 357–64.

Notcutt WG, Knowles P, Kaldas R (1992) Overdose of opioid from patient-controlled analgesia pumps. *Br J Anaesth* 69: 95–97.

Oxman AD & Guyatt GH (1991) Validation of an index of the quality of review articles. *J Clin Epidemiol* 44: 1271–78.

Ready LB, Oden R, Chadwick HS et al (1988) Development of an anesthesiology-based postoperative pain management service. *Anesthesiology* 68: 100–06.

Schug SA & Torrie JJ (1993) Safety assessment of postoperative pain management by an acute pain service. *Pain* 55: 387–91.

Werner MU, Søholm L, Rotbøll-Nielsen et al (2002) Does an acute pain service improve postoperative outcome. *Anesth Analg* 95: 1361–72.

Abbreviations and acronyms

ACOG	American College of Obstetricians and Gynecologists
ADEC	Australian Drug Evaluation Committee
AERD	aspirin-exacerbated respiratory disease
AIDS	acquired immunodeficiency syndrome
ALA	adrenaline [epinephrine], lignocaine [lidocaine], amethocaine
AMH	*Australian Medicines Handbook*
ANZCA	Australian and New Zealand College of Anaesthetists
ASA	American Society of Anesthesiologists
ASRA	American Society of Regional Anesthesia and Pain Medicine
CAM	complementary and alternative medicines
CFNB	continuous femoral nerve blockade
CI	confidence interval
CNS	central nervous system
CPAP	continuous positive airway pressure
CPNB	continuous peripheral nerve blockade
CR	controlled-release
CRPS	Complex Regional Pain Syndrome
CSE	combined spinal epidural
DNA	deoxyribonucleic acid
DRG	dorsal root ganglion
DSP	distal symmetrical polyneuropathy
ECG	electrocardiogram
ENT	ear, nose and throat
FDA	Food and Drugs Administration (US)
FPM	Faculty of Pain Medicine, ANZCA
HIV	human immunodeficiency virus
IASP	International Association for the Study of Pain
ICU	intensive care unit
IM	intramuscular

IN	intranasal
INR	International Normalised Ratio
IR	immediate-release
IV	intravenous
JCAHO	Joint Commission on Accreditation of Healthcare Organisations (US)
LMWH	low molecular weight heparin
M3G	morphine-3-glucuronide
M6G	morphine-6-glucuronide
mGluR	metabotropic glutamatereceptor
MLAC	minimum local anaesthetic concentration
MS	methionine synthetase
N_2O	nitrous oxide
NCCPC-PV	Non-Communicating Children's Pain Checklist-Postoperative Version
NCCPC-R	Non-Communicating Children's Pain Checklist
NHMRC	National Health and Medical Research Council
NICS	National Institute of Clinical Studies
NK1	neurokinin-1
NMDA	n-methyl-D-aspartate
NNH	number-needed-to-harm
NNT	number-needed-to-treat
NO	nitric oxide
NPC	National Pharmaceutical Council (US)
NRS	numeric rating scale
NSAID	non-steroidal anti-inflammatory drug
OSA	obstructive sleep apnoea
OTFC	oral transmucosal fentanyl citrate
PAG	periacqueductal grey
PCA	patient-controlled analgesia
PCEA	patient-controlled epidural analgesia
PCINA	patient-controlled intranasal analgesia
PCNBA	patient-controlled nerve block analgesia

PCRA	patient-controlled regional analgesia
PDPH	post dural puncture headache
PGH	prostaglandin endoperoxide
PHN	post-herpetic neuralgia
prn	as needed
QOL	quality of life
RACP	Royal Australasian College of Physicians
RCA	Royal College of Anaesthetists (UK)
RVM	rostroventromedial medulla
SACD	subacute combined degeneration
SAD	substance abuse disorder
SC	subcutaneous
SF-36	Short Form 36 of Medical Outcomes Study
SIGN	Scottish Intercollegiate Guidelines Network
SIP	Sickness Impact Profile
SL	sublingual
SPID	summed pain intensity difference
SR	slow-release
SSRI	selective serotonin re-uptake inhibitors
SUNCT	short-lasting unilateral neuralgiform headache attacks with conjunctival injection and tearing
TCA	tricyclic antidepressant
TENS	transcutaneous electrical nerve stimulation
THC	tetrahydrocannabinol
TOTPAR	total pain relief
TTH	tension type headache
VAS	visual analogue scale
VASSPID	visual analogue scale summed pain intensity difference
VASTOTPAR	visual analogue scale total pain relief
VDS	verbal descriptor scale
VNRS	verbal numerical rating scales

Index

INDEX

INDEX

INDEX

INDEX

INDEX

INDEX

INDEX